Fats that Heal
Fats that Kill

Fats that Heal
Fats that Kill

by Udo Erasmus

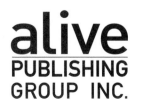

alive
PUBLISHING
GROUP INC.

Note to Readers:

The information in this book is presented for educational purposes. It is not intended to replace the services of healing professionals for conditions that require them.

Published by:

Alive Books, 7432 Fraser Park Drive, Burnaby BC Canada V5J 5B9

Tel: (604) 435-1919 • 1-800-663-6580

www.alive.com

Illustrations: Janet Sephton
Cover Design: William Stockmann
Layout & Typography: Sheila Adams

18   19   20

First Edition *(Fats and Oils):*
  First Printing – August 1987
  Second Printing – March 1988
  Third Printing – January 1989
  Fourth Printing – February 1991

  Second Edition *(Fats That Heal Fats That Kill):*
  First Printing – December 1993
  Second Printing – August 1994
  Third Printing – March 1995
  Fourth Printing - September 1996
  Fifth Printing - September 1997
  Sixth Printing - April 1998

Second Edition *(continued):*
  Seventh Printing - December 1998
  Eighth Printing - April 1999
  Ninth Printing - June 1999
  Tenth Printing - March 2001
  Eleventh Printing - June 2001
  Twelfth Printing - November 2001
  Thirteenth Printing - May 2002
  Fourteenth Printing - September 2002
  Fifteenth Printing - May 2004
  Sixteenth Printing - September 2005
  Seventeenth Printing - January 2006
  Eighteenth Printing - November 2006

Translated into Dutch and Danish

Canadian Cataloguing in Publication Data

Erasmus, Udo
  Fats that Heal, Fats that Kill

  Previously published as: Fats and Oils.
  Includes bibliographical references and index.
  ISBN 0-920470-40-8 (bound).   ISBN 0-920470-38-6 (pbk.)

  1. Lipids in human nutrition. 2. Oils and fats, Edible. 3. Fatty acids - Physiological effect.
  4. Cholesterol. I. Title. II. Title: Fats and oils.

TX553.L5E73 1993   641.1'4   C94-910027-7

Printed and bound in Canada.

For my children T'ai, Usha, and Rama.

May understanding of health be the starship of the next generation.

May the worship of diseases die with us.

Comments on the First Edition

Reviewers:

"I have never been so delightfully surprised by a book that should *be boring and pedantic. Udo Erasmus has put together all the current information about fats and oils and laid it out for all the world to see."*
Lendon Smith, MD, "The Children's Doctor", author of best-sellers *Feed Your Kids Right,* and *The Encyclopedia of Baby and Child Care.*

"I have gone over the manuscript very carefully, and think that Udo Erasmus has done a marvellous job of summarizing almost everything one needs to know about fats and oils.'
Abram Hoffer, MD, PhD, researcher, editor of the *Journal of Orthomolecular Medicine,* author of *Orthomolecular Medicine for Physicians.*

"Udo Erasmus has taken a complex topic and made it understandable. In fact, he has gone far beyond the scope of the title and also given a broad insight into nutrition and health in general. I highly recommend it."
Jonn Matsen, Naturopathic Physician, author of best-selling book *Eating Alive.*

"An excellent guide to a subject which is proving of the greatest importance for human health."
David Horrobin, MD, editor of *Clinical Uses of Essential Fatty Acids.*

"Udo Erasmus has written a very timely and important book . . . filled with interesting and accurate information concerning . . . fatty acids in nutrition and health. An excellent contribution to the field of clinical nutrition."
Jeffrey Bland, PhD, President *Health Comm*

Lay Readers:

"I really love your book on fats and oils. I recently graduated from Phys Ed and took a number of "nutrition" courses, but your book certainly is an eye opener."
M.M., Fredericton, NB

"The remarkable thing about your book is that it seems to exist in a vacuum. The new edition of Earl Mindell's Vitamin Bible *and* Fit for Life II *remain unenlightened on the subject of fats. It is so nice for the minority of us who will listen that there's information available which is powerfully life-changing."*
S.M., Denver, CO

"After all the confusion about the fatty acids, your book is amazingly clear and concise.
L.C., Pine City, MN

"I found your presentation so clear, even I could grasp the chemical concepts.
D.T., Ojai, CA

"We applied the principles, and between the two of us we were able to greatly reduce a case of acne, and control eczema, arthritis, and hypertension. Although the topic was technical, your light writing style made it a pleasant read.
D.S., Washington, DC

"I am off insulin, blood pressure pills, and have a cholesterol of 140-160. I weigh 50 pounds less than I did. Proudly, I'm in size 34 pants – the first time since high school. My zest for life has truly doubled. My mental attitude is astonishingly upbeat. All in all, I am truly a walking miracle. I owe much to you . . . "
R.C., Los Angeles, CA

"A most informative book on fats and oils. I am now much more careful about the oils I buy . . ."
L.M., Vancouver, BC

"After experimenting with different health diets and wrestling with macrobiotics and food combining, then feeling more confused than ever, I bought your book. It was a real eye opener and a delight to read. The medical profession scared me into thinking all fats and oils were bad and I was afraid I'd get cancer, so my whole family (2 small children included) weren't allowed a touch of oils, fats, nuts, seeds, etc. I only wish I knew of these healthy oils sooner."
C.C., Edmonton, AL

"It fills a tremendous gap in health literature."
J.K., New York, NY

". . . addresses one of the basic problems of the average diet. You have done a great service to the public, and to humanity by writing your book."
D.W., Lakewood, CO

". . . contains many hints and tips that would be useful to people with allergic and other health problems. It is highly recommended."
B.S., Wellington, New Zealand

"I wish there were more people like you who were willing to look under the "rocks" and tell us what they have found hidden there, and who also possessed the ability to communicate it so well."
J.B., San Francisco, CA

Professionals:
"Your book is not only unusually well written, but it fills a near vacuum of published material relating to this important subject."
G.L., MD, Vancouver, BC

"Relates to cardiovascular disease, many forms of cancer, diabetes, high blood pressure, plus other fatty degenerative diseases. Very clearly written and logically presented. Also very interesting to read – not dull and pedantic – stayed up most of one night reading this, once started. Undoubtedly the most complete book on this vital subject."
J.L., Clinical Nutritionist, San Diego, CA

"Your book really opened my eyes and I am using its information actively almost every day – I am a nutritional consultant."
C.D., Ottawa, ON

"Since the 1988 Surgeon General's report, there has been a demand for more information concerning the effect of fats on health. I recommend your book as a resource for all my clients who wish to change their diet and commit to a healthier life-style."
B.G., Nutrition Consultant, Philadelphia, PA

"I think your book is way ahead of its time. Your book is explicit, concise, and obviously the result of painstaking research. Of particular use to me have been explanations of cholesterol; saturated/unsaturated fats; fish oils; fatty acids in cell membranes; general nutrition."
G.W., Licensed Massage Therapist, Eugene, OR

"Anyone who has any degree of nutritional sense seems to be very familiar with your book."
M.J., MD, Clarksville, TN

"Your excellent detail and simplicity in your book have enabled me as a doctor to finally understand the basic underlying concepts and importance of the field of fats and oils and to be able to apply them therapeutically in my office as well as my own home. Results with degenerative and non-responsive cases of the past are now remarkable. Thanks to you, my office is now preventing future illnesses rather than just treating the immediate problems."
D.G., Chiropractor, Pepperell, MA

"With so many nutrition books on the market, I am very pleased to read one that has real scientific explanations to back it up."
M.L., Optometrist, Wyomissing, PA

"Should be required reading for all students of the health care professions. . . . I especially appreciated your chapter on flax seed and immediately added it to my own diet, and I've begun encouraging patients to do the same."
K.P., DC, Pasadena, CA

"An excellent reference manual for physicians, RNs, teachers and nutritionists – in fact for anyone concerned about the consequences of high consumption of fats and oils. I am thrilled to discover a book that addresses this most pertinent topic at a time when research clearly points to the important link between diet and degenerative disease. The book is clear on what our alternatives are and how they can be implemented."
L.F., RN, Vancouver, BC

PLEASE NOTE:

Recently there has been a trend to show the symbol for Omega 'w' in 'n-' form, rather than 'w'. While this practice is still in the transition stage, the publisher has already made the changes on the diagrams.

Prostaglandins are now usually called eicosanoids. Eicosanoids include prostaglandins, prostacyclins, thromboxanes, and leukotrienes.

Contents

SECTION EIGHT
Toward Total Health – Live Long and Feel Fat-astic   397

List of Figures

SECTION FOUR
The Fire Inside Each Cell   **154**

SECTION FIVE
Quality of Products   **206**

SECTION SIX
Therapeutic Oils   **252**

SECTION SEVEN
Effects of Killer Fats on Health   **324**

List of Tables

Preface and Acknowledgements

This book began with a personal disaster. I was poisoned by the careless industrial application of pesticides on a job I held for three years, could not get help from medical doctors, and came to three inescapable conclusions: first, that *my* health is *my* responsibility; second, that our drug-oriented medical approaches *cannot* lead us to health; and third, that foods and nutrition are the *primary* options for self-help in health. I became extremely interested in the relationship of foods and essential nutrients to health. While information on proteins, minerals, and vitamins was readily available, the area of fats and oils was poorly covered, and I found it frustratingly contradictory and confusing. Knowing that the poisons I had been exposed to were carcinogenic and that cancer often involves fats, I needed clear, accurate, factual information.

I buried my head in research journals and, having pored through thousands of research entries, I began to organize what I found relevant to health into what has become this book. It took three years full-time and three years part-time to write.

The sources of information for this book include:
- Textbooks outlining the basic principles of physics, chemistry, biochemistry, physiology, biology, and nutrition, as well as medicine;
- Technical books and research journals in nutrition, biochemistry, orthomolecular medicine, lipids (fats, oils, and cholesterol), agricultural science, and processing technology;
- Books that correlate traditional diets with human health;
- Clinical reports of the use of nutrition to reverse degenerative conditions;
- Personal accounts of others; and
- My own experiences.

I am grateful for the efforts and contributions that researchers and clinicians have made to our understanding of fats, oils, cholesterol, nutrition, and human health. Dr. David Horrobin first explained the biochemistry of essential fatty acids and prostaglandins to me at a trade convention. Siegfried Gursche introduced me to Johanna Budwig's work, which further sparked my interest in the field, and inspired me to search the journals for several years to gather information and to explore the field of nutrition and health.

Many people and events continued to conspire to keep me going whenever I felt like quitting over the course of the six long years it took to gather and organize the information contained in this book.

Christoph Quest invited me to Germany to study and to teach. Many people in Europe and North America reported their experiences with the use of fresh, unrefined oils containing essential fatty acids. The positive effects of these oils on their health gave me the practical assurance to push ahead with my writing.

Rees Moerman shared with me the tribulations of the road warrior.

This book is a family affair as well as a community effort. Senta Erasmus provided the support that made it possible for me to write the first edition (*Fats and Oils*). Gerd Erasmus introduced me and my material to grade 9 to 12 students and their teachers in Nechako Valley Secondary School, and boosted my confidence in my ability to explain this complex field in an understandable way.

Several people helped to transform the concept of the book into reality. Norma Smith turned an impossible rough draft into a workable first manuscript. Evelyn Mielke made illustrations out of illegible scribbles. Steven Carter and Carolyn Zonailo masterminded the first edition called *Fats and Oils*.

Major revisions, rewrites, and additions were made to produce this second edition – *Fats That Heal Fats That Kill.* Joy Hemphill did the initial copy editing. Janet Sephton drew new diagrams, and typed editing changes from convoluted hand-written inserts and corrections without losing her ability to smile. Sheila Adams typeset, formatted, and did final copy editing and proofreading. Bill Stockmann co-ordinated the cover design. Ron Crompton co-ordinated technical production and generally cracked the whip (*his* words). Gisela Temmel did substantive editing and expertly guided the project. As publisher, Siegfried Gursche made the project possible. The result of the efforts of these people is the book you hold in your hands. Their diligent efforts and assistance deserve a special note of gratitude.

Finally, I wish to acknowledge those people who, by following wholesome eating habits, have set a model for us to follow and those who, by changing from mistaken eating habits to healthy ones, have shown us the healing power of nutrients and foods.

Introduction

Recently, exhausted Asian refugees were rescued from boats adrift for months on the open sea. To escape political oppression and chaos, they had left family, home, culture, and possessions for an uncertain life in an unknown world, risked life and limb for the hope of a stable future. When they were found, they had only the clothes on their backs and small containers that they were unwilling to leave behind. Rescuers who opened these containers found them filled with rancid, stinking fat. When questioned, the refugees explained that this was their most precious possession. Of all the things to take with them into the new world, they chose fat. The extreme circumstances in which they drifted had destroyed the treasure they bore, but they knew the importance of fat to their health, and valued it above all other worldly goods.

Most of us do not share the view of these Asian immigrants on the value of fat. This is largely due to our having been misinformed.

Popular books on nutrition that tackle fats, oils, and cholesterol contain many contradictory statements of 'fact'. The reason is that most writers are not knowledgeable in this field. Some of their 'facts' tell only half the story, the part about the fats that kill. Some of their 'facts' about fats and oils are the half-truths that industries disseminate in order to market fat and oil products for profit. Also, authors often copy each others' mistaken 'facts' because they have not invested the time and effort required to extract truths from the research literature. This book departs from that lazy practice.

Easy Reading

To keep the language simple and make the story easy to follow, I took on the challenge of translating 'technicalese' into plain English. Judging from letters of both technically untrained readers and professionals, I succeeded in explaining fats, foods, and health in ways that someone with little scientific training can follow, yet without losing accuracy. I tested my explanations on 14- to 17-year-old high school students, who were able to understand me. I have included graphics for readers with a background in biochemistry. They can be passed over without losing the story.

All aspects of how fats, oils, cholesterol, and essential nutrients affect our health are covered in this book, including:

- the properties of fats, fatty acids, sugars, and cholesterol;
- the healing and the killing fats;
- how fats and oils are made into marketable consumer products;
- the health effects of applying technical skills (processing) to foods without regard to human health;
- the body's ways of dealing with fats and foods;
- fats and cholesterol found in foods;
- how food preparation affects health;
- research findings;
- how to make and use oils with human health in mind;
- new and therapeutic products;
- other important nutrients;
- degenerative diseases;
- the politics of health; and
- a consideration of the basis of human health.

You will end up with a broad understanding of the topic, have specific, detailed information at your fingertips, and gain insights that will make it easier to optimize health and avoid degenerative diseases. This book separates fact from advertising fiction, and equips you to assess future developments in the field.

Organizing the Story

I divided the story of fats, foods, cholesterol, and human health into sections that follow a logical sequence, continuity, and progression. Each chapter is a complete story, cross-referenced with other relevant chapters to avoid repetition.

The book can be read in several ways. If you want the whole story, read it from cover to cover. If you want a handy reference on how fats, oils, cholesterol, and essential nutrients affect our health, you will find this information under separate headings. If you like to follow specific topics in fats, nutrition, processes, degenerative diseases, and health, you can skip from section to section.

I hope your interest will be sparked to read the entire book. Fats, oils, essential nutrients, and foods hold most major keys to successful prevention and treatment of degenerative conditions.

Accurate information enables us to make better choices in our quest to purchase food products that support our health. To a large extent, these choices determine the health (or illness) of those affected by our choices: ourselves, our children, and our fellow humans.

Expanded Second Edition

The first edition of this book, a much shorter version (59 instead of the present 91 chapters) that we called *Fats and Oils* was published in 1986. Much has happened in the field since then. More research has been done on essential fatty acids; refined and unrefined oils; hormone-like prostaglandins; and the effects of fats, oils, cholesterol, and nutrients on health. This recent research has been incorporated into the new book. We named it *Fats That Heal Fats That Kill* in order to make the key point about fats and oils in human health right from the beginning.

New ways of making oils with human health in mind were pioneered as a result of the publication of the first edition. I was intimately involved with their conception and development, and report here on their progress. These new oils made in new ways have been clinically used with excellent therapeutic benefits. Flax has risen from obscurity to prominence in human nutrition, a development that I championed. It is getting serious research attention and will become the wonder grain of the 21st century. New oils have been pioneered, such as kukui nut and hemp. Hemp oil is particularly exciting, and got its own chapter. The benefits of unrefined (virgin) olive oil have been put on a firmer research foundation.

Additional information on the natural treatment of degenerative conditions, which is one of the most rapidly growing areas of consumer interest, has been added. Widespread misinformation on how to feed infants prompted a chapter on infants and oils. Athletes and pets each got a chapter on the usefulness of certain oils on performance and health. Erucic acid and canola oil had to get a second hearing. Tropical fats also needed attention because of the bad press they've received since 1988. Medium chain triglycerides also got some space. The processes of fractionation (used in chocolates and confections) and transesterification have been described.

In addition, a chapter on the importance of balancing oxidation with protection by antioxidants has been added.

You'll like the chapters on snake oil, the biological basis of natural therapies, and alkylglycerols. The politics of health got a chapter, because of its powerful restricting influences on the availability of health care in affluent nations.

The section on degenerative conditions was broken out into a dozen separate chapters. Much has been learned about natural treatments that help alleviate and reverse these conditions.

Enjoy the journey!

A Broader Context

We begin by introducing the topic of fatty degeneration – the family of great killer diseases of our time, whose members include cardiovascular disease, cancer, diabetes, multiple sclerosis, and many more.

After making a case for the importance of fats, we outline the foundations of human health and the broader stage upon which all fats must play their roles.

Essential substances, including healing fats, must be obtained in optimum quantities to build optimum health. Surveys show that the majority of the members of affluent populations are obtaining too little of many essential substances, leading to sub-optimal, deteriorating health which in turn leads to degeneration due to malnutrition, which ultimately kills two-thirds of the population.

History tells us that past populations suffered less physical degeneration than we do, and a smaller percentage of them died of cancer, cardiovascular disease, and diabetes. Reversal of degenerative conditions is possible in most cases. 'Incurable' diseases can usually be cured!

Fatty Degeneration **1**

The Importance of Fats

Degenerative diseases that involve fats prematurely kill over two-thirds of the people currently living in affluent, industrialized nations. Sixty-eight percent of people die from just three conditions that involve fatty degeneration: cardiovascular disease (43.8%), cancer (22.4%), and diabetes (1.8%). These deaths are the result of eating habits based on ignorance and misconceptions.

Controversy and Misinformation about Fats and Oils

Butter and margarine have been controversial for years. There is continuing debate about why polyunsaturates, which are essential, also cause cancer. There is talk of 'bad' beef fat and 'good' fish oils. We hear rumors about hydrogenation and processed oil products. There are stories about fried fats. There's the scary topic of cholesterol. These stories have generated more heat than light.

Simplistic and inaccurate half-truths that serve advertising and sales efforts have created confusion. We need clear, factual information, in simple English.

Information (or misinformation) has trickled down to us through the grapevine as rumors, hearsay, advertising copy, popular articles by reporters and amateurs without training or clarity in this complex topic, doctors untrained in nutrition, and industry's 'experts'. Everyone I meet in my travels has heard conflicting stories about how fats, oils, cholesterol, and nutrients affect human health. People are interested but confused, and they want clear, practical answers.

Medical failings. Medical doctors, to whom we have entrusted our health because we have not yet learned to care for it ourselves, studied disease rather than health in medical school. Their curriculum included little on nutrition, lots on pharmaceutical drugs, and nothing about the effects of processing fats and oils on human health.

Since we are natural biological organisms, we must attain, maintain, and regain good health through *natural* approaches – through foods and life-styles in keeping with the biological needs that nature genetically built into us. Each of us

3

must learn to care for our own body, since we alone live in it, we alone feed and direct it, and we alone bear the direct consequences of eating habits and life-styles out of line with our natural biological requirements.

Drug and high-tech approaches to disease management are slowly yielding to overwhelming amounts of new research evidence that supports the importance of foods and nutrients in healing. But doctors steeped in drug-oriented medical practices (crisis intervention, symptom control, and disease management) remain skeptical about natural approaches to health. Beyond advising us to heed woefully inadequate pronouncements about the 'four daily food groups' (our changing times have seen three, five, and seven food groups recommended by the same regulating bodies), such doctors fail those who struggle toward improved health through natural means based on improved nutrition – including healing substances that come from fats and oils.

Nutrition Research

Accurate information about the importance of nutrients to health is gathering dust, buried in research journals written in the boring style of scientific writing, hidden under a technical language that most readers have not been taught. Information on fats, oils, and cholesterol now numbers in the thousands of volumes.

Healing fats and killing fats. The fact is that some fats are absolutely required for health, while others are detrimental. Some fats heal, and others kill. Whether a fat heals or kills depends on several factors: What kind of fat is it? How has it been treated – is it fresh, has it been exposed to light, oxygen, heat, hydrogen, water, acid, base, or metals like copper and iron? How old is it? How has it been used in food preparation? How much was eaten? What balance of different fats do we get?

If we get the right kinds of fats in the right amounts and balances, and prepare them using the right methods, they build our health and keep us healthy. The wrong kinds of fats, the wrong amounts or balances, or even the right kinds of fats wrongly prepared cause degenerative diseases that we call *diseases of fatty degeneration*. Other nutrients can also cause fatty degeneration, and so can *lack* of certain essential nutrients. We can reverse diseases of fatty degeneration by making appropriate changes in fat choices, preparation, and consumption, and by supporting these important changes with attention to other nutrients in our food supply.

The Roots of Fatty Degeneration

If we want to get at the root of fatty degeneration, we must investigate all aspects of fats, oils, fatty acids, and cholesterol: What are they? How do they work? What do they do in our body? Where do we get them? How does our body use them? How do we process and alter them? Which ones can produce illnesses? How do we avoid the 'killer fats'? Which ones enhance our health? Where do we find and how do we use the fats that heal?

We have gathered and published enough research information in scientific journals, developed enough biochemical understanding, documented enough clinical experience, and studied enough food traditions around the world to tell the whole story. This story should be known by everyone. It must not be allowed to gather dust in the ivory towers of higher academic education.

In order to maintain health, avoid disease, and regain health once we have lost it, we need to change our consumption of fats, oils, and other fatty substances. If we want to avoid premature death from cardiovascular disease, cancer, diabetes, and other diseases of fatty degeneration, and if we want to avoid the suffering of arthritis, obesity, premenstrual syndrome, and certain types of mental illness, we need to take this last and least well-understood area of human nutrition into full account in our food choices. To do so, we must become informed.

Fats Do Not Act Alone

Fatty degeneration involves many substances other than fats, oils, and cholesterol. It is, therefore, absolutely essential that we understand the broader context into which the story of the fats that heal and the fats that kill must fit. The next chapter presents that broader context in a general form.

Foundations of Human Health 2

From the *broadest* possible perspective, a universal energy created nature by processes that are still largely unknown to us. *How* this energy uses simple substances to form the complex organizations we call plants, animals, and humans is the realm of physics, chemistry, and biology. In this realm we will find the natural state we call health.

Foods Make Bodies

We have discovered a few of the secrets of our creation by asking questions, making observations, and doing research. A few useful truths have emerged from these efforts. Most fundamental to health is the fact that *the entire human body is made from foods, water, air, and light.*

This simple statement is the basis of a revolution in health care that is sweeping the globe – the foundation upon which the entire field of work that links nutrition to human health is built. From this basic truth follows everything that is part of how we must understand human health and the products and methods we must use to care for it.

The fact that our entire body is made from foods, water, air, and light establishes that these four must be the *primary* determinant of physical health. Food, water, air, and light properly chosen for nutrient content, purity (absence of interfering substances that we call toxins or poisons), biological compatibility (determined by each individual's genetic and biochemical uniqueness) and naturalness, must constitute *primary* (not alternate or complementary) health care.

We have little control over the biochemical processes that take place after we swallow, breathe in, or expose ourselves. We *can* choose *what* we swallow, breathe in, or expose ourselves to. Our health depends on our choices.[1]

Proteins, carbohydrates, and fats are the major components of the foods from which our body is made – the 'pillars of nutrition'. A substantial amount (15 to 20%) of our calories should come from fats.

Some Substances We've Got to Have

We cannot get our nutrients by eating rocks, sand, and soil, or by drinking sea water. We cannot live on carbon dioxide or argon. We cannot survive on our own wastes. We cannot use petroleum or nylon for food. These obviously ridiculous dietary options point out limits to what our body can digest, absorb, and process into body structures, or into energy to move these structures.

Research has discovered about 50 essential factors (of which about 45 are nutrients) that must come from our environment. They include:

- essential nutrients: 20 or 21 minerals; 13 vitamins; 8 amino acids (10 for children, 11 for premature infants); and 2 essential fatty acids;
- a source of energy (most commonly starch or glucose);
- water;
- oxygen; and
- light.

Our body cannot *make* these 50 factors, but it *must have them* to live, function properly, and be healthy. The 50 factors must therefore come from outside, from our surroundings.

In addition to the 50 essential factors, several substances that are not considered essential are also required for good health. Among these are *fiber* and *friendly bacteria* that keep our intestines healthy, and *hydrochloric acid, bile,* and *digestive enzymes* that digest the foods we eat.

In this book, we spearhead the importance of nutrition to human health by focusing on the two essential fatty acids. They are uniquely sensitive to destruction by light, air, and heat. All other essential substances (except water) can be easily stabilized through drying and powdering.

---

[1] In addition to the physical components – the building blocks – of human bodies, physical activity and rest, emotional and mental states, and life-styles and environments are also important for health. We will give these topics more attention later.

Too Little, Too Much, or Just Right?

For each essential factor, there is a 'too little' (deficiency), a minimum, a maximum, a 'too much' (excess), and a Goldilocks 'just right' (optimum) daily amount.

These measures differ for each of the different factors, for different individuals, and under different physical, mental, and environmental situations such as gender, pregnancy, lactation, infancy, growth, adolescence, intense physical activity, and senescence. They also differ during stress, illness, infection, and convalescence.

'Too little' or complete absence of an essential factor *must* inevitably bring about increasing physical deterioration (degeneration), ending in death if the factor is not reintroduced in minimum to optimum quantities. 'Too much' may result in toxicity symptoms, which can be reversed by decreased intake of the factor. Degeneration from deficiency is far more common than toxicity from excess.

Progressing deficiency of essential nutrients results in a progressive deficiency syndrome characteristic of the nutrient that is lacking. More difficult to identify is a mixture of syndromes resulting from multiple deficiencies of essential nutrients. For each of the essential fatty acids, either too little or too much can lead to disease.

Degeneration has Causes and Cures

Most healers agree that *degeneration can have only two causes: malnutrition and/or internal pollution (poisoning, toxicity)*. Malnutrition results mainly from deficiencies, but may also be due to imbalances (or, rarely, excesses) of nutrients, poor digestion, and poor absorption.

Internal pollution results from environmental poisons taken in with foods (pesticides, heavy metals, toxic synthetics, disease-producing organisms), water (chlorine, trihalomethanes, soil-water-air pollutants), and air (dust, smog, ozone, nitrous oxide, molds, bacteria); from street and pharmaceutical drugs and food additives; from synthetic substances used in paints, carpets, tiles, countertops, and adhesives; from tobacco and alcohol; from toxic allergic reactions; and from normal metabolic functions.

Malnutrition and internal pollution can be reversed by natural interventions such as nutrient enrichment (or restriction), pollution control, and detoxification.

Inherited (genetic) defects cannot be as easily fixed, but better diet, lifestyle, and detoxification can bring substantial improvements.

It has been estimated that 60% of the population gets too much of one essential fatty acid, and that 95% of the population gets too little of the other. Almost all of us get too many chemically altered, toxic fatty acids.

Deficiencies are Common

Large U.S. government-sponsored surveys have shown that *over 60% of the population is deficient in one or more essential nutrients*. The surveys measured *minimum* requirements for healthy adults (U.S. Recommended Daily Allowances), not *optimums* for best of health, or increased requirements for abnormal or stressful circumstances. The surveys tested for only 13 of about 45 essential nutrients. They found that deficiency ranged from 10 to 80% of the population for each of 12 essential nutrients, with low rates of deficiency for the remaining one. Other surveys and estimates indicate that 10 to 95% of the population obtains less than the minimum required for health of each of another 11 essential nutrients (see Chapter 13, Essential Nutrients).

Therefore, of about 45 essential nutrients, at least 23 are lacking in the foods eaten by a substantial portion of the population. Remember that deficiency leads to progressive degeneration (degenerative diseases), ending in death if adequate quantities of the lacking nutrients are not returned to the diet.

When the lacking nutrients are returned, deficiency symptoms are reversed and the deficiency disease is cured.

Degeneration Kills

The 1988 Surgeon General's Report on Nutrition and Health concluded that 15 out of every 21 deaths (more than two-thirds) in the U.S. involve nutrition. Conditions with malnutrition as at least part of their cause (and the percentage of deaths attributable to each) include: cardiovascular disease – heart disease, stroke and atherosclerosis – (43.8%), cancer (22.4%), and diabetes (1.8%), accidents (4.4%), lung diseases (3.7%), pneumonia and flu (3.2%), suicides (1.4%), and liver diseases (1.1%). All 10 leading causes of death in the U.S. are included in this list. They account for 81.9% of all deaths, which total just over 2 million people each year in the U.S.

Deficiencies, excesses, or imbalances in fats are involved in 70% or more of all U.S. deaths. Reliable statistics for degeneration due to internal pollution are not as readily available.

Degeneration Has Not Always Killed So Many

In 1900, only 1 in 7 people died of cardiovascular disease, and only 1 in 30 people died of cancer. Between that time and today, something basic and critical to health has drastically changed. This span of history includes processed foods becoming a mega-industry; the introduction of pesticides; the rising use of pharmaceutical drugs; increased industrial pollution of our soil, water, and air; chlorination of water; car exhaust; tobacco smoke; and indoor pollution through the use of synthetic chemicals for everything – cleaners, paint, carpets, furniture.

All of these factors were rare before 1900. All are factors we introduced into our own biology. All are factors we could remove from our environment and our body. Major changes have also been made in this century in the kinds of fats we eat, the amounts we consume, and how we process them.

Degenerative Conditions are Reversible

Malnutrition can be corrected by improved nutrition, by using nutrient-rich whole foods; fresh vegetable and fruit juices rich in minerals, vitamins, and enzymes; specialty foods super-rich in nutrients; and nutrient supplements.

Internal pollution (poisoning) can be avoided, and much toxicity can be reversed by detoxification. Indoor pollution can be avoided by using natural materials and removed by the use of filters for water and air. Outdoor pollution requires political will, coming less from politicians than from an informed public demanding change.[2]

By correctly addressing malnutrition and pollution, cardiovascular disease, cancer, type II diabetes, arthritis, multiple sclerosis, asthma, hypoglycemia, and many other degenerative conditions can often be completely reversed. Changing the kinds and quantities of fats we eat, as well as how we process and use them is part of addressing both malnutrition and internal pollution.

There is a Point of No Return

When vital organs are damaged beyond their ability to function or to recover, reversal of degeneration is no longer possible. No one knows when that point has been reached, therefore no patient should be automatically written off.

Degenerative diseases are a serious matter that we should take very seriously – preferably before they occur – by learning and applying principles of health. The same seriousness of purpose applies to issues involving mental, social, and environmental degeneration.

Limitations of Natural, Nutritional Approaches

Not *all* health problems and degenerative conditions can be cured by foods and life-style changes. Specific genetic conditions, which affect a total of about five per 1000 individuals, may not be curable but can still be helped with improved nutrition and detoxification.

Eventually, the human body naturally wears out. This inevitable fact is one that we must come to terms with. It can help remind us to examine our priorities for living – to make our choices with the inevitable fact of our own end in mind.

Natural nutritional approaches *are* effective for reversing degenerative diseases that result from eating habits and life-styles out of line with nature. These degenerative conditions, which affect the majority of affluent people in the world, *can* be reversed.

The following 89 chapters provide an array of useful information about

---

[2] A 'leadership' elected by popular vote is not leadership but the rule of the average, the mediocre. Real leaders are pioneers. They go ahead, in front, on the basis of understanding and inner convictions, even if they have to go alone.

how foods and essential nutrients affect human health, with special focus on fats, oils, and cholesterol. This information will help consumers better understand human health and make food choices for better health, and to lessen their reliance on drugs. Doctors and healers can use this information as a powerful ally in healing degenerative conditions.

Face Fats!

Components of Fats, Oils, and Cholesterol

N on-technical readers might find the next two chapters a bit dry. Skip them, or nibble. Or challenge yourself to walk through them. Even if you are new to molecules, the chapters are easy to follow and understand. At the very least, you'll get a sense of the molecular level, where the birth of our health takes place.

I would have preferred to put these chapters at the back of the book, but I couldn't figure out how to talk about unknown molecules without first describing and naming them. So here they are, at the front.

In this section, we tackle the important task of looking at molecules that are the basis of the effects that solid fats, liquid oils, and cholesterol have on human health. We must do this because health is very precisely defined and built on the level of molecules, and *all* diseases are rooted in the behavior of molecules – on the molecular level.

The fats that heal have different molecular structures than those that kill. Their healing or killing potential rests in these molecular differences – differences that make them behave differently in our body.

After an overview and an introduction to their names, we look at the different kinds of building blocks (fatty acids), starting with the simplest ones. A chapter on sugars is included because they too can turn into fats. We end the section with a chapter that rounds out the picture of nutrition by introducing the essential nutrients that come from proteins, minerals, and vitamins.

Before we begin, a short list of the most common definitions is in order (a longer glossary of terms is found at the back of the book). *Fats, oils, cholesterol,* and several other fat-like substances (such as *sphingolipids* and *ceramides* that are not discussed in this book because they are made by the body and are relatively unimportant in nutritional self-care) are collectively called 'lipids' by chemists. Lipids also include *fatty acids,* the main building blocks of fats and oils; *phospholipids,* from which the barrier (membrane) that surrounds and protects our cells is made; and *alkylglycerols* that are briefly described in Section Six.

Fats are solid while oils are liquid, because fats and oil molecules contain different fatty acids with different properties. Chemists call fats and oils *triglycerides* because they consist of three (tri) fatty acid molecules joined to a glycerol (glyceride) molecule.

Chemists call the lipids found in cell membranes *phospholipids* because a chemical arrangement of the elements phosphorus and oxygen called phosphate (phospho), and two fatty acids (lipids) are attached to glycerol.

With these short definitions, let us step into the ring of molecules: the components of fats, oils, and cholesterol. We will see what they look like in their natural state before we discuss how processing can turn natural molecules into unnatural molecules that cause disease.

Fatty Acids Overview **3**

Fatty acids are members of several different families. This chapter introduces these families of fatty acids. There is no need to remember all their names and characteristics. You will get to know them intimately as we wind our way through the book. Diagrams are included for those readers with training, or an interest in biochemistry. They can be ignored without losing the story.

Fats, Oils, and Fatty Acids

A molecule of any *solid* fat or *liquid* oil is always made up of one molecule of glycerol (which is best known for its use in glycerin soap) to which three fatty acid molecules are attached.

Fatty acids come in many different shapes and sizes. They are the key building blocks of all fats and oils (lipids) both in our foods and in our body. Fatty acids are the main components in neutral fats (triglycerides) carried in our bloodstream. They are also the main components of fats stored in our fat (adipose) cells, which serve as important sources of stored energy.

Fatty acids are also the main components of membranes that surround all cells and, within cells, surround subcellular organelles (see Chapter 10, Phospholipids and Membranes). Fatty acids play key roles in the construction and maintenance of all healthy cells.

We'll look at phospholipids and triglycerides in later chapters. Here, we'll focus on the fatty acid building blocks.

Structure of Fatty Acids

A fatty acid molecule is shaped like a caterpillar. It is so tiny that 100 quintillion (or 100 followed by 18 zeroes) are present in a single drop of oil. Each tiny caterpillar is composed of two parts: a *fatty chain* at one end, and an *acid group* at the other end.

The **fatty chain** of the molecule is a water-insoluble ('hydrophobic', which means 'water-hating'), oil-soluble, non-polar chain of variable length. This means that it dissolves in oil but not in water, an important property for fatty acid functions in our body. This fatty chain is made entirely of carbon and hydrogen

Families of Molecules

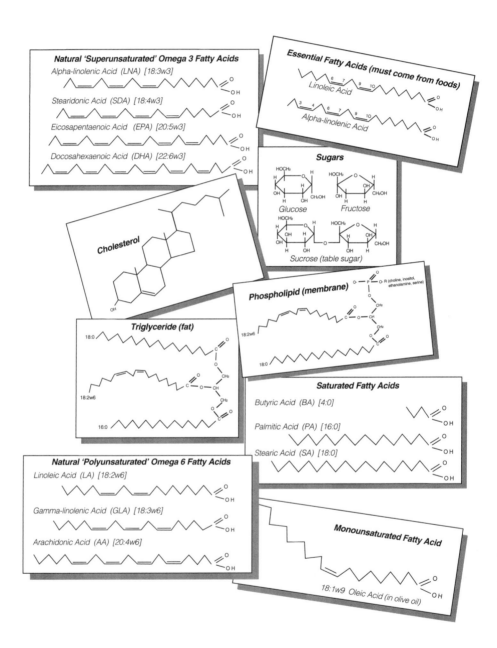

Fats, oils, fatty acids, sugars, and cholesterol.

atoms, and ends in a methyl (-CH3) group.

The **acid end** of the molecule is a water-soluble ('hydrophilic', which means 'water-loving'), polar, weak organic acid known as a carboxyl (-COOH) group, which dissolves in water but not in oil. As we will soon see, this structure gives properties to fatty acids that are important for their functions. Figure 1 shows what a fatty acid looks like.

Chain length. Fatty acids can have any number of carbon atoms in their fatty chain, but the most common lengths range between 4 carbons (butyric acid, found in butter) and 24 carbons (found in fish oils and brain tissue). Formic acid with 1 carbon (bee sting and ant bite) and acetic acid with 2 carbons (vinegar) are also part of this family of compounds, but are not usually included among fatty acids because their fatty chains are so short that they behave as water-soluble acids. Figure 2 shows two fatty acids commonly found in nature.

To make it easier to talk about where chemical reactions take place in a fatty acid, chemists assign numbers to the carbon atoms in fatty acid chains. The numbering system we use in this book is called the omega (w) system, illustrated in

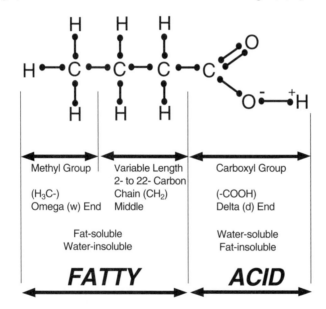

Methyl Group	Variable Length 2- to 22- Carbon	Carboxyl Group
(H$_3$C-)	Chain (CH$_2$)	(-COOH)
Omega (w) End	Middle	Delta (d) End
Fat-soluble Water-insoluble		Water-soluble Fat-insoluble
FATTY		*ACID*

- ● Electron
- ●—● Bond formed when 2 electrons from different atoms are shared
- H Hydrogen Atom
- C Carbon Atom
- O Oxygen Atom

Figure 1. Basic structure of a (saturated) fatty acid.

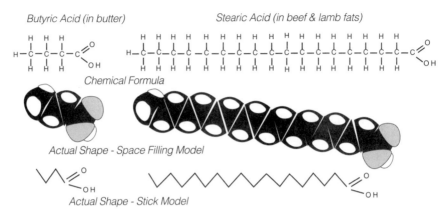

Butyric Acid (in butter)   Stearic Acid (in beef & lamb fats)

Chemical Formula

Actual Shape - Space Filling Model

Actual Shape - Stick Model

Figure 2. Two saturated fatty acids commonly found in nature.

Figure 3. This system numbers carbon atoms in sequence, starting from the methyl end.[1]

Bonds. A bond between lovers, which begins with attraction ('good chemistry') between them, may be expressed by holding hands. It is similar in the chemistry that bonds atoms. Carbon and hydrogen atoms in the fatty acids shown in Figure 2 are linked by sharing electrons (holding hands) with one another. Each shared pair of electrons forms what is known as a single bond, which joins carbon to carbon. Fatty acids whose carbons are joined by single bonds are called saturated. Each carbon atom forms four bonds (because that is the nature of carbon) and, in addition to bonds with other carbons, holds as many hydrogen atoms as it can (three on the end carbon, and two on all others). There are no carbon-to-carbon double bonds in these molecules.

Double bonds. Plant and animal cells can modify saturated fatty acids. They 'insert' one or more double bonds (like lovers holding both hands) into the chain by removing two hydrogen atoms.[2] This process produces *unsaturated* fatty acids, which differ from saturated fatty acids in shape, physical properties (e.g., melting point), and chemical properties, such as the ability to react with water, oxygen, hydroxyl (-OH) and sulphydryl (-SH) groups, and light. Unsaturated fatty acids are less stable and more active chemically than saturated fatty acids,

---

[1] The other commonly used system, called the delta (d) system, starts at the acid end and numbers the carbon atoms in reverse direction. To avoid confusion, we will not use the delta system in this book.

[2] Unlike humans, however, carbon has four 'hands' (electrons) that can form bonds. The fact that carbon has four electron 'hands' makes it capable of forming a wide range of molecules with different forms, shapes, and properties – exactly what is required to form the molecules of life – proteins, fats, carbohydrates, vitamins, hormones, enzymes, etc., which are all built around carbon.

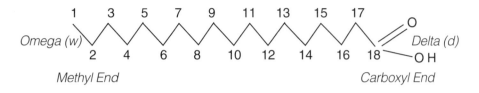

Figure 3. The w (omega) numbering system for fatty acids.

which are relatively stable and inert.

Double bonds can occur between any two carbons in a carbon chain. Plants insert double bonds at different points in fatty acid chains than do animals. This has extremely important implications for nutrition and health (see Chapter 8, The Healing Essential Fatty Acids). Human beings, for instance, rarely (if ever) insert double bonds into fatty acids with less than 16 carbon atoms in their chain. Likewise, human enzymes *cannot* insert double bonds into positions closer than seven carbons from the methyl (w) end. Plants, on the other hand, insert double bonds as close as 3 and 6 carbons from the methyl end. This ability enables plants to produce two 'families' of fatty acids known as the omega 3 (abbreviated as w3 throughout this book) and omega 6 (w6) families, respectively. We call these two fatty acids *essential* because both are vital to human health but cannot be made by our cells and must, therefore, be provided by foods.

Unsaturated fatty acids in nature have from one to as many as six double bonds in their chain. These double bonds change the properties and biological functions of fatty acids that contain them. Figure 4 shows the three most common unsaturated fatty acids found in nature.

Unsaturated fatty acids with two or more double bonds are known as *polyunsaturated* ('poly' means many – or more than one) fatty acids, but market use of this term usually refers to w6 fatty acids found in popular vegetable oils (safflower, sunflower, corn, sesame). The members of the w3 family (polyunsaturated because they also have more than one double bond) are better called *superunsaturated* fatty acids to distinguish them from the w6 fatty acids. This distinction is important because w3 and w6 fatty acids have opposite effects in our body, which powerfully affect our health.

If two or more double bonds are present in the fatty chain of a naturally occurring oil, these double bonds usually start 3 carbon atoms apart. This spacing of double bonds is called *methylene interrupted*. Figure 5 shows methylene interrupted double bonds in a superunsaturated w3 fatty acid. The box at the right illustrates 'conjugated' double bonds, which always start two carbons apart. These are common in many molecules found in nature, but not in fatty acids. A double-bond shift from methylene interrupted to conjugated greatly changes the chemi-

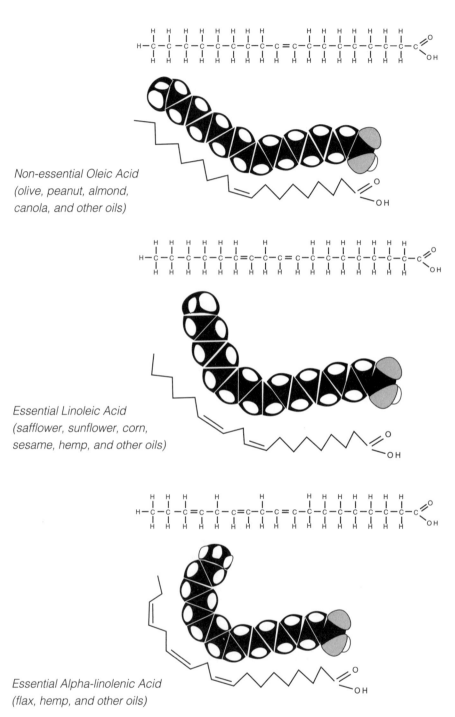

Non-essential Oleic Acid
(olive, peanut, almond,
canola, and other oils)

Essential Linoleic Acid
(safflower, sunflower, corn,
sesame, hemp, and other oils)

Essential Alpha-linolenic Acid
(flax, hemp, and other oils)

Figure 4. Unsaturated fatty acids commonly found in nature.

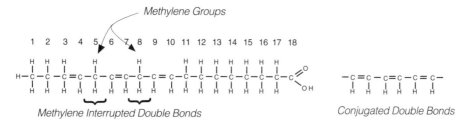

Figure 5. Methylene interrupted double bonds in a fatty acid.

cal properties of a fatty acid.

Cis- and Trans- configurations. To add further complexity and precision, nature arranges double bonds in naturally occurring, nutritionally important fatty acids in what is called the *cis-* configuration. In this configuration, both hydrogen atoms on the carbons involved in the double bond are on the same side of the molecule. The hydrogen atoms repel one another, and the fatty carbon chain kinks to take up some of the empty space on the side of the molecule opposite the hydrogen atoms. The kink changes the caterpillar-like molecule to a bent shape, altering its properties, behavior, and functions in our body.

A double bond in the fatty acid chain can also be in the *trans-* configuration. In this arrangement, we find the hydrogen atoms of the carbons involved in the double bond on opposite sides of the molecule. *Trans-* fatty acids are more stable than *cis-* fatty acids. The molecule straightens out, altering the fatty acid's properties and biological functions (see Chapter 18, Margarines, Shortenings, and *Trans-* Fatty Acids). Even though they are unsaturated, they behave like saturated fatty acids because their shape has been unkinked. Figure 6 shows *cis-* and *trans-*configurations.

Functions of Fatty Acids

Fatty acids in body fat under our skin and around our organs provide insulation and absorb shock.

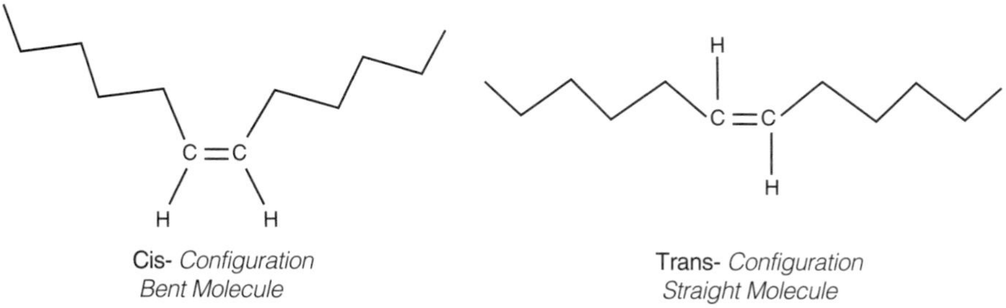

Cis- *Configuration*
Bent Molecule

Trans- *Configuration*
Straight Molecule

Figure 6. Cis- and trans- *configurations around a double bond.*

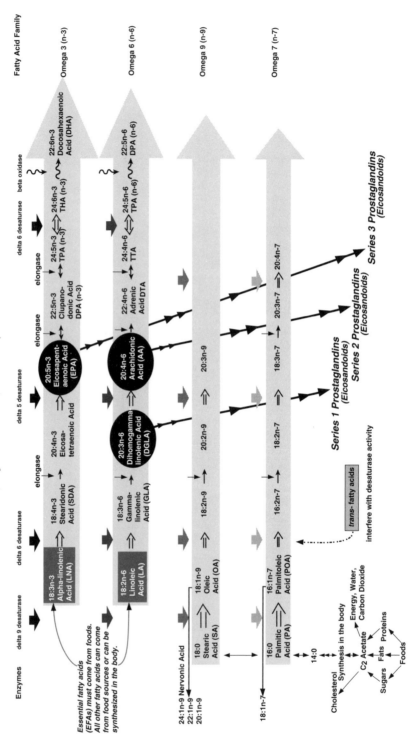

Figure 7. Overall schematic of fatty acid metabolism in human beings.

20

Saturated fatty acids containing less than 16 carbon atoms provide energy, calories, and heat. The shorter the saturated fatty acid, the more readily it 'burns' (oxidizes), and the more easily we can digest it. Our liver must process (metabolize) the fats and oils we eat. Poor digestion of fatty foods, and feeling tired, heavy, or nauseous after fat-containing meals can be symptoms of liver malfunction. Shorter-chain fatty acids are less taxing on our liver than longer ones, and are preferable for people with impaired liver function.

Our body uses saturated fatty acids containing 16 or 18 carbons to generate energy, construct membranes, or make unsaturated fatty acids. It can also store them in fat tissues for future use.

Although all fatty acids produce 9 calories of energy per gram, our body prefers to save the important w3 and w6 *essential* fatty acids for vital hormone-like functions.

Our body uses unsaturated and essential fatty acids to construct membranes, create electrical potentials, and move electric currents. It can also burn them to produce energy if the more vital roles that these fatty acids play have been adequately fulfilled.

Our body can lengthen (elongate) unsaturated and essential fatty acids, and insert more double bonds (desaturate). The resulting highly unsaturated molecules serve functions in all cells, and are especially key in the most active tissues of our body: brain, sense organs, adrenal glands, and testes. Highly unsaturated fatty acids attract oxygen, help generate electrical currents, and help transform light energy into electrical energy, and then into nerve impulses.

Enzyme-controlled and extremely precise processes in our body can change essential fatty acids into derivatives that, in turn, can be partially oxidized by other enzyme-controlled processes to produce hormone-like substances that regulate many functions of all tissues (see Chapter 58, Prostaglandins).

Figure 7 sketches an overall scheme of fatty acid metabolism in human cells, and sums up the generation and conversions of dietary fats and oils in our body. It identifies (in boxes) two essential fatty acids that must come from foods, and shows (in ellipses) three essential fatty acid derivatives from which prostaglandins are made.

Food Sources of Fatty Acids

Short-chain saturated fatty acids are especially abundant in butter and tropical fats. In minor quantities, they are present in all fats and oils.

Long-chain fatty acids are found in all fats and oils. We will list below those food sources in which they make up a large part of the total fatty acid content.

Superunsaturated W3 Family

• **Alpha-linolenic Acid** (LNA), improperly called linolenic acid by some writers (see Chapter 4, What's in a Name?), is found in flax, hemp seed, canola, soy bean, walnut, and dark-green leaves. Flax seed is the richest source, containing over 50% of its fatty acids as LNA. Chia and kukui (candlenut) oils contain about 30% LNA. Hemp seed oil contains about 20% LNA. Pumpkin seed oil may contain as much as 15% LNA, or as little as none. Canola oil contains up to 10%, and walnut oil contains between 3 and 11% LNA. Soybean oil usually runs about 5 to 7% LNA. Other seed oils contain less LNA than these, or none. Dark green leaves contain only a little oil, but this oil is over 50% LNA.

- **Stearidonic Acid** (SDA) is found in black currant seeds, whose refined oil is available in capsules. It is also found in several kinds of wild seeds that have not been commercialized.
- **Eicosapentaenoic Acid** (EPA) and **Docosahexaenoic Acid** (DHA) are found in the oils of cold water fish and marine animals. Salmon, trout, mackerel, sardines, and other cold water marine animals are rich sources of these fatty acids, containing up to 30% combined EPA and DHA. Among land animals, brain, eyeballs, adrenal glands, and testes are rich in EPA and DHA. Primitive tribes prized these tissues highly, and ate them raw immediately after a kill because, as science found out centuries (or millennia) later, these highly nutritious oils deteriorate and spoil rapidly after an animal dies. Chinese water snake oil is the richest source of EPA at 20% (see Chapter 56, Snake Oil and Patent Medicines). From EPA, our body makes series 3 prostaglandins with many beneficial effects on health.

Polyunsaturated W6 Family

- **Linoleic Acid** (LA) is found in safflower, sunflower, hemp, soybean, walnut, pumpkin, sesame, and flax. Safflower and sunflower are the richest source of LA, but new genetic varieties of 'high oleic safflower' and 'high oleic sunflower' seeds contain only small quantities of LA.
- **Gamma-linolenic Acid** (GLA) is virtually absent from mothers' milk, contrary to advertising claims. Borage is the richest source of GLA (20%+), followed by black currant seed oil (15%). Evening primrose oil contains 9% GLA. Several other seeds also contain GLA.
- Mothers' milk does contain **Dihomogamma-linolenic Acid** (DGLA) from which our body makes series 1 prostaglandins with many beneficial effects on health.
- **Arachidonic Acid** (AA) is found in meats and other animal products. From AA, our body makes series 2 prostaglandins that mediate survival as well as disease functions. AA is not present in peanut oil, contrary to popular belief.

Monounsaturated W9 Family

- **Oleic Acid** (OA) is found in large quantities in olive, almond, avocado, peanut, pecan, cashew, filbert, and macadamia oils. Land animal fats and butter are other sources of OA. OA and other members of this family are produced in our body.

Monounsaturated W7 Family
- **Palmitoleic Acid** (POA) is found in tropical oils, especially coconut and palm kernel. Our body converts POA into several other members of the w7 family.

Saturated Family
- **Stearic Acid** (SA) is found abundantly in beef, mutton, pork, butter, cocoa butter, and shea nut butter.
- **Palmitic Acid** (PA) is found in large quantities in tropical fats: coconut, palm, and palm kernel.
- **Butyric Acid** (BA) is found in butter.
- **Arachidic Acid** – not arachidonic acid – is present in peanuts.

All oils contain varying proportions of different fatty acids (see Chapter 50, Oils in Seeds).

What's in a Name? 4

Naming Fatty Acids

Like people, fatty acids go by several names. A fatty acid may have a nickname, and it always has a proper name. Its molecular structure may be drawn in several ways. It also has a shorthand name. We'll describe the different naming systems. Some of them will be used in the book, and if you are familiar with them, it will make the text easier to follow. Once you know the names, they're quite simple.

Nicknames
The scientist who discovers a fatty acid may give it a nickname, and the name may be as eccentric as the scientist. If he knows Greek or Latin word roots, the name may reflect his erudition. Perhaps he will name it for the animal or plant from which he isolated it, or perhaps some other whim will move him to name his new discovery.

For example, butyric acid was so named because it was found in butter. Caproic, caprylic, and capric acids were found in goat's milk (the same Latin root is also found in the sun sign Capricorn, the goat). Oleic acid got its name from the olive oil in which it is found, and linoleic and linolenic acids got theirs from the Latin name for flax, which is *Linum*. Stearic acid comes from the Greek root word for fat, which is *stea-;* lauric acid comes from laurel; palmitic acid comes from palm; and vaccenic acid, a fatty acid found in cow's milk, got its name from the Latin word for that animal, which is *vacca*.

However, nicknames fail to show us the structure of the fatty acid: what it looks like and what it can do, therefore each fatty acid has another name that gives us more of this information.

Proper Names

The proper name for a fatty acid contains all the information that a chemist needs in order to draw its structure and know its properties, even if he has never seen this fatty acid before. Proper naming follows strict rules laid down by chemists at meetings.

These meetings are like christenings. The chemists – parents, aunts, uncles, and friends of a new chemical – attend. They discuss names for their new baby, and afterwards they often celebrate. They agree on a naming system for future additions to the chemical family so they can discuss the structures and behaviors of molecules with one another. Whenever a new group of chemical compounds is found or synthesized, another christening party is held to decide how and what to name the new chemical children.

For example, the proper name for palmitic acid is hexadecanoic acid. Hexadeca means 16; -oic acid is the name for a fatty acid. All together, the name tells us that this is a fatty acid with 16 carbons in its chain. Simple.

The proper name for linoleic acid (Figure 4) is a little more complicated, because the molecule has more character. It is called: all *cis*- w6,9-octadecadienoic acid, where:

- -oic acid = a fatty acid;
- octadeca = 18 carbons.
- di = 2,
- 'en' = double bonds;
- w6,9 describes where in the chain the double bonds are located: they start on carbons 6 and 9, counting from the w (methyl) end and go to the next carbon (i.e., there is a double bond between w carbons 6 and 7, and another double bond between w carbons and 9 and 10);
- all *cis*- means that both hydrogen atoms on the carbons involved in each double bond are on the same side of the molecule.

That's not too difficult, but molecules can get quite complicated.

Recently, I came across 1-(1-(2cyanoaziridinyl)isopropyl)aziridin-2-carboxylic acid amide. I was lost on that one, so I looked at a picture of the structure of its molecule instead. This brings us to the third kind of name.

Structural Formula

When we use a structural formula to make one of our chemical children known to others, we draw a picture of the entire molecule, showing which atoms are joined. A picture of the chemical 'child' allows people to see for themselves what a particular molecule looks like.

For example, here is the structure of the saturated palmitic acid, also known as hexadecanoic acid:

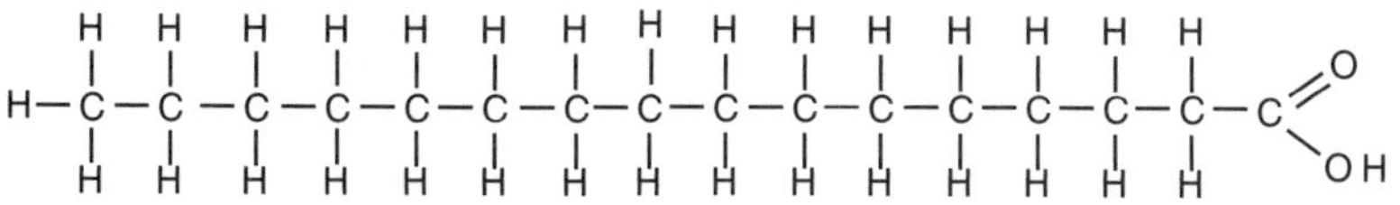

Here is the structural formula of linoleic acid (*cis, cis*- w6,9-octadecadienoic acid):

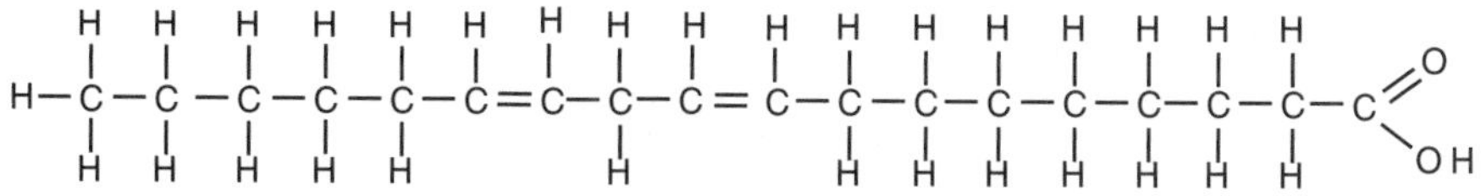

As you can see, a structural formula makes it easy to picture the molecule being talked about. Drawing the structural formula, however, is slow and cumbersome, (on a typewriter, usually impossible), so a shorthand system has been developed to overcome these limitations.

Shorthand Names

The shorthand used to name fatty acids is most convenient. We'll use examples to illustrate it.

Butyric acid (Figure 2) is the nickname. The structure looks like this:

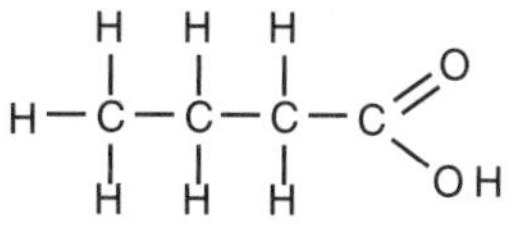

The shorthand name is 4:0, where:
- 4 = the number of carbon atoms in the fatty-acid chain;
- 0 = the number of double bonds.

There is a methyl group (-CH3) at one end, and an acid group (-COOH) at the other, because this is true for all fatty acids.

Let's take another example. Alpha-linolenic acid (LNA) (Figure 4) is the nickname. The proper name is all *cis*- w3,6,9-octadecatrienoic acid. The structural formula is:

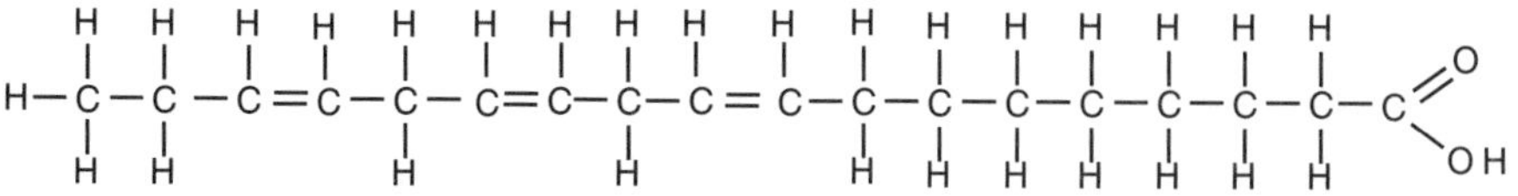

The shorthand name is 18:3w3, where:
- 18 = the number of carbon atoms;
- 3 = the number of double bonds;
- w3 = the position, from the methyl end, of the carbon atom at which the

first double bond starts.

Scientists know (and we have already learned) that double bonds in natural fatty acids are methylene interrupted. From this, we know that the second double bond starts at carbon 6, and the third double bond starts at carbon 9. The first double bond unites carbons 3 and 4; the second double-bond unites carbons 6 and 7; and the third double-bond unites carbons 9 and 10. We also learned that natural fatty acids have all their double-bond hydrogens in the *cis-* configuration, on the same side of the molecule.[1] Once you know the agreed-upon rules and get some practice, shorthand becomes simple.

We can also do it the other way around. 18:2w6 means: an 18-carbon chain; 2 double bonds (methylene interrupted and in *cis-* configuration), where the first double bond starts at the w6 carbon, the sixth carbon from the w (methyl) end. The second bond must start at carbon w9. Therefore, the structure of 18:2w6 is:

The shorthand name 22:6w3 means: 22 carbon atoms; 6 double bonds (methylene interrupted and in *cis-* configuration), where the first double bond is on carbon 3, counting from the w (methyl) end. There is always the carboxyl (-COOH) acid at the right end. Therefore the structure of 22:6w3 is:

First we made 22 Cs. To the carbon at the left end, we added three hydrogens to make the methyl end. To the carbon at the right end, we added =O and -OH to make the acid group. Then we put in the double bonds. The first double bond goes between carbons 3 and 4; the others go between C6 and 7, C9 and 10, C12 and 13, C15 and 16, and C18 and 19. Then we put the hydrogens of both carbons involved in each double bond on the same side of the molecule, and we connected all remaining carbons with one bond each. That's how far we got in the drawing. When we add the remaining hydrogens (2 per carbon, 1 on each side of the molecule), we get the structural formula for 22:6w3.

We will use shorthand designations, structural formulas, and common names throughout the book. The following 2-page reference list of names and structures of the important common fatty acids should be helpful.

---

[1] If a double bond in a fatty acid is in the *trans-* configuration, that is specified by a t in the nickname. For instance, t18:1w9 has 18 carbons with a *trans-* double bond between carbons 9 and 10.

Saturated Fatty Acids

Butyric Acid (BA) [4:0]

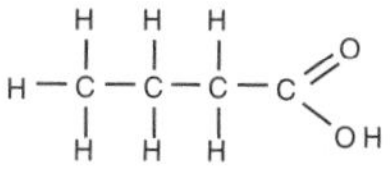

Caproic Acid [6:0]

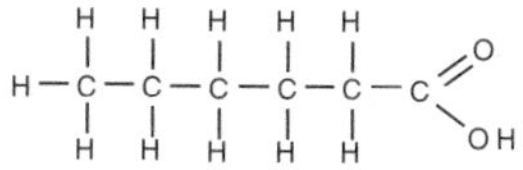

Caprylic Acid [8:0]

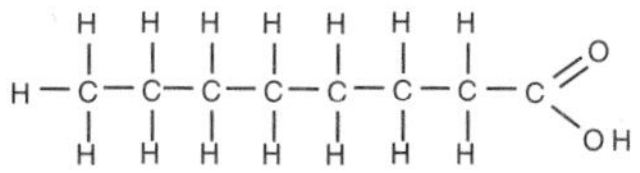

Capric Acid [10:0]

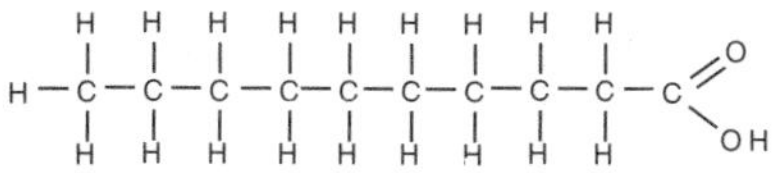

Lauric Acid [12:0]

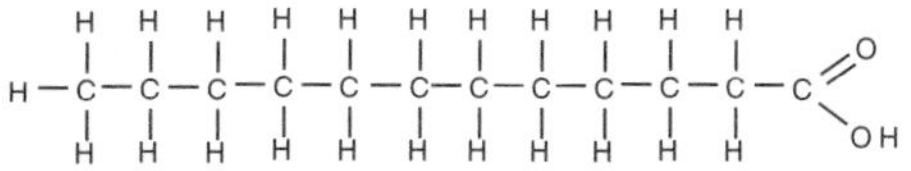

Myristic Acid [14:0]

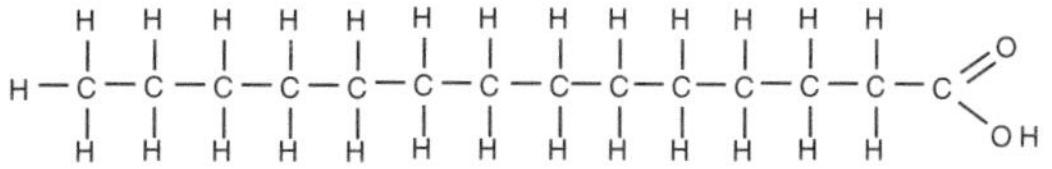

Palmitic Acid (PA) [16:0]

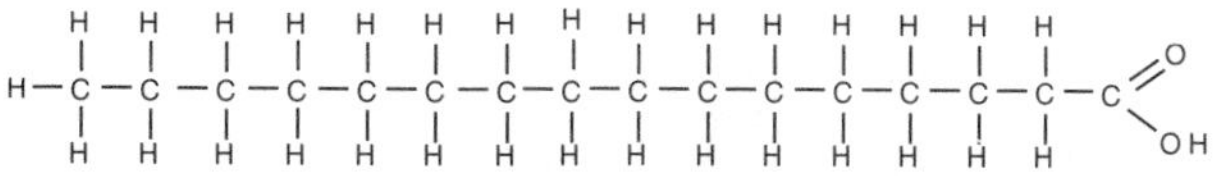

Stearic Acid (SA) [18:0]

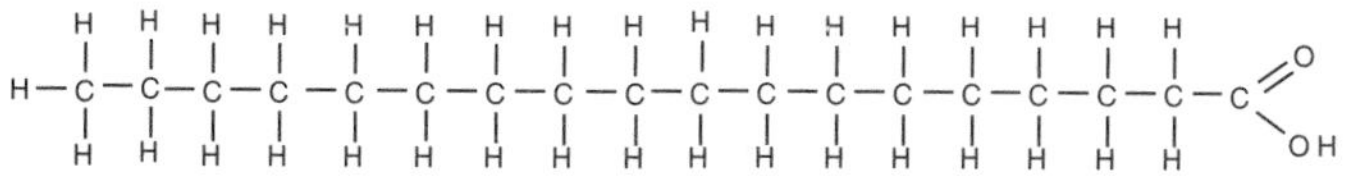

Arachidic Acid [20:0]

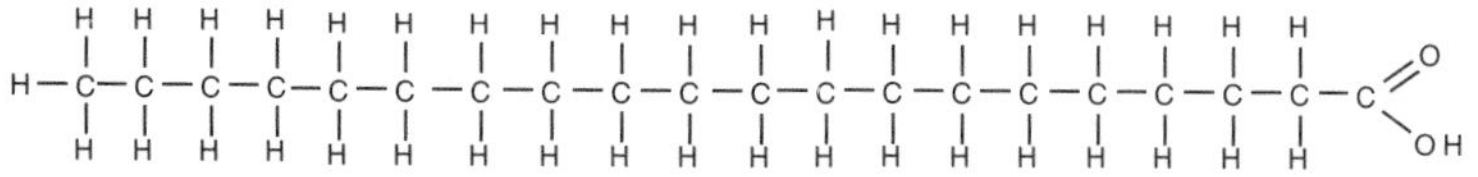

Unsaturated Fatty Acids

Nickname (abbreviation) [shorthand]	Structural Formula

Monounsaturated Fatty Acids

Palmitoleic Acid (POA) [16:1w7]

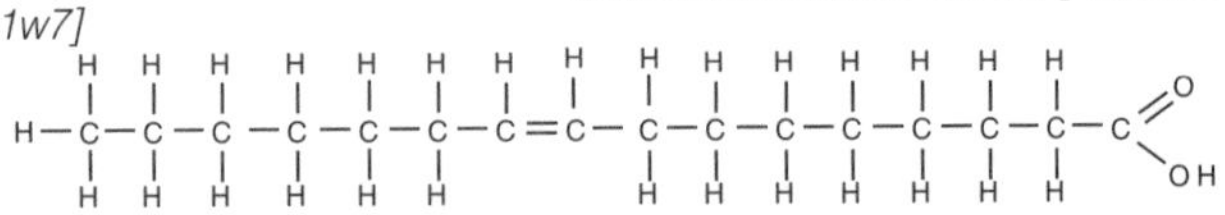

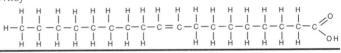

Oleic Acid (OA) [18:1w9]

Essential Fatty Acids

Linoleic Acid (LA) [18:2w6]
'polyunsaturated'

Alpha-linolenic Acid (LNA) [18:3w3]
'superunsaturated'

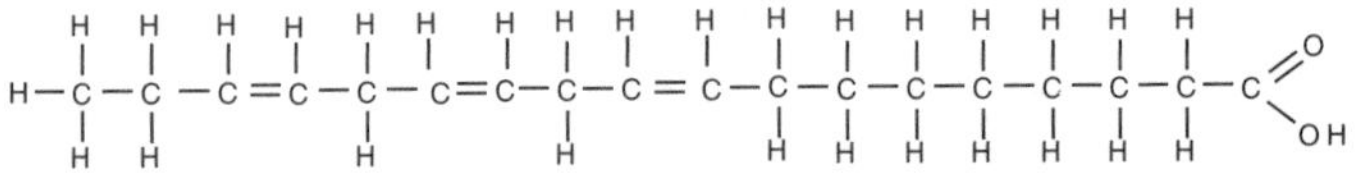

Omega 6 Derivatives
'polyunsaturates'

Gamma-linolenic Acid (GLA) [18:3w6]

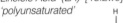
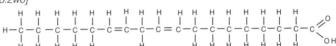

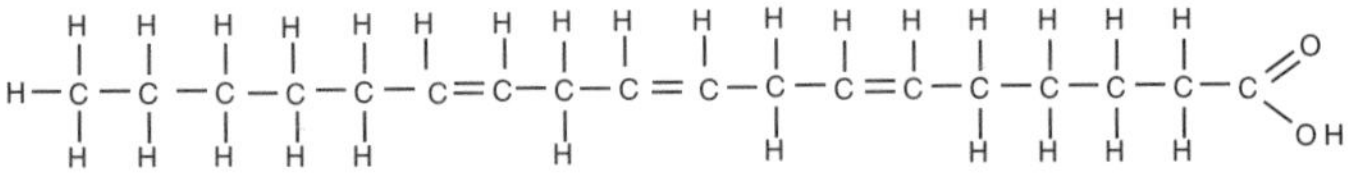

Arachidonic Acid (AA) [20:4w6]

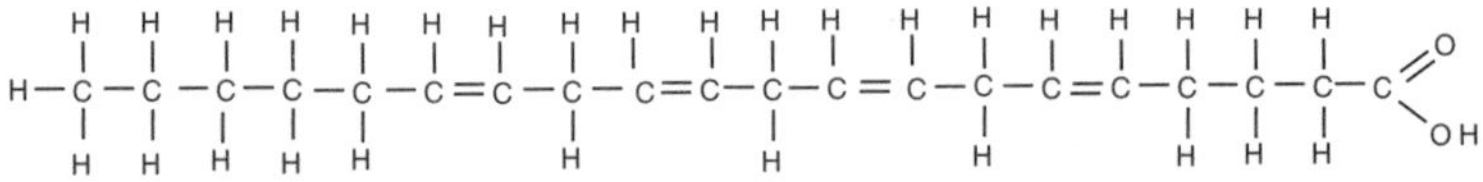

Omega 3 Derivatives
'superunsaturates'

Stearidonic Acid (SDA) [18:4w3]

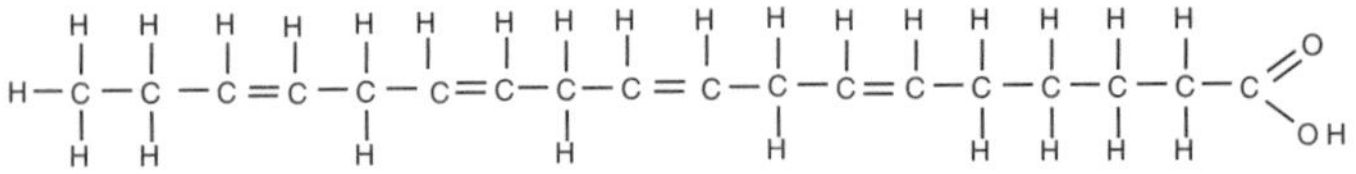

Eicosapentaenoic Acid (EPA) [20:5w3]

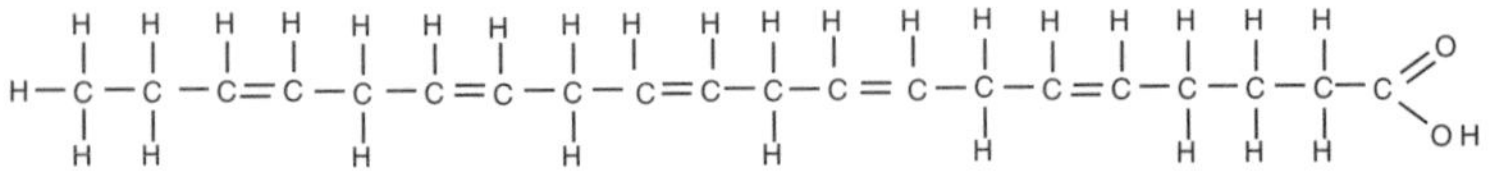

Docosahexaenoic Acid (DHA) [22:6w3]

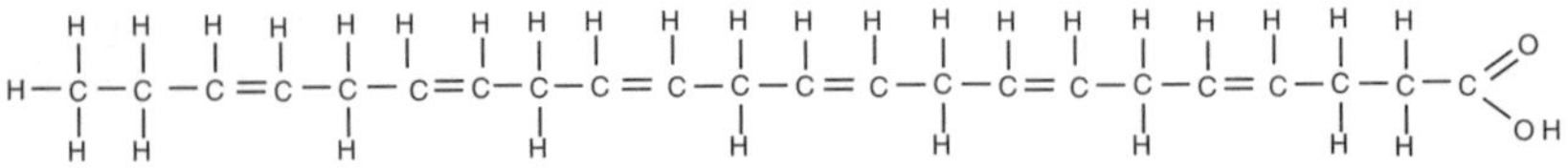

Hard Fats and
Saturated Fatty Acids (SaFAs) 5

Saturated fatty acids (SaFAs) are found in all food fats and oils, but are especially abundant in hard fats. An *excess* of SaFAs can cause health problems for our heart and arteries.

SaFAs are the simplest fatty acids. They carry the carboxyl (acid) group at one end and the rest of the molecule is fatty material. The fatty material is an arrangement of carbon atoms chained together, and each of the remaining positions on the carbon atoms are taken up by hydrogen atoms. Since SaFAs carry as many hydrogen atoms as they possibly can, they are *saturated* with them. Figures 1 and 2 in Chapter 3 illustrated saturated fatty acids.

General Properties

SaFA carbon chains can be from 4 to 28 carbon atoms long. They are straight, have no kinks, contain no double bonds, are slow to react with other chemicals, and carry no electric charges. The acid group of SaFAs reacts readily, either with glycerol to produce fats and membranes, or with strong bases to make soaps. Essentially, SaFAs are sluggish molecules, uninteresting in comparison to unsaturated fatty acids that we consider later (see Chapter 7, Liquid Oils and Unsaturated Fatty Acids).

Melting Points

The length of a SaFA carbon chain determines the SaFA's melting point and its solidity. The acid part of the molecule is usually hooked up to a glycerol molecule. The fatty part, on the other hand, wants to aggregate. Fat likes to dissolve in fat and hates water, so the fatty parts of the molecules tend to stick together. The longer the fatty part of the molecule, the greater its tendency is to aggregate. A 'sticky' molecule means it is harder and has a higher melting point. Table A1 lists chain lengths and melting points of common SaFAs.

Short-Chain Saturated Fatty Acids

Short-chain SaFAs (4:0 to 6:0) make up less than 10% of the total fatty acids found in butter and milk fat. Some short-chain SaFAs are also found in coconut and palm kernel oils.

Up to a length of 8 carbons, SaFAs are liquid at room temperature. Up to 10 carbons, they are liquid at body temperature (37°C; 98.6°F). Above 10 carbons, they are solid at body temperature.

Our body uses SaFAs up to 12 carbons long mainly to produce energy. They are easy to digest, and people suffering from liver and digestive ailments

29

Table A1. Chain lengths and melting points of saturated fatty acids.

Name of Fatty Acid	Number of Carbon Atoms	Melting Point
butyric (4:0)	4	-8°C (18°F)
caproic (6:0)	6	-3°C (27°F)
caprylic (8:0)	8	17°C (63°F)
capric (10:0)	10	32°C (90°F)
lauric (12:0)	12	44°C (111°F)
myristic (14:0)	14	54°C (129°F)
palmitic (16:0)	16	63°C (145°F)
stearic (18:0)	18	70°C (158°F)
arachidic (20:0)	20	75°C (167°F)
behenic (22:0)	22	80°C (176°F)
lignoceric (24:0)	24	84°C (183°F)

should include them in their diets. Butyric acid (4:0) helps feed the friendly bacteria that keep our colon healthy. Caprylic acid (8:0) is used to inhibit the growth of yeasts and candida in our intestines. It appears to be incorporated into the membranes of yeast cells and then these membranes rupture, killing the yeast cell.

Butyric acid (4:0), the shortest SaFA, dissolves in water. Caproic (6:0) and caprylic (8:0) acids are partially water-soluble. SaFAs with chains longer than 8 carbons do not dissolve in water, but dissolve readily in oil. As the oil-soluble chain lengthens, the water-soluble acid group makes up a decreasing part of the molecule, which explains both the decreasing water solubility and the increasing ability of the SaFA molecule to dissolve in oily, organic or non-polar solvents that carry no electrical charge.

Medium-Chain Saturated Fatty Acids

Medium-chain SaFAs contain 6 to 12 carbon atoms – but mainly 8 and 10 – in their chains. Our body metabolizes medium-chain SaFAs the same way it metabolizes short-chain SaFAs: to produce energy. It does not store them as fat. For this reason, they are used as medium-chain triglycerides (MCTs) in diets of people with digestive and liver problems.

As MCTs, medium-chain SaFAs are also popular with athletes, who use them as a source of energy before workouts. Too many MCTs can produce an unpleasant, scratchy sensation at the back of the throat (see Chapter 65, Medium-Chain Triglycerides), so only one or two tablespoons should be used for this purpose.

Long-Chain Saturated Fatty Acids

Our cells use long-chain SaFAs to build cell membranes (see Chapter 10, Phospholipids and Membranes). The tendency of SaFAs to aggregate balances the tendency of unsaturated fatty acids to disperse (see Chapter 7, Liquid Oils and Unsaturated Fatty Acids). Both kinds of fatty acids are found in membranes.

By keeping unsaturated fatty acid chains physically separated from one another, SaFAs may prevent unsaturated fatty acids in membranes from taking part in unwanted chemical reactions with one another.

Long-chain SaFAs are solid at body temperature. They are insoluble in water and form crystal structures, sticking together (aggregating) to form droplets. Their tendency to aggregate involves long-chain SaFAs in one of the major health problems related to human nutrition: sticky platelets that can readily form blood clots in an artery.

By making platelets more sticky, the aggregating tendency of long-chain SaFAs plays a role in cardiovascular disease which plagues populations whose diets are high in beef, mutton, pork, dairy products, and other food products containing a large amount of long-chain SaFAs.[1] They can be deposited within cells, organs, and arteries along with proteins, minerals, and cholesterol (a non-polar, very sticky, and extremely hard fatty substance that melts at 149°C [300°F]). Diets high in refined sugars can also create cardiovascular problems, in part because our body converts excess sugar into SaFAs (see next chapter).

The Sugar-Fat Connection 6

A book on fats and oils would not include a chapter on sugars and starches, except for the fact that these carbohydrates are – I was going to say kissing cousins, but their relationship is even closer – the hidden parents of the fats that can kill us. Refined dietary sugars almost always turn into fats, and starches can also turn into saturated fats. Let's see how sugars and starches can keep us healthy and make us sick, and can even kill us. Figure 8 shows illustrations of several carbohydrates.

Sugars

The sugars category includes all refined sugars and syrups. These are: *simple sug-*

---

[1] The stickiness of saturated fats and cholesterol is only one factor in cardiovascular disease. The *complete* story is more complex. There is injury to the lining of the artery, due to toxic free radicals, oxidized LDL cholesterol, oxidized triglyceride fatty acids, etc. This is followed by attempts at repair that involve thickening the arteries by repair proteins apo(a) and fibrinogen, along with fats and cholesterol. The combination of thickened (narrowed) arteries *and* sticky platelets sets the stage for heart attacks, strokes, and emboli.

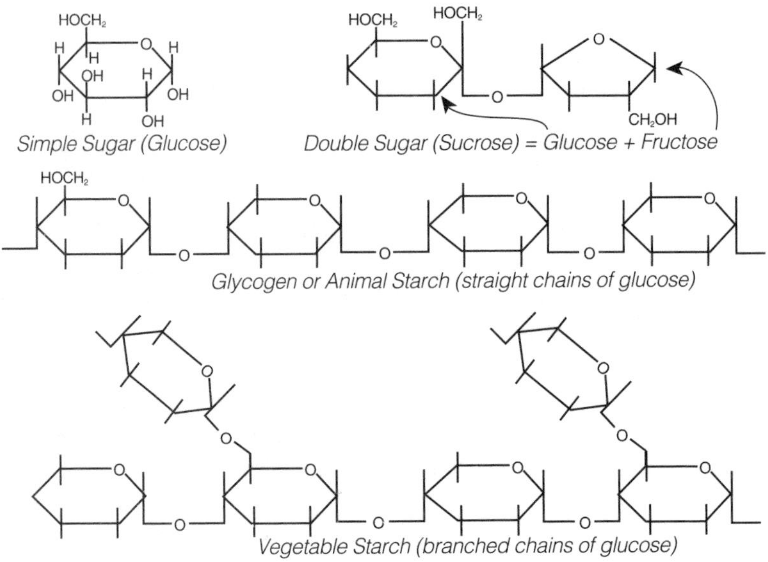

Figure 8. Sugars and starches = carbohydrates.

ars: glucose (or dextrose), fructose (or levulose), and galactose; *double sugars:* sucrose (table sugar), maltose (in beer), and lactose (in milk); *dextrins* and *dextrans;* and *syrups* made from sugarcane, sugar beets, sorghum, and maple. Even *honey* and *maple syrup* are included. Our body digests and absorbs these concentrated sources of sugars rapidly, and quickly turns them into saturated fatty acids. This is described in more detail a little later.

Starches

Starches are sugar (glucose) molecules bonded together. Enzymes in our body must break the bonds between the glucose molecules, gradually turning (digesting) starches into glucose, the primary fuel for all cells in our body. Starches are preferable to sugars because they are digested more slowly, and therefore absorbed more slowly over an extended period of time. Refined starchy foods – white flour, white rice, pasta, enriched flours (both white and dark), corn starch, tapioca, breakfast cereals, and products made with these ingredients – are more likely to turn into fats than starches from whole grains, which contain more fiber and are digested even more slowly.

Products that contain hidden sugars and/or starches include soft drinks; cakes, cookies, and pies; candies and confections; many canned fruits and juices; ice creams and shakes; jams and jellies; and desserts. Ketchup contains a huge amount of sugar.

Many meat and sausage products are extended with refined starch. Protein-starch mixtures are more difficult to digest than either protein or starch by itself.

When poorly or incompletely digested, such mixtures can lead to bloating, intestinal pain, and gas.

Whole grains do not usually present problems. They contain more fiber, and are digested and absorbed more slowly than sugars and refined starches. They are also rich in mineral and vitamin co-factors that enable our body to completely burn them for energy. Complex carbohydrates can fatten us only if we live sedentary lives without exercise, eat for social reasons when we're not hungry, or eat compulsively for psychological reasons. Complex carbohydrate foods include grains, corn, and starchy vegetables such as broccoli and cauliflower. Potatoes and yams contain starch that is quickly broken down, and can increase blood sugar levels rapidly.

Sweet fruits contain starches, but also large amounts of sugar, and can lead to fat production when they form more than a small part of our diet. In nature, fruit is available mainly in the fall. Wild animals such as bears eat fruit in the fall in order to build up their fat. These fat stores are used up during the bears' mostly foodless winter hibernation. When we eat sweet fruit year-round (an unnatural situation in temperate climates), we can get fat on it year-round.

Carbohydrates and Health Problems

If we are active and healthy with competent digestive function and no food allergies, we can eat natural complex carbohydrates (vegetables and grains, a little fruit) without getting fat. In fact, complex carbs are the best sources of slowly released glucose, which is the best fuel for providing the energy we live on.

Complex carbohydrates contain fiber and other materials that are digested slowly. Their starches are only slowly converted into glucose, which is then burned (oxidized) in body functions at the same rate at which it is produced. Therefore, complex carbs do not provide excess energy that turns into fat. Complex carbs also contain vitamins and minerals (co-factors) that enable our body to burn them cleanly into carbon dioxide, water, and energy.

People who spend most of their working day sitting in an office and their evenings as couch potatoes, or people whose diet contains a lot of refined starches and sugars, are likely to have a weight problem (really a fat problem). Males may die from the results of cardiovascular disease (CVD) or diabetes as early as their late 30s to early 60s. Women are protected from CVD during their reproductive years due to hormones (resulting in menstrual iron loss).[1]

Children who lead inactive, TV-addicted lives while consuming popular,

---

[1] It has recently been proposed that excess iron, a powerful pro-oxidant, initiates the oxidation of fats and cholesterol that lead to arterial damage and atherosclerosis. Women's monthly loss of iron-containing blood protects them against cardiovascular disease before menopause by preventing them from building up an excess of iron. If this is true, men could live longer by donating blood on a regular basis.

33

sugar-laden, nutrient-poor junk food diets often have weight and cardiovascular problems beginning at an early age, and may already have severely blocked arteries by the time they become teenagers. How does this happen?

Refined sugars need no digestion and are absorbed rapidly. They lack the co-factors, and our body cannot burn them properly. Glucose floods our blood and cells. High blood glucose is a dangerous condition that can result in diabetic sugar shock (hyperglycemia), coma, and death. Such a condition must be prevented.

Excess Glucose

Our body deals with excess glucose in two ways:

1. It stores excess glucose from times of feasting – as fat – for use in future times of famine. This economical method, designed by Nature during a past of regular food shortages, is maladaptive in affluent, developed nations.
2. It spills excess glucose into our urine (a common symptom of diabetes). Our body uses this method only if the first method fails, due to overload or failure of sugar-regulating mechanisms (see Refined Carbohydrates and Disease, below).

Nature did not equip our body to deal with *continued* excess. We must therefore avoid the health problems caused by consuming excess refined carbohydrates by making wiser food choices, eating only when we are hungry and stopping when our hunger is satisfied (even if our plate is not empty); working off caloric indulgences by physical activity; and/or examining our psychological reasons for overeating.

If we have made poor food choices, stuffed ourselves on refined sugars, and overloaded on glucose, our body responds in the following way: high blood glucose triggers our pancreas to secrete insulin, which moves glucose into our cells. Here, glucose is fed into the energy-producing (Krebs) cycle within the mitochondria in our cells. Glucose in excess of our cells' energy requirements stimulates the production of fatty acids. Three fatty acids, hooked to a glycerol molecule, make a fat molecule (triglyceride). These fat molecules are deposited in our cells and organs, or transported by our blood to fat (adipose) tissues for storage. Sugar consumption leads to high blood triglyceride levels, which are associated with cardiovascular disease.

Healing and killing fatty acids. Some fatty acids found in nature can heal degenerative conditions; others can kill us. Killer saturated long-chain fatty acids, which are sticky and therefore increase our chances of stroke, heart attack, clogged arteries, and diabetes, are produced from refined sugars.

Our body can insert double bonds into these sticky, saturated fatty acids, making them unsaturated. Unsaturated fatty acids can oxidize and damage arteries if our diet lacks antioxidants. The latter are removed from many foods when they are processed. Both saturated and body-made unsaturated fatty acids can serve as sources of energy for our body, but neither type is essential. Neither type can fulfill our body's need for essential fatty acids, or help cure deficiency (see

Chapter 8, The Healing Essential Fatty Acids). On the contrary, fatty acids made from sugars interfere with essential fatty acid functions, and increase the likelihood of diseases of fatty degeneration. An excess of refined sugars can also increase cholesterol levels in our blood.

Sugars Turn Sour and Vinegar Becomes Fat

How does our body convert sugar molecules into fats and cholesterol? When our cells' furnaces (mitochondria) break down a 6-carbon glucose molecule to produce energy, one of the steps involves the creation of 2-carbon acetates (vinegar). These acetates are building blocks for both cholesterol (see Chapter 12, Cholesterol) and saturated fatty acids. If acetates are produced faster than they can be burned by our body into carbon dioxide, water, and energy, they pressure enzymes in our cells to hook them end to end to make saturated fatty acids and cholesterol. This process prevents the metabolic problems that excess acetates would cause in our cells if they were allowed to accumulate. In the short term, excess vinegar in our cells is more toxic than excess fats and cholesterol.

But not fat back to sweet. Our body can turn excess sugars into fat, but it cannot turn fat back into sugars. It must burn off the fat through activity. Fat burn-off can take place in most of our organs, because they can use fat as energy-producing fuel. Our brain, however, is more fussy about its fuel supply. It demands glucose, glutamic acid, or ketones to function. It cannot use fat. If no glucose is present in our diet, our body must make it. Since our body is unable to use fat to make glucose, it converts protein to the brain fuel glucose.

People intolerant of, or allergic to certain grains[2] must eat extra protein. For them, proteins must perform double duties: providing building materials for enzymes and body structures; and providing materials for making brain fuel.

Refined Carbohydrates and Disease

Refined sugars are digested and absorbed into our bloodstream with uncanny speed, and raise blood glucose levels too high. This is hyperglycemia, one symptom of diabetes. Insulin does its job of removing excess glucose from our bloodstream with amazing efficiency. Then our glucose levels may fall too rapidly or too low. The result is hypoglycemia, with symptoms that may include depression, dizziness, crying spells, aggression, insomnia, weakness, and even loss of consciousness.

When blood glucose falls too low, our adrenal glands kick in to mobilize the body's stores of glycogen,[3] and also stimulate the synthesis of glucose from proteins and other substances present in our body.

---

[2] Wheat and corn allergy, for instance, are quite common.

[3] Glycogen, also called animal starch, and stored in liver and muscle, consists of many glucose molecules hooked end to end in a chain.

A diet of refined carbohydrates catches our pancreas and adrenal glands in a biochemical see-saw, overworking them. If our pancreas weakens, it secretes less insulin. Blood glucose remains high, and diabetes (hyperglycemia) may result, with glucose spilling into our urine. Cardiovascular complications that develop from excess glucose and/or fats kill many diabetics. In addition, hard fats interfere with insulin function, leading to 'insulin insensitivity'. If our adrenal glands give out, adrenal exhaustion – the inability to respond biochemically to stress – results. Stress-caused diseases occur. Overworked adrenal glands fail in their blood sugar-raising function, resulting in low blood sugar (hypoglycemia) from the action of insulin. Hypoglycemia gives rise to craving for sweets. The rapid absorption of sugar in sweets eaten in response to this craving starts another vicious hyper-glycemia-hypoglycemia-sugar-craving cycle.

If our body is unable to use all of the extra fats and cholesterol produced from sugar, it must dump the additional load. Fats can be deposited in the cells of our liver, heart, arteries, fat tissues, kidneys, muscles, and other organs.

One aspect of fatty degeneration is the deposition of visible fat in places where it is not normally found in healthy people. Atherosclerosis, fatty liver and kidneys, some tumors, obesity, and some forms of diabetes belong to this group.

More Problems

Saturated fatty acids decrease oxygen supply to our tissues (hypoxia), choking them by making red blood cells stick together, less mobile, and less able to deliver oxygen to cells. By increasing our body's load of these unnecessary fatty acids, refined sugars cause tissue hypoxia. Hypoxia is common to many degenerative conditions and to fatty degeneration (see Chapter 1, Fatty Degeneration).

Sugars inhibit the functions of our immune system, and increase diseases caused by poor immune function, such as colds and flu. Sugars also support the development of food allergies with symptoms that include colitis, asthma, behavioral disorders, joint pain and deterioration, and muscle pain. Food allergies can lead to auto-immune diseases, which attack and destroy our own tissues.

Sugars increase our body's production of adrenaline by four times, which puts the body into a state of 'fight or flight' stress, without anything to fight or flee from, except the consumption of sugar. This stress reaction increases the production of both cholesterol and cortisone. Cortisone inhibits immune function.

Sugars lack the vitamins and minerals required for their own metabolism, and must draw on our body's stores of these nutrients. As these are depleted, our body becomes less able to carry out other functions that require minerals and vitamins to be present: to metabolize fats and cholesterol; to convert cholesterol into bile acids for removal from our body through the stool; or to burn-off excess fats as heat or increased activity. As a result, our cholesterol level rises; our metabolic rate goes down; fats burn more slowly; we feel less like exercising, and we may become obese. Obesity increases the risk of diabetes, cardiovascular disease, and cancer. Decreased metabolic rate is also involved in aging, arthritic diseases, cancer, and cardiovascular disorders, and is another general symptom of degenerative diseases.

And Still More

Sugars feed candida (yeasts), fungi, other pathological (toxin-producing) organisms, and cancer cells.

Sugars interfere with the transport of vitamin C, because both use the same transport system. Vitamin C's immune, virocidal, bacteriocidal, collagen- and elastin-building, and tissue 'glue' (mucopolysaccharide) forming functions are inhibited by sugar.

Sugars cross-link proteins, leading to aging and wrinkles even in young skin. Hard fats, those made from sugars and those that come from foods, encourage the production of pimples. Teenagers beware!

High blood sugar inhibits the release of linoleic acid (LA, 18:2w6) from storage in fat tissues, and thereby contributes to essential fatty acid deficiency. LA present in our body remains stored, unable to fulfill its functions. In spite of the presence of adequate LA within us, we may be *functionally* deficient in LA.

Finally, lack of fiber in refined carbohydrates slows down the speed at which foods pass through our digestive tract. They remain in our colon too long, serve as food for harmful bacteria that produce gas and toxins, and can cause our colon to become inflamed (diverticulitis) and ballooned (diverticulosis). Lack of fiber also causes constipation – it is so consistent in this effect that white (fiber-poor) bread was used in the 1800s to stop diarrhea because of its reliability in plugging up the colon. Lack of fiber also results in liver-weakening toxin reabsorption, hemorrhoids and varicose veins, and encourages the development of bowel cancer. Fiber helps remove excess cholesterol and bile acids from our body, preventing their reabsorption and recirculation. Fiberless refined sugars are of no help in this matter.

Sugars thus play a considerable role in causing fatty degeneration and degenerative diseases by contributing to the fat and cholesterol our body must carry; by depleting our body's stores of vitamins and minerals; by interfering with essential fatty acid, adrenal gland, and immune system functions; and by their lack of bulk and fiber.

Identifying the Culprit

Many researchers consider sugars to be the major dietary cause of degenerative diseases. Some of their effects are due to the fats (triglycerides) into which our body converts excess sugars. Triglycerides produced from sugars can create major health problems for our body, especially when they have been oxidized due to lack of antioxidant minerals and vitamins.

If one compares changes in total sugar consumption, total fat consumption, and consumption of altered vegetable fat substances with the vast increase in degenerative disease over the last 100 years, one finds the *best* correlation between altered vegetable fat substances and disease, a less strongly positive correlation between sugar consumption and disease, and an even less strongly positive correlation between total fat consumption and disease. All three, however, do show positive correlations to degenerative disease.

Historical Perspectives

The sugar monster – a historical (hysterical) anecdote. When refined white sugar first appeared on the market, so a story goes, people did not want to use this pure white stuff, because they were unfamiliar with it and therefore did not trust it. The producers set about changing peoples' perceptions.

An artist in an advertising department invented and drew an *imaginary* 'bug-monster.' The ad showed a big picture of this 'bug-monster' and the copy read: "White sugar never contains *any* of these." The ploy worked. The rest is history. Sugar consumption increased from 5 pounds to 135 pounds per person per year.

Paying for the industrial revolution. Before the industrial revolution, only rich people could afford to eat white, fiberless flour. It had to be hand-sifted, which was slow, hard work. As a result, degenerative diseases that result from deficiencies of nutrients and fiber afflicted mainly the wealthy: kings, noblemen, aristocrats. The poor ate whole grains.

'Refined' people ate 'refined' products. The common man's foods were 'crude', like his upbringing and manners. Poor people struggled to become 'refined'. To be able to afford 'refined' foods was a sign of upward mobility. The connection between refined foods and degenerative diseases was overlooked. The fact that 'refined' foods are actually 'nutrient-impoverished' (and should be so named) escaped peoples' notice. Their perspective on foods and health was wrong.

In Japan too, this misconception about refined foods is widespread. Popular opinion holds that only poor people eat *brown* rice.

The processing technology invented during the industrial revolution made 'refined' foods available to everyone. Now everyone can eat the foods once restricted to the privileged minority, and all can suffer the degenerative conditions once confined to the world's elite.

If that is the price of privilege, perhaps we should strive for poverty?

Liquid Oils and Unsaturated Fatty Acids (UFAs) 7

The fats that heal contain unsaturated fatty acids (UFAs), which makes them liquid oils. UFAs differ from saturated fatty acids (SaFAs) in only one respect. They contain one or more double bonds between carbon atoms in their fatty carbon chain, and for each double bond, they have given up two hydrogen atoms. Aside from this difference, they are identical in structure. Like saturated fatty acids, they have a methyl end and an acid end, and have carbon chains of varying lengths. Figure 9 shows the formation and structure of a UFA.

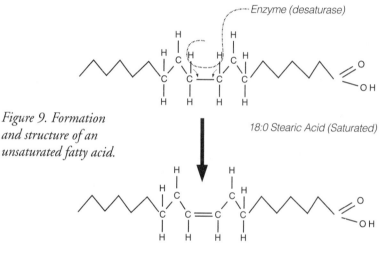

Enzyme (desaturase)

18:0 Stearic Acid (Saturated)

Figure 9. Formation and structure of an unsaturated fatty acid.

18:1w9 Oleic Acid (Unsaturated)

Properties of the Double Bond

The presence of this small difference in structure – the double bond – drastically changes an UFA's properties. Because of the way the hydrogen atoms are placed on the carbons involved in the double bonds,[1] the chain is bent at the double bond position. Whereas SaFAs and *trans-* fatty acids look like straight-bodied caterpillars, UFAs look like bent caterpillars. This so-called *cis-* configuration and the resulting kink in the molecule was illustrated in Figure 6. The kinks created by *cis-* double bonds in fatty acids make them difficult to align. Therefore UFAs aggregate poorly, and melt at lower temperatures (are more liquid) than SaFAs.

---

[1] This placement of hydrogen atoms is called the cis- configuration. Both hydrogens on the carbons involved in the double bond are on the same side of the carbon chain. The other way of placing the hydrogens on the double bond carbons is called the trans- configuration.

A double bond produces a slight local negative charge because it has a pair of extra electrons. Since like charges repel one another, UFA chains repel one another and tend to spread out over surfaces. Thus, while SaFAs tend to aggregate, UFAs tend to disperse, to move apart, to be anti-sticky. The more double bonds there are, the greater their tendency is to disperse. Figure 10 compares some properties of different fatty acids.

These properties of UFAs help provide the fluidity needed in cell membranes. Fluidity allows molecules within our membranes the freedom to swim and dive, to make and break contacts with one another, and to fulfill important chemical and transport functions.

Monounsaturated Fatty Acids (MUFAs)

MUFAs are unsaturated fatty acids with one double bond. The length of their carbon chains can vary. The shortest MUFAs are 10-carbon (C10) chains. C12 and C14 MUFAs are also found, appearing in small quantities in milk. Their double bonds are found in various locations along the chain. However, C12 and C14 MUFAs are of minor importance in nutrition.

More important is a MUFA with a 16-carbon chain and a double bond between carbons 7 and 8. It is called *palmitoleic acid* (POA, 16:1w7) and occurs in larger quantities in milk, and also in coconut and palm oils. An excess of this MUFA can lead to health problems by interfering with the chemical conversion of essential fatty acids (see Chapter 8, The Healing Essential Fatty Acids) into hormone-like prostaglandins (see Chapter 58, Prostaglandins).

The most important MUFA in nutrition has an 18-carbon chain, and its double bond is always between carbons 9 and 10. It is called *oleic acid* (OA, 18:1w9). OA is found in olive, almond, peanut, pistachio, pecan, canola, avocado, hazelnut, cashew, and macadamia oils, in the membranes of plant and animal cell structures, and in the fat deposits of most land animals. OA's fluidity (it melts at 13°C [55°F]) helps keep our arteries supple. It resists damage by oxygen and is therefore fairly stable. OA is the major fatty acid found in the oils produced by our skin glands. Our body can also *make* OA from saturated fatty acids. In excess, however, OA can interfere with essential fatty acids and prostaglandins.

MUFAs with double bonds in positions other than between carbons 9 and 10 are also known. Many different kinds exist, but they have no special significance in human nutrition.

Unsaturated Fatty Acids with More Than One Double Bond

These are the most interesting fatty acids. Several chapters will consider their structures, functions, and health effects in more detail. Here is a preview.

The most important unsaturated fatty acids with more than one double bond contain 18 carbon atoms in their chains. Two of these 18-carbon UFAs are known as essential fatty acids (EFAs). They are extremely important in nutrition,

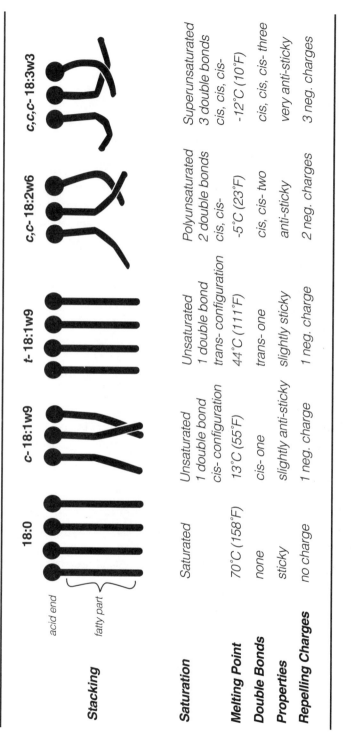

	18:0	**c- 18:1w9**	**t- 18:1w9**	**c,c- 18:2w6**	**c,c,c- 18:3w3**
Stacking					
Saturation	Saturated	Unsaturated 1 double bond cis- configuration	Unsaturated 1 double bond trans- configuration	Polyunsaturated 2 double bonds cis, cis-	Superunsaturated 3 double bonds cis, cis, cis-
Melting Point	70°C (158°F)	13°C (55°F)	44°C (111°F)	-5°C (23°F)	-12°C (10°F)
Double Bonds	none	cis- one	trans- one	cis, cis- two	cis, cis, cis- three
Properties	sticky	slightly anti-sticky	slightly sticky	anti-sticky	very anti-sticky
Repelling Charges	no charge	1 neg. charge	1 neg. charge	2 neg. charges	3 neg. charges

Figure 10. Some properties of different types of fatty acids.

and are vital to health (see Chapter 8, The Healing Essential Fatty Acids).

One – the w6 EFA called *linoleic acid* (LA, 18:2w6) – has two double bonds. It is often referred to as 'polyunsaturated'. Members of the w6 group of fatty acids also include *gamma-linolenic acid* (GLA, 18:3w6) found in borage, hemp, and evening primrose oils, and *arachidonic acid* (AA, 20:6w4) found in animal products. Both play important roles in our body.

The other – the w3 EFA called *alpha-linolenic acid* (LNA, 18:3w3) – has three double bonds. It is sometimes referred to as 'superunsaturated' to distinguish it and its family of w3 derivatives from the polyunsaturated w6 family. LNA is abbreviated as ALA in some research publications, and is also called ALENA by w3 researchers. W3 UFAs include *eicosapentaenoic acid* (EPA, 20:5w3), and *docosahexaenoic acid* (DHA, 22:6w3). Both are found in fish oils, and play vital roles in our body (see Chapter 55, Oils from Fish and Seafoods). EPA has also vindicated the much maligned snake oil salesman. (see Chapter 56, Snake Oil and Patent Medicines).

Within the w6 and w3 groups of UFAs, we also find other intermediates in our body's conversion of these essential fatty acids to derivatives. These intermediates have 18, 20, or 22 carbon chains, and 3, 4, or 5 double bonds.

Natural and Unnatural

W6 'polyunsaturated' fatty acids are abbreviated to PUFAs. Natural w6 PUFAs are vital to our body's health, but there are also non-natural and man-made w6 PUFAs, which interfere with biological functions (see Chapter 25, Polyunsaturates and Superunsaturates).

The same is true for w3 'superunsaturated' fatty acids (SUFAs). They also come in beneficial, natural, vitally important kinds, and man-made, toxic forms which are artifacts of processing.

Converts

Our body converts EFAs into the longer and more highly unsaturated, above-named EFA derivatives, which have important functions in brain cells, nerve endings (synapses), sense organs, adrenal glands, sex glands, and all cells. Our body uses some of these derivatives to make prostaglandins, which have hormone-like regulating and communicating functions in our cells. These are extremely important to health (see Chapter 58, Prostaglandins).

Some of these EFA derivatives can be supplied by plant seeds, seed oils, fish, snakes, and marine animals.

If all this sounds complicated, take heart. We will devote the entire next chapter to w3 and w6 EFAs, and develop their story more clearly. Our life and health depend on these two families of healing fatty acids.

The Healing
Essential Fatty Acids (EFAs) 8

In our frenzy to avoid killer fats, we can easily forget the fats that heal – those fats that we *must obtain* from foods in order to be healthy. The key components of healing fats are the essential fatty acids (EFAs), which were introduced in the previous chapter. Their names are *linoleic acid* (LA) and *alpha-linolenic acid* (LNA).

Linoleic Acid

The proper scientific name for LA is: all *cis-* w6,9-octadecadienoic acid, abbreviated to 18:2w6. To review, the abbreviation 18:2w6 means that there are 18 carbon atoms in the chain, there are 2 double bonds, the double bonds are methylene interrupted, the first double bond starts at carbon atom number 6 counting from the methyl end, and the double bonds are in the *cis-* configuration (see Chapter 4, What's in a Name?). LA is the w6 *polyunsaturated* fatty acid abundant in safflower, sunflower, corn, sesame, and other oils. It looks like a caterpillar bent in two places as shown in Figure 4 on page 18.

Alpha-Linolenic Acid

The proper scientific name for LNA is all *cis-* w3,6,9-octadecatrienoic acid, abbreviated to 18:3w3. LNA has three double bonds, the first of which is on carbon atom number 3, counting from the methyl end. LNA, the w3 EFA, is sometimes called *superunsaturated* to distinguish it from the w6 EFA. The distinction is important because, although they *appear* quite similar, many of the *effects* of w6s and w3s in the body are opposite in nature. LNA looks like a caterpillar bent in three places, as shown in Figure 4. Figure 11 shows stick models of both EFAs.

18:2w6 Linoleic Acid

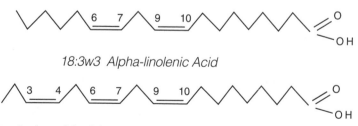

18:3w3 Alpha-linolenic Acid

Figure 11. Stick models of the essential fatty acids (EFAs).

Both LA and LNA are EFAs for humans (fish require LNA, but LA is not essential for them, because they can make it from LNA). This means that our body must have them, but cannot make them. It must therefore get LA and LNA from foods. A third fatty acid, called arachidonic acid (AA, 20:4w6), was thought to be essential in the past, but our body can make it from LA, and therefore AA is not an EFA, but an EFA derivative. If either LA or LNA is missing or deficient in the diet, cells deteriorate and, inevitably, deficiency symptoms *will* gradually develop.

LA Deficiency Symptoms
The symptoms of LA deficiency include:
- eczema-like skin eruptions;
- loss of hair;
- liver degeneration;
- behavioral disturbances;
- kidney degeneration;
- excessive water loss through the skin accompanied by thirst;
- drying up of glands;
- susceptibility to infections;
- failure of wound healing;
- sterility in males;
- miscarriage in females;
- arthritis-like conditions;
- heart and circulatory problems; and
- growth retardation.

Prolonged absence of LA from the diet is fatal. All of the deficiency symptoms (except death) can be reversed by adding LA back to the diet from which it was missing.

LNA Deficiency Symptoms
Symptoms of LNA deficiency include:
- growth retardation;
- weakness;
- impairment of vision and learning ability;
- motor incoordination;
- tingling sensations in arms and legs; and
- behavioral changes.

These symptoms can be reversed by adding LNA back to the diet from which it was missing. Other symptoms that can result from LNA (or w3) deficiency include:
- high triglycerides;
- high blood pressure;
- sticky platelets;
- tissue inflammation;
- edema;
- dry skin;

- mental deterioration;
- low metabolic rate; and
- some kinds of immune dysfunction.

These are not considered 'classic' symptoms of w3 deficiency, but often respond remarkably well to w3 supplementation.

Experts have recently begun to suggest that EFA deficiency (especially of the w3 EFA) is far more widespread than was formerly believed. Its symptoms closely resemble some of the symptoms of diseases of fatty degeneration. It comes as no surprise, therefore, that tissue and/or blood levels of people with these diseases are often low in w3 EFAs; nor is it surprising that this set of diseases responds well to dietary increases in EFAs, and to improvements in the dietary intake of the essential minerals and vitamins required for EFA metabolism.

Chemical Nature of Essential Fatty Acids

The usefulness of LA and LNA in our body results from their chemical properties.

EFAs attract oxygen. This property made EFA-rich oils useful to the paint industry as 'drying' oils, which dry and harden when exposed to air. Oils commonly used for this purpose were safflower oil: 80% LA; linseed oil: 50% LNA, 20% LA; and hemp oil: 55% LA, 20% LNA, and 2% GLA. Fresh, these oils are excellent nutritional oils. Because they are chemically reactive, they increase oxidation and metabolic rate. Flax oil (the undenatured version of linseed oil) and hemp oil are nutritionally superior to safflower oil because they contain both EFAs (safflower contains only LA) and are chemically more active – they contain more double bonds in an equal number of oil molecules.

EFAs absorb sunlight. Their absorption of light energy increases about a thousandfold their ability to react with oxygen. This makes them chemically very active indeed.[1]

Carrying slight negative charges, EFA molecules repel one another. This means that they do not easily aggregate, so they keep membranes fluid, a property that is important in membrane functions. Their tendency to disperse, called surface activity, gives biological systems the power to carry substances such as toxins to the surface of the skin, intestinal tract, kidneys, or lungs, where these substances can be discarded. The surface activity of EFAs also helps to disperse concentrations of substances that react with or dissolve in these fatty acids.

Their negative charge also makes the EFAs weakly basic (as opposed to acidic), and able to form weak hydrogen bonds with weak acid groups such as the sulphydryl groups found in proteins. Sulphydryl groups are important in oscillating reactions that take place between them and the double bonds of EFAs. They

---

[1] Saturated fatty acids, though able to react with oxygen, do so at a rate very much slower than the rate of reaction of essential fatty acids. They react at 1/125th and 1/25th of the rate of reaction of LNA and LA, respectively.

allow the one-way movement of electrons and energy in molecules to take place. The chemical reactions on which life depends require this one-way movement.

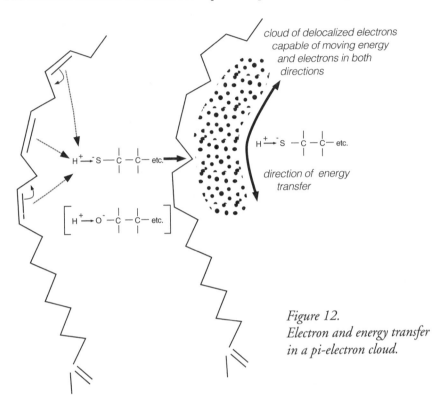

Figure 12.
Electron and energy transfer
in a pi-electron cloud.

Because of their special arrangement, electrons involved in the double bonds of essential fatty acids can be induced to become loose and move as so-called delocalized pi-electrons that resemble clouds floating along the fatty acid chain. This concept is illustrated in Figure 12.

EFAs can form phase boundary potentials, like charges of static electricity in a capacitor, which are caught between the water within and outside cells, and the oils within the membranes. These charges can produce measurable bio-electric currents, like the zap when static electricity discharges, which are important in nerve, muscle, heart, and membrane functions.

Functions of LA and LNA

Much is still unknown about the functions of EFAs in our body. Of the two, LA has been studied far more extensively than LNA. Both are difficult to work with, because they are easily destroyed, but LNA is five times more sensitive to destruction than LA.

Energy production. There is still a lot of work to be done before LNA's activities are fully understood (this is also true for all other essential nutrients – vitamins, minerals, trace elements, and amino acids). However, a list of functions in which they are involved can be given, based on scientific studies, clinical experience, and understanding of their chemical nature. Overall, EFAs are involved with producing life energy in our body from food substances, and moving that energy throughout our systems. They govern growth, vitality, and mental state. They hook up oxygen, electron transport, and energy in the process of oxidation. Oxidation, the central and most important moment-to-moment living process in our body, is the 'burning' of food to produce the energy required for life processes.

Oxygen transfer. LA and LNA are thought to be involved, in ways not well understood, with the transfer of oxygen from air in our lungs, through the thin lung tissue (alveolar) membranes, through capillary walls into the watery fluid in which our blood cells are suspended (blood plasma), across the membranes of our red blood cells to hemoglobin, which then carries oxygen to all our cells. At the cell end, they apparently help transport oxygen from our red blood cells through plasma, across the walls of our capillaries, across cell membranes and, in our cells, to precise location(s) in our mitochondria which use it in oxidation reactions to produce energy.

EFAs can be likened to oxygen 'magnets' that pull oxygen into our body similar to the way in which a magnet pulls iron filings. Figure 13 illustrates the attraction between oxygen and EFAs.

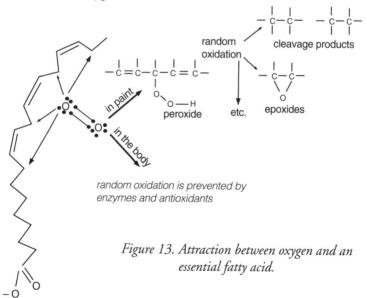

Figure 13. Attraction between oxygen and an essential fatty acid.

LA and LNA appear to hold oxygen in our cell membranes, where the oxygen acts as a barrier to viruses, fungi, bacteria, and other foreign organisms that cannot thrive in its presence.

Hemoglobin production. LA helps produce red blood pigment (hemoglobin) from simpler substances. Both EFAs are involved in a process that makes oxygen available to our tissues by 'activating' (or opening) oxygen molecules by way of free radicals or electrostatic forces, regulated by sulphur-containing proteins.

Membrane components. EFAs are part of all cell membranes. They help hold proteins in the membrane by the electrostatic attractive forces of their double bonds, and thus they are involved in the traffic of substances in and out of our cells via protein channels, pumps, and other special mechanisms. Figure 14 suggests a relationship between EFAs and sulphur-containing proteins in membranes. EFAs help maintain the fluidity of membranes. They also help create electrical potentials across membranes which, when stimulated, generate bioelectric currents that travel along cell membranes to other cells, transmitting messages.

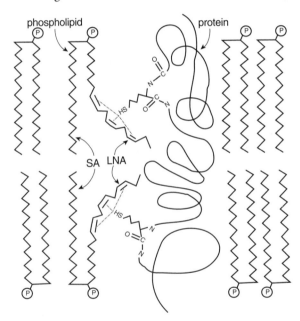

Figure 14. Possible relationship between EFAs and sulphur-containing proteins.

EFAs are also structural parts of the membranes of subcellular organelles or 'small organs' within our cells. These include:

- *endoplasmic reticulum* where protein synthesis takes place;
- *Golgi apparatus* which is involved in the secretion of substances within each cell;
- *vesicles* that transport substances into and out of our cells;
- *mitochondria,* little factories within each cell which burn (or oxidize) food molecules to release the sunlight stored in them for use in our life functions, on both the biochemical level and the human activity level;

- *nucleolus,* which stores products made by the nucleus; and
- *nucleus* which contains chromosomes that carry the master plan according to which our whole body is constructed, and control the sequences of biochemical events that we know as development and cell function, beginning at conception and continuing constantly until death.

Information carried on our chromosomes determines eye color, hair color, body type, gender, and so on. Figure 15 shows a cell with its organelles. Figure 16 shows fatty acids commonly found in membranes, including EFAs and their derivatives.

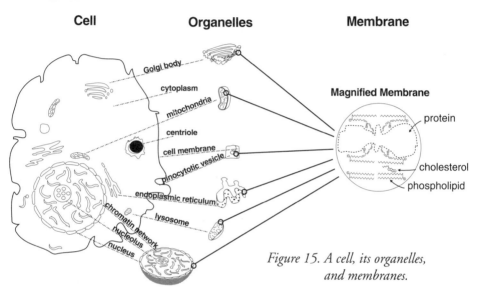

Figure 15. A cell, its organelles, and membranes.

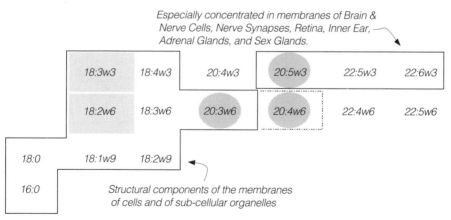

Figure 16. Fatty acids commonly found in membranes.

Recovery from fatigue. LA and LNA substantially shorten the time required for fatigued muscles to recover after exercise. They facilitate the conversion of lactic acid to water and carbon dioxide. This is especially important to athletes and others involved in intense activity. LA and LNA are also involved in making the secretions of both juice-producing (exocrine) and hormone-producing (endocrine) glands.

Prostaglandins. EFAs are precursors of prostaglandins, three families of short-lived, hormone-like substances that regulate many functions of the cells in all tissues on a moment-to-moment basis. Some prostaglandins affect the tone of smooth (involuntary) muscles in our blood vessels, some lower blood pressure, some relax coronary arteries, and some inhibit platelet stickiness. Others have opposite effects, and a delicate balance exists in our bodies between these opposing effects, which determines the state of physical health of our cardiovascular and other systems (see Chapter 58, Prostaglandins).

EFAs are precursors for even longer and more (5 and 6 times more) unsaturated fatty acids needed by the most active, oxygen-requiring, energy- and electron-exchanging tissues: brain, retina, adrenal, and testicular tissues. These highly unsaturated fatty acids carry the high energy chemical reactivity required by these tissues and ensure high oxygen availability.

Growth. EFAs are growth-enhancing. At levels above 12 to 15% of total calories, they increase the rate of metabolic reactions in our body, and the increased rate burns more fat into carbon dioxide, water and energy (heat), resulting in fat burn-off and loss of excess weight.

In ways that are poorly understood and require further study, EFAs seem to be involved in electron and energy transport. EFAs are involved in the transport (esterification) of cholesterol. LNA and its derivatives can lower elevated blood fats (serum triglycerides) by up to 65%.

EFAs help keep body fats fluid. They help generate the electrical currents that make our heart beat in orderly sequence. Heart tissue requires LA for proper functioning.

Cell division. EFAs are found around the hereditary material (chromatin) in our chromosomes, where they may play a part in maintaining chromosome stability, and may have functions in starting and stopping gene expression. EFAs help energize and govern the movement of chromosomes during cell division by their functions in spindle fiber development, and they form part of the new cell membranes that separate the daughter cells after a cell has divided. EFAs help our immune system resist and fight infections, and prevent allergies from developing.

EFAs can buffer excess acid as well as excess base in our body and are the richest source of energy in nutrition. In short, essential fatty acids govern every life process in our body. Life without them is impossible. When our foods are EFA-poor, we can expect a diversity of health problems.

Other LNA functions. LNA produces smooth, velvety skin, increases stamina, speeds healing, increases vitality, and brings a feeling of calmness. LNA reduces inflammation, water retention, platelet stickiness, and blood pressure. It also inhibits the growth of tumors. LNA enhances some immune functions, reduces the pain and swelling of arthritis, and completely reverses premenstrual syndrome in some cases. Remember however, that LNA can unfold its important functions only as part of a complete program that contains *all 50* essential factors.

LNA kills malaria (animal studies), and has been used successfully to treat bacterial (staph) infections.

Brain development. In children, LNA is required for brain development. In animals, deficiency of LNA during fetal development and early infancy results in permanent learning disabilities.

Co-factors to EFA Functions

To unfold some of their functions, LA and LNA must first be converted into EFA derivatives, or into prostaglandins. These conversions require vitamins B_3, B_6 and C and the minerals magnesium and zinc. Other vitamins and minerals may also modify conversion.

This means that a deficiency of any of the above five essential nutrients may mimic the degenerative symptoms of EFA deficiency, and that such a condition, looking like EFA deficiency, could eventually be fatal even if we are getting the EFAs we need for health.

Daily Requirement of Essential Fatty Acids

Linoleic acid. Of about 45 known essential nutrients, linoleic acid (LA, 18:2w6) is the one with the highest daily requirement, but the *exact* amount required each day is still being debated. LA requirement also varies from time to time for the same person. It depends on the level of physical activity and stress, nutritional state, and individual differences. Because of hormonal differences, males may require more than females.

One to two percent of calories (3 to 6 grams per day) is enough to prevent symptoms of deficiency in most healthy adults. An optimum amount might be in the range of 3 to 6% of calories, or 9 to 18 grams (about half an ounce or 1 table-spoon) of LA per day. Obese people and those on diets high in saturated fatty acids and olive oil may require even more. In animal studies, as much as 28.5% of calories (that would be over 60 grams, or 2 ounces per day) has been given as LA without problems in long-term feedings, as long as enough vitamin E was also included (about 1 part vitamin E for 1500 parts LA). Eighteen grams of LA per day would require less than 30 International Units (IU) of vitamin E. Other nutrients required for LA to properly perform its functions in our body are vita-mins C, B_3 and B_6, and the minerals magnesium and zinc. Vitamin A, or its pre-cursor carotene, is also important. To build optimum health, a nutritional pro-gram must include optimum amounts of all essential nutrients, every day.

51

Alpha-linolenic acid. The optimum amount of alpha-linolenic acid (LNA 18:3w3) needed for health is perhaps between one-fifth and one-half of that of LA, or between 2 and 9 grams (1 or 2 teaspoons) per day. Estimates suggest 2% of daily calories as LNA. Our body's content of LNA is less than that of LA, usually around 2% of body fat in healthy people.

Nutrients that help LNA perform its functions in our body include antioxidant vitamins, and the minerals and vitamins that have already been listed as necessary for LA functions: vitamins C, B$_3$, and B$_6$, and magnesium and zinc.

Body Content and Sources of EFAs

An average adult carries a total of about 10 kilograms of body fat. About 10% of that, or 1 kilogram (2.2 pounds) is LA. Vegetarians contain up to 25% of their total body fat as LA. People with degenerative diseases average about 8% of their fat tissue as LA.

LNA at 2% of body fat makes up about 200 grams (half a pound). In our brain, LA and LNA are present in about equal amounts.

Plants make enzymes that 'insert' a double bond into (desaturate) fatty acids at positions w3 and w6 to make w3 and w6 fatty acids, but humans do not produce these enzymes. This means that LA and LNA are not essential to plants because plants can make them, but they *are* essential to us because we cannot make them ourselves. They must therefore be present in our foods if we are to be healthy, and they usually come from plant sources.

Our richest source of LNA is flax oil. Safflower oil is our richest source of LA. Hemp seed oil contains w6 and w3 essential fatty acids in an ideal long-term ratio of 3:1. Other seed and nut sources of EFAs can be found in Table D7 of Chapter 50, Oils in Seeds.

W6:W3 Ratio

W3 consumption has decreased to one sixth the level found in our food supply in the 1850s. W6 consumption has doubled in that time, drastically changing the ratio of w6 to w3 in our food supply. This change is reflected in the makeup of our tissue fats and in our health.

Flax, our richest source of w3s, provides a quick way to make up for long-standing, widespread w3 deficiency. W3 deficiency can be reversed by a dozen 250 mL (8.5 ounce) bottles of good-quality flax oil consumed over the course of a few months.

Long-term exclusive use of flax oil can result in w6 deficiency symptoms, because flax oil contains four times more w3s than w6s. One can expect w6 deficiency symptoms from exclusive use of flax oil within 16 months to 2 years.

Over the long term, what ratios would be healthy? W6:w3 ratios found in diets varies from 1:2.5 (Inuit diets), through 6:1 (other traditional diets), to 20:1 (contemporary safflower and corn oil diets). Inuit are relatively healthy, but many of them suffer strokes, probably due to deficiency of vitamins C and E, and osteoporosis due to high protein intake, which leaches calcium from bones. Other traditional diets keep users free of degenerative diseases. Contemporary diets cause degenerative conditions.

The w6:w3 ratio in the brain is about 1:1. The ratio in our fat tissue is about 5:1. Other tissues are about 4:1. Our enzymes convert w6s only one-fourth as quickly as they convert w3s. To get equal conversion then, the ratio in foods should be 4:1, but because w6s mediate degenerative conditions, the ratio should favor w3s.

Such ratios can be developed by blending w3-rich oils with w6-rich ones to arrive at the appropriate ratio. Hemp oil, which contains three w6s (LA) for each w3 (LNA) and also 1.7% GLA, giving w6 conversion a head start in making beneficial PG1 prostaglandins, could be used in such blends, along with flax and other w6-rich oils.

As you may know, hemp is marijuana. The oil is legal, as are the steamed (unsproutable) seeds. Eating hemp seeds or drinking hemp seed oil will not produce any intoxicating effects, since both oil and seeds contain very little THC (tetrahydrocannabinol, which causes the intoxication, but traces of THC may be present, enough to show up in urine drug screens, leading to the loss of jobs).

Caring for Essential Fatty Acids

LA and LNA are essential to our health. They are also very temperamental. Light, air, and heat destroy them. Nature packages these oils in seeds that keep out light, air, and heat. In nature's package, these oils will sometimes keep for years without spoiling.

When we extract the oil from such seeds, we need to make sure that light, air, and heat are kept from the oil from before pressing until the oil is consumed. Special care needs to be taken in processing, packaging, and storing oils rich in EFAs. To set such conditions is expensive, and the necessary care is not usually taken (see Chapter 16, From Seed to Oil, and Chapter 28, Making Oils with Human Health in Mind).

Light, the greatest enemy of EFAs, produces free radicals in oils, and speeds up the reaction of oils with oxygen from the air by 1000 times, resulting in rancid oil. Light can induce cross-linking of fatty acid molecules into dimers and polymers that are rubber-like substances. Light-induced free radical chain reactions (see Chapter 21, Light, Free Radicals, and Oils) can break EFAs down into many different kinds of products, including aldehydes, ketones, and other toxic and non-toxic components. Light destroys the vital biological properties of the EFAs.

Oxygen, even in the absence of light, breaks down EFAs. The result is what we know as rancid oil, which has a scratchy, bitter, fishy, or painty taste, or a characteristic unpleasant smell, like a parking lot in August heat. Dozens of breakdown products form, with toxic or unknown effects on our body's functions.

Heat, used in deodorizing, hydrogenation (to make margarines and shortenings), and commercial frying and deep-frying used to make consumer items, destroys EFAs by twisting their molecules from a natural *cis-* shape to an unnatural *trans-* shape (see Chapter 18, Margarines, Shortenings, and *Trans-* Fatty Acids). Frying and deep-frying in the home also twist the molecules (see Chapter 22, Frying and Deep-frying).

Fresh EFA-rich oils should be pressed and packaged in the dark, in the absence of oxygen, and with minimal heat, then stored in *opaque containers* to prevent contact with light and oxygen. They should be *shelf-dated*. If they are frozen solid (which does not damage them), oils remain unspoiled for a long time. They should be shipped directly by manufacturer to retailer or consumer without stops along the way, to reach consumers quickly.

9   *Triglyceride Fats* (TGs)

Triglycerides (TGs) are the main kind of body fat. All fats and oils are mixtures of TGs (see Chapter 50, Oils in Seeds), and they make up 95% of the fats we eat. Most of the stored fat we carry around in our bodies is composed of TGs. TGs are also carried in our bloodstream, and high blood TGs are one risk factor for cardiovascular disease. When sugars turn into saturated fatty acids, these fatty acids are also carried as triglycerides.

TGs are the main form in which living organisms store energy for future use. Edible oils from seeds, egg yolks, and fat deposits (depot fats) of animals are also mainly TGs. Fats normally carried in our bloodstream include TGs. Triglycerides also serve as our body's reserve of the vital essential fatty acids, LA and LNA.

Structure of Triglyceride Fats

Figure 17 shows the way a triglyceride is built. A glycerol molecule is the backbone, and from each of its three carbon atoms hangs a free-swinging fatty acid, making a molecule that looks like a three-pronged fork. Each fatty acid is hooked to a glycerol carbon by an ester bond.

In oils found in nature, the two outside carbons of glycerol prefer to hold a saturated fatty acid (SaFA), whereas the middle position prefers an essential fatty acid (EFA). This arrangement is brought about by enzymes specifically designed to keep just this arrangement.[1] The preference is not 100% however, and so one also finds the positions switched. The type of oil or fat in question helps determine which fatty acids will be found in which position. Beef fat, for instance, is made of triglycerides that carry mostly saturated and monounsaturated fatty acids

---

[1] Industrial processes are sometimes used to randomize fatty acid attachments on triglycerides by transesterification or interesterification.

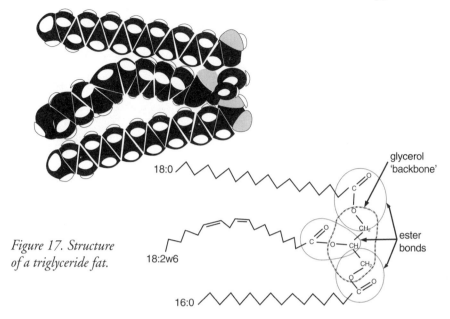

Figure 17. Structure of a triglyceride fat.

in all positions (it contains hardly any EFAs).

Completely hydrogenated fats carry almost 100% SaFAs in *all* positions. Flax oil and safflower oil must carry EFAs in outside positions, because both of these oils contain more than 70% EFAs. Only one-third (33.3%) of these can fit in the middle position. The rest *must* go to outside positions on glycerol.

The fatty acids attached to a glycerol molecule to make a TG can be short or long. Butter contains many short-chain SaFAs between 4 and 14 carbon atoms in length. Tropical fats contain mostly SaFAs 16 carbons or less in length. Most plant seed oils and animal depot fats have mainly 18-carbon fatty acids in their TGs. Fatty acids in the TGs of fish oils are up to 22 carbons long.

The number of possible combinations and arrangements of fatty acids in TGs is large, since there are 3 positions, at least 7 different degrees of saturation (saturated, monounsaturated, twice unsaturated, etc., up to six times unsaturated), and at least 10 different possible carbon chain lengths (4 to 22 carbon atoms, even numbers only). In addition, odd-numbered and unusual types of fatty acids are also found in TGs.

Figure 18 shows examples of possible combinations of fatty acids on TGs.

In nutrition, the arrangement of fatty acids on the glycerol molecule appears less important than the total amount of each kind of fatty acid present, because our body separates fatty acids from glycerol by means of digestive enzymes, then recombines the parts back into triglycerides by means of other enzymes, according to its specific needs. It burns short-chain, and saturated and monounsaturated 16- and 18-carbon fatty acids for energy, while preserving EFAs for their more important structural and metabolic functions in our body.

4:0	6:0	12:0	18:0	18:1w9	12:0	18:2w6	18:3w3
18:1w9	16:1w7	8:0	18:0	18:3w3	18:2w6	18:2w6	18:3w3
10:0	4:0	14:0	18:0	18:0	18:1w9	18:0	18:2w6

18:2w6	18:0	16:1w7	12:0		outside position
18:2w6	18:2w6	18:3w3	18:2w6	*etc.*	middle position
18:2w6	18:0	18:1w9	16:0		outside position

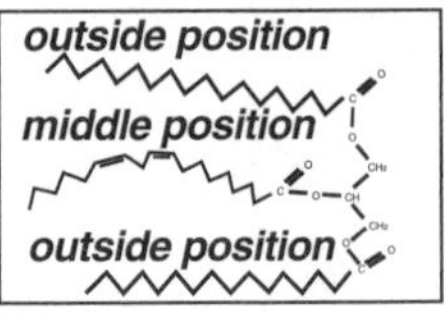

Figure 18. Some possible arrangements of fatty acids in triglycerides.

Functions of Triglyceride Fats

TGs have several functions. They are excellent insulation material. They form a layer around our body just under our skin which, especially in cold surroundings, conserves heat. Without this layer, more food consumption, more digestion, more absorption, and increased metabolism would be required to keep body temperature constant. It is more efficient and less wasteful to conserve heat than to keep producing it, just as it is more efficient to put on a jacket than to heat the whole house. In the heat of summer, this excellent insulation often makes overweight people feel uncomfortably hot.

Body fat (adipose) is singularly effective at dampening shock waves that could injure delicate tissues. The fat layer around our body and internal organs protects us from shock and injury when we bump into things and every time we take a step, walking or running. The fat pad under our heel takes up a tremendous amount of shock each time our heel hits pavement. We can still feel the shock wave travel up through our body at every step, but in much reduced intensity.

Mainly, fat tissues store energy reserves on which our body can draw between meals, during increased physical exertion, while asleep, while pregnant, or during famine. Humans living in nature were subjected to extremes of feasts and famines. Body fat developed to mellow out the fluctuations. Plants did not evolve fat tissue, and stop growing and being active when sunshine and warmth fade. Maintaining activity in cold weather requires a warm body that can use internally stored energy.

Our body converts a toxic excess of the sugars required for brain function into less harmful TGs. Thus, in addition to being energy reserves, TGs provide a safety mechanism for our body.

Fatty acids from TGs are fuel for all organs except our brain, which requires glucose (which can be made from glycerol), glutamic acid (which comes from protein or is supplied in the form of glutamine), or ketones (breakdown products from incomplete fat metabolism). TGs, since they are made from fatty acids and glycerol, store emergency brain fuel.

TGs store our body's reserves of EFAs. These are required both for structure and functions of our membranes, and serve as precursors of prostaglandins (see Chapter 58, Prostaglandins) and highly active, very highly unsaturated fatty acids required for our brain cells, synapses, retinas, adrenal glands, and testes to function.

Triglycerides and Disease

Excess TGs can cause problems. High blood TG levels increase our risk of heart disease. They are produced by overeating and by high dietary intake of refined sugars, sticky saturated fats, and too few antioxidants. Under these conditions, TG fatty acids oxidize and damage the insides of our arteries. High blood TG levels may also increase the tendency of blood cells to clump together.

Excess stored triglyceride fats (in overweight or obese people) correlate with high blood cholesterol and triglyceride levels. All increase our risk of cardiovascular disease, high blood pressure, heart and kidney failure, cancer, and other degenerative diseases.

Protection

Diets high in fats but also rich in minerals and vitamins lessen the danger of degeneration. Antioxidant vitamins C and E, and carotene, sulphur, selenium, zinc, and manganese are important for preventing fatty acids from oxidizing. Vitamin B_6 should be increased on a high-fat diet. It is necessary for metabolizing the fatty acids.

A diet rich in w3 fatty acids, LNA (18:3w3) from flax or EPA (20:5w3) and DHA (22:6w3) from fish and marine animal oils (see Chapter 55, Oils from Fish and Seafoods), can lower serum triglyceride levels by up to 65%. People eating w3-rich, nutritionally balanced diets remain free of cardiovascular and other degenerative diseases longer than those on w3-poor diets. People who begin to take w3 oils sometimes show remarkable reductions in their blood TG levels. Their cholesterol levels may also decrease by as much as 25%.

Exercise lowers blood TG levels by burning up excess fats to produce energy. Normal blood TG levels are about 100 milligrams per deciliter (mg/dl). The levels in 25% of North American, European, and other affluent populations are far enough above that to cause concern.

10 Phospholipids (PLs) and Membranes

'Skins' (membranes) surround our cells, organelles, blood fats, and cholesterol. Made from what we eat, these skins play vital roles in our health.

Phospholipids (PLs), also known as phosphatides, are the second major class of lipids (besides triglycerides). They make up less than 5% of the total lipids found in foods and our body. They are major structural components of cells and intracellular membranes in all living organisms.

Structure of Phospholipids

PLs are similar to triglycerides (TGs) in that two fatty acids (usually 16- or 18-carbon chains) are attached to a glycerol backbone. They differ from TGs in that, whereas the third position on the glycerol of TGs holds a third fatty acid, this position in phospholipids holds a phosphate group. This phosphate group completely changes the properties of the molecule.

TGs are water-insoluble and fat-soluble, and aggregate into oil droplets. The phosphate group of PLs is polar and water-soluble, while its fatty acids are oil-soluble. As a result, PLs spread out in a thin layer over surfaces of water, and naturally form thin membranes. Figure 19 shows the structure of a phospholipid molecule.

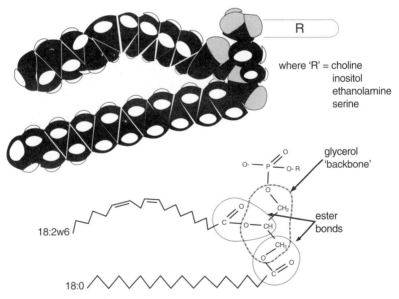

where 'R' = choline
inositol
ethanolamine
serine

glycerol 'backbone'

ester bonds

18:2w6

18:0

Figure 19. Structure of a phospholipid.

58

Phospholipid Function and Biological Membranes

PLs form double-layered membranes, the skin that surrounds every living cell of all living organisms: bacteria, plants, animals, and humans. Figure 20 shows the structure of a biological membrane.

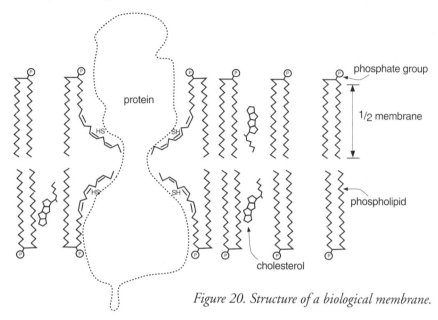

Figure 20. Structure of a biological membrane.

PLs also form skins around little organs within our cells (organelles). They surround mitochondria, nucleus, nucleolus, lysosomes, and other intracellular factories, and form the membranous structures of Golgi and endoplasmic reticulum.

Phospholipids have many functions within our membranes. They form a barrier that keeps the outside world outside, and the inside world inside, each cell. Along with proteins, PLs determine which substances can drift or be pulled into cells from outside, and which substances from within cells will drift or be pushed out (membrane selectivity). Fat-soluble toxic substances such as alcohol, barbiturates, drugs, and carcinogens can exert toxic effects because they dissolve in and pass through our cells' PL membranes, into our cells. Obviously, toxins can disrupt cell functions and change cell metabolism only if they can get in, and toxic effects vary, depending on the extent to which the toxins penetrate the cell.

PLs help hold proteins in place in membranes to fulfill structural, enzymatic, and transport functions.

The middle carbon of glycerol molecules in PLs usually holds an essential fatty acid (EFA) which, being highly unsaturated, is bent and cannot be tightly packed. It takes up more space than a straight saturated fatty acid (SaFA) molecule, and keeps membranes from hardening. Figure 21 illustrates this point. Thus, phospholipids fluidize cell membranes, enabling proteins within them to move

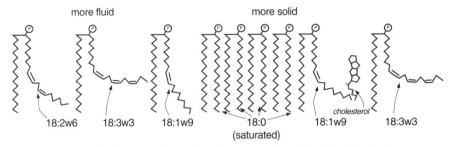

more fluid   more solid

18:2w6   18:3w3   18:1w9   18:0 (saturated)   cholesterol   18:1w9   18:3w3

cholesterol and saturated fatty acids make membranes more solid
unsaturated fatty acids make membranes more fluid

Figure 21. How membranes become more fluid or more solid.

freely around the surface of the cell to perform vital functions. PLs also store each cell's supply of EFAs, which are required to make prostaglandins that regulate cell activities (see Chapter 58, Prostaglandins).

EFA molecules attract oxygen, which discourages infectious organisms (bacteria, fungi such as candida, and viruses) from thriving. In this way, PLs help protect our cells from invasion by foreign organisms.

A SaFA or monounsaturated fatty acid is usually found on the outside carbon of glycerol in PLs. The SaFA provides membrane rigidity, and also separates highly unsaturated fatty acids from one another, preventing them from reacting (cross-linking) with one another, which would not be conducive to life.

The water-loving phosphate group ensures that each molecule of phospholipid lines up in the same direction on a water surface, with the precise regularity required to form the membrane.

Several other chemical groups – choline, inositol, serine, or ethanolamine – can be attached to phosphate groups. For instance, phosphatidyl choline is a phospholipid with a choline group attached to its phosphate group.

Besides PLs and proteins, our membranes contain cholesterol, which fine tunes membrane fluidity under constantly fluctuating conditions of food fat intake (see Chapter 12, Cholesterol). A diet rich in EFAs (which are fluid) means that more cholesterol (which is rigid) will be built into membranes – one reason why EFAs lower blood cholesterol levels – to balance their fluidity. A diet rich in SaFAs (which are hard) means more cholesterol will be removed from membranes back into our blood – one reason for the ability of SaFAs to raise blood cholesterol levels. Membranes also contain vitamins E and carotene, which help protect them from destruction by free radicals (see Chapter 21, Light, Free Radicals, and Oils). Attached to the inside of our membranes is sulphur-containing glutathione, which helps snag free radicals that make it across the membrane and into a cell.

Single-Layered Membranes

Phospholipids are also important in the single-layer membranes that form the envelopes that surround the fats and cholesterol (as well as vitamins E and A, and carotene) being transported from our intestines to our liver, from our liver to our cells, and from our cells back to our liver. The main types of these single-layered carrying vehicles are shown in Figure 22.

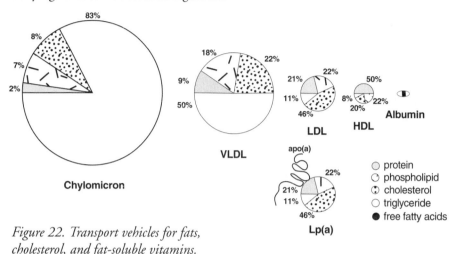

Figure 22. Transport vehicles for fats, cholesterol, and fat-soluble vitamins.

Chylomicrons, made in our intestinal cells, carry food fats. *Very low-density lipoproteins* (VLDL) are made in our liver. *Low-density lipoproteins* (LDL) carry fats, cholesterol, and fat-soluble vitamins from our liver to our cells. *High-density lipoproteins* (HDL) carry cholesterol and fats from our cells back to our liver (see Chapter 41, Blood Cholesterol). The relationships between these carriers are complex (see Chapter 33, Digestion of Fats, Oils, and Cholesterol). The newest addition to these carrier vehicles – *lipoprotein(a)* [Lp(a)] – also has a single-layered membrane as its envelope.

Single-layer PL membranes keep water-insoluble fats, cholesterol, and vitamins soluble in the watery bloodstream. If PLs did not surround them, fats and cholesterol would coalesce, form 'greasy' bubbles in our blood, and rise within us in the same way that cream rises to the top of a bottle of milk, turning us (literally) into fat-heads. Our head and shoulders would be a 'cream' of fats, oils, cholesterol, and other fat-soluble substances, and the rest of us, protein and water. PLs prevent such a disaster from happening.

Phospholipids and Disease

PLs are extremely well regulated by body mechanisms because of their importance. They are so important to life that no diseases are associated with them. Any genetic defect in an organism's ability to make or use PLs kills that organism during early prenatal development, because the structures and functions of all cells would be completely disrupted due to membrane defects, right from the beginning.

11 *Lecithin*

Lecithin is a phospholipid (PL) supplement that can help improve both our digestion and our health. The name 'lecithin' was derived from the Greek word for egg yolk from which it was first isolated, and it is the best known member of the phospholipids (see Chapter 10, Phospholipids). Figure 23 shows a molecule of lecithin.

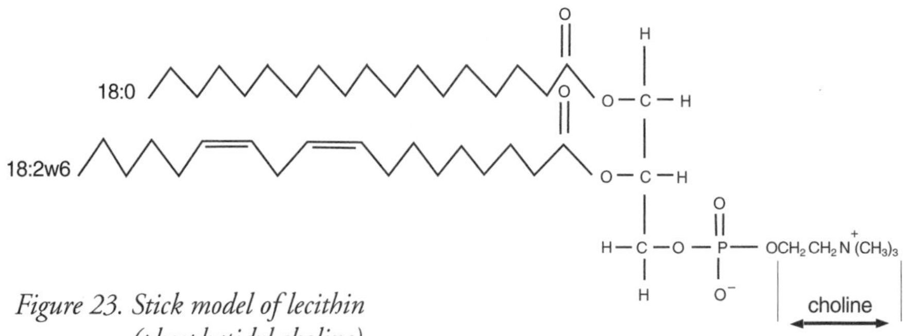

Figure 23. Stick model of lecithin (phosphatidyl choline).

Biological Value of Lecithin

Lecithin's nutritional value rests on several factors. It supplies *choline*, which is necessary to make the neurotransmitter acetylcholine. Acetylcholine is required for brain and nerve function. In our liver, choline also helps our body utilize fats properly. It is a 'fat-loving' (lipotropic) factor in this function.

Lecithin is also valuable because it is usually made from soybean oil containing both *essential fatty acids* (EFAs). Commercially made lecithin was one of the few reliable sources of small amounts of the w3 essential fatty acid until flax and hemp oils became available.

Lecithin is also valuable as an *'edible detergent'*, which breaks up fats into suspensions of smaller droplets ('emulsifies' fats). As we will see a little later, the emulsifying action of lecithin is extremely important.

All unrefined seed oils contain some lecithin. The richest commercial source of lecithin is unrefined (crude) soybean oil, of which 2% or more is lecithin containing both essential fatty acids – 57% linoleic acid (LA, 18:2w6), and 5 to 7% alpha-linolenic acid (LNA, 18:3w3). Lecithin from most other oils contains only LA. Lecithin is removed when oils are refined (see Chapter 16, From Seed to Oil).

Commercial Changes

Because EFAs – especially LNA – spoil rapidly, breeding experiments are being carried out to develop genetic strains of soybeans with only 3% LNA instead of the higher amounts found in natural strains. When oils and lecithins from these new strains become commercially available, their shelf-life will be longer, but nutritional quality will be lower. We sacrifice nutritional quality for convenience. The price we pay in diminished health is not considered by manufacturers and marketers.

Similar changes occur when food animals are raised on artificial, man-made feeds. In order to increase feed shelf life, EFAs are largely removed. More stable but non-essential oleic acid (OA, 18:1w9) replaces the missing EFAs.

The EFAs present in eggs, chickens, and meats must come from the feeds the animals consume. Eggs and meat from animals raised on commercial feeds contain low-EFA fats and lecithins, which provide insufficient EFAs for optimum human health (see Chapter 49, Eggs).

Functions of Lecithin

Lecithin helps keep cholesterol soluble. In a food like eggs, which contain a large amount of cholesterol, it is especially important that lecithin be of high quality.

Lecithin keeps cholesterol isolated from arterial linings, protects it from oxidation, and helps prevent and dissolve gall and kidney stones by its emulsifying action on fatty substances.

Lecithin is necessary in our liver's detoxification functions, which keep us from slowly being poisoned by breakdown products of metabolic processes that take place in our body. Poor liver function is a common forerunner of cancer. According to some healers, cancer *always* involves the liver. Deficiency of either choline or EFAs can induce cancer in experimental animals, and is likely involved in causing some human cancers.

Lecithin increases resistance to disease by its role in our thymus gland. Here, EFAs are precursors of several prostaglandins (see Chapter 58, Prostaglandins), as well as being vital as part of the ammunition made by our immune cells to kill bacteria (fatty acid peroxides are used to produce bacteriocidal hydrogen peroxide).

Lecithin is a phospholipid that makes up 22% of both the high density (HDL) and low density lipoprotein (LDL) cholesterol-carrying vehicles in our blood. These vehicles keep cholesterol and triglyceride fats in solution in our bloodstream and carry them to and from all parts of our body.

Lecithin is an important part of membrane PLs that are involved in electric phenomena, membrane fluidity, and other functions for which EFAs are responsible (see Chapter 8, The Healing Essential Fatty Acids).

Finally, lecithin is an important component of bile. Its function in digestion is to break food fats into small droplets (emulsify them), to increase their surface area, speeding up the digestion of fats by enzymes (see Chapter 33, Digestion of Fats, Oils, and Cholesterol).

Lecithin is not an essential nutrient. Our body can make it, provided that sufficient EFAs, choline, and phosphate are present in the foods we eat.

12 *Cholesterol*

Cholesterol plays both vital and detrimental roles in our health. There is no nutritional substance as controversial as cholesterol, and no substance about which there is more confusion. There is no other substance as widely publicized by the medical profession – and no bigger health scandal. Cholesterol can strike terror into the minds of misinformed people. The cholesterol scare is big business for doctors, laboratories, and drug companies. It is also a powerful marketing gimmick for vegetable oil and margarine manufacturers who can advertise their products to be 'cholesterol-free' (see Chapter 24, Advertising and Jargon).

The fact is that 999 out of every 1000 people (or 499 out of every 500, depending upon which expert source you read) can control their cholesterol level and, more importantly, their cardiovascular health, by nutritional means alone. The remaining 1 in 1000 people can also benefit from nutritional improvement. Medical professionals that are untrained in nutrition cannot help us reach this objective.

A hard, waxy lipid substance that melts at 149°C (300°F), cholesterol is essential for our health, but we do not need to obtain it from foods. Our body can manufacture it from simpler substances (2-carbon acetates) which it derives from the breakdown of sugars, fats, and even proteins, especially when our total intake of these foods supplies us with calories in excess of our body's requirement. Figure 24 shows the structure of cholesterol.

The more excess calories we consume – especially from sugars, and saturated and other non-essential fatty acids – the more pressure there is on our body to make cholesterol. In addition, the more stress we are under, the more cholesterol our body makes, because cholesterol is the precursor of stress hormones.

Before we get into the supposed evils of cholesterol, let's look at the natural and vital functions of cholesterol in our body – cholesterol's good side.

Vital Functions of Cholesterol

One function of cholesterol is to *compensate for changes in membrane fluidity,* keeping it within the narrow limits required for optimal membrane function. This function is so important that nature has equipped each cell with the means to synthesize its own membrane cholesterol.

Our intake of dietary fatty acids – building material for membranes – varies from day to day. More highly unsaturated fatty acids make membranes more

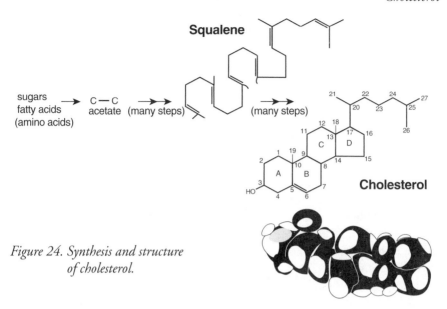

*Figure 24. Synthesis and structure
    of cholesterol.*

fluid, and more saturated fatty acids harden membranes. Cholesterol made by our cells is the regulating factor – it is added to stiffen a membrane that is too loose, and it is removed to fluidize a membrane that is too stiff.

Our body makes *steroid hormones* from cholesterol. The male and female sex (steroid) hormones develop and maintain the delightful differences between the genders. The three best known of these hormones are the female hormones estrogen and progesterone, and the male hormone testosterone.

Anabolic steroids used by athletes are synthetically made male steroid hormones. They have serious side effects like liver, brain, kidney, ligament, and joint damage. They can also cause cancer. Steroids masculinize the women who use them, resulting in bone growth (square jaws), muscle growth, facial hair, a lower voice, and clitoral enlargement.

Our body also makes *adrenal corticosteroid hormones* from cholesterol. These hormones include aldosterone, which regulates water balance through our kidneys, increasing sodium retention by our renal tubules; and cortisone, which promotes the synthesis of glucose to prepare our body for fight or flight in response to stress, and also suppresses inflammation. Doctors use large doses of cortisone to suppress inflammatory reactions.[1]

Our body makes *vitamin D*, the sunshine vitamin that regulates calcium and phosphorus metabolism, from cholesterol.

Bile acids are derived from cholesterol. Through bile acids, cholesterol per-

---

[1] The pharmacological doses used, much higher than what the body itself normally manufactures, produce powerful side effects that include water retention and immune system suppression, and are not recommended for prolonged use.

forms vital functions in our digestion and absorption of fats, oils, and fat-soluble vitamins from foods. Our body discards excess cholesterol that it no longer needs as bile acids.

Cholesterol is secreted by glands in our *skin.* It covers and protects our skin against dehydration, cracking, and the wear and tear of sun, wind, and water. In its capacity as skin covering, cholesterol also helps heal skin tissue and prevents infections by foreign organisms.

Cholesterol may also pinch-hit as an *antioxidant* (AO) when our body's supply of mineral and vitamin AOs is low. High levels of oxidized cholesterol are found in low-density lipoprotein (LDL) and high-density lipoprotein (HDL) transport vehicles when our body lacks food-borne AOs. Some of these AOs, including vitamins C, E, B_3, and carotene, as well as the elements selenium, sulphur, and zinc/copper, can lower cholesterol. Chromium, though not an AO itself, can be combined with vitamin B_3 to lower cholesterol in 50% of people with high serum levels. The combination of chromium with niacin molecules has been patented as a cholesterol-lowering agent.

Sources of Cholesterol

Cholesterol can be made in our body, or it can come from foods.

Homemade cholesterol. Our cells manufacture the cholesterol they need for their membrane requirements in response to demand. For instance, when we drink alcohol, it dissolves in and fluidizes our membranes. In response, cells build more cholesterol into the membrane, and thereby bring the membrane back to a normal (less fluid) state. As the alcohol wears off, the membrane hardens, and some membrane cholesterol is removed to reestablish normal (greater) membrane fluidity. The extra cholesterol is hooked up (esterified)[2] to an essential fatty acid (EFA) and shipped via our bloodstream to our liver to be changed into bile acids, as long as the vitamins and minerals necessary for this change are present. Our liver dumps bile acids into our intestine to help with fat digestion, and then removes them from our body with solid wastes, as long as our foods contain sufficient fiber and bowel action is regular enough to prevent bile acids in our intestine from being reabsorbed and recycled.

Besides our cells' production of cholesterol, our liver, intestine, adrenal glands, and sex glands all make cholesterol for the other functions in which cholesterol is involved. During pregnancy, the placenta also makes cholesterol, from which it manufactures progesterone, which keeps pregnancy from being terminated.

Making homemade cholesterol. Our body makes cholesterol by hooking 15 two-carbon acetates (vinegars) end to end to make a 30-carbon chain. Through many steps involving different enzyme catalysts, this chain is cyclized,

---

[2] Vitamin B_6 is required for this step.

and finally 3 carbons are clipped off to produce the 27-carbon cholesterol molecule. The process is complex and interesting for biochemists, but the important *nutritional* question is to find the source of the 2-carbon acetates.

When our cells break down fatty acids, sugars, starches, or amino acids in our energy-producing mitochondria, they clip off 2-carbon acetates at each step. Alcohol also provides acetates for cholesterol production.

Proteins and EFAs. Our body conserves proteins as much as possible for building structures and enzymes, so proteins are burned for energy only in extreme circumstances: fasting, some disease states, and after consumption of excessive amounts of protein.

Our body also conserves EFAs for non-fuel functions. Since EFAs are conserved by the body for other vital functions, saturated and monounsaturated fatty acids are the main sources of acetate fragments from fats.

Foods rich in refined carbohydrates also produce an excess of acetates in our body, which 'push' increased cholesterol production. High cholesterol levels in people living in 'processed foods nations' often involve excessive calorie intake.

Stress also increases homemade cholesterol production.

Cholesterol from food sources. Only foods from animal sources contain cholesterol – plant foods are cholesterol-free. Cholesterol is found in eggs, meat, dairy products, fish, and shellfish. One egg, 1/4 pound of liver, and 1/4 pound of butter each contain about 250 mg of cholesterol; fish and shellfish contain somewhat less.

The average North American adult consumes about 800 mg of cholesterol daily, of which about 45% comes from eggs, 35% from meat, and 20% from dairy. About half of the dietary cholesterol is actually absorbed. The rest passes through unused.

For 70% of the affluent populations of the world, increased cholesterol *consumption* decreases cholesterol *production* within their body by means of a regulating feedback system that protects them. The other 30% of the population may not have adequate feedback, and are wise to limit their cholesterol consumption. What is not clear is to what extent drugs (some of which are known to increase our body's cholesterol production) and other toxic molecules from foods, water, air, and the environment play a role in making the feedback system ineffective. A good topic for research!

Body Content of Cholesterol

The average person's body 'owns' about one-third of a pound (150 grams, or 150,000 mg [5 ounces]) of cholesterol. Most of this is found in membranes, and about 7 grams is carried in our blood. The daily turnover of cholesterol is about 1100 mg, or just over 1 gram. These figures vary depending on diet, state of health, and body size. The daily cholesterol turnover on a strict vegetarian diet (who does not eat meat, eggs, or dairy products) is less than 1 gram; bodies of meat eaters turn over more cholesterol as cholesterol consumption increases, but less as fiber consumption decreases.

Removal of Cholesterol

Cholesterol is unique in that our body can make it but, once made, cannot break it down. By contrast sugars, fatty acids, amino acids, and nucleic acids can all be taken apart and turned into carbon dioxide, water, and ammonia. As a result of this peculiarity, cholesterol must (and can only) be removed from our body through our stool (in the form of bile acid and cholesterol molecules).

The removal of cholesterol is increased by dietary fiber. If fiber is absent, up to 94% of the cholesterol and bile acids are reabsorbed and recycled. This is one of the reasons why low-fiber diets increase blood cholesterol levels.

Atherosclerosis

About two-thirds of the North American, European, and affluent populations world-wide suffer from atherosclerotic deposits to some degree. These deposits, made of proteins, fats, cholesterol, and minerals, narrow arteries and slow down blood flow. In addition, cholesterol and saturated or denatured fatty acids make our platelets sticky, increasing the risk of a clot forming. The combination of atherosclerosis and clots may completely block an artery, cutting off oxygen and nutrients to the cells of the part of our body supplied by that artery. These cells then die.

If an artery to our brain is blocked, a stroke occurs and, depending on the size and location of the blocked artery, the stroke may be minimal or fatal. Narrowed arteries to our heart produce chest pains (angina pectoris) on exertion or after a meal high in fats that makes blood thicker and less capable of supplying oxygen. Blockage of an artery supplying our heart results in a heart attack (coronary occlusion).[3] If a clot blocks an artery in our lungs, pulmonary embolism occurs. A blocked artery to our legs results in impaired circulation that can lead to gangrene. Blindness and deafness can occur when arteries supplying sense organs are blocked.

Atherosclerotic deposits also 'harden' our arteries, resulting in raised blood pressure because the arteries' resilience, which normally takes up the pressure generated by each heartbeat (contraction), is lost. This results in a heavier load on our heart and kidneys which, when prolonged, leads to water retention (edema) and heart and kidney failure.

Controversy About Cholesterol

Since making cholesterol requires energy, some researchers suggest that having

---

[3] Depending on which source supplies the statistics, between 20 and 60% of first heart attacks are fatal.

cholesterol in our diet is an evolutionary advantage, and claim that meat, egg, and dairy eaters are better adapted for survival than vegetarians. However, the fact that so many people have cholesterol-containing deposits in their arteries has led other researchers to provide different explanations:

(1) that humans cannot metabolize large amounts of dietary cholesterol effectively;

(2) that the mechanism which regulates our body's cholesterol levels does not compensate well for dietary cholesterol; or

(3) that high meat diets contain too little cholesterol-removing fiber.

More topics for further research. Proponents of orthomolecular nutrition (see Chapter 37, Orthomolecular Nutrition) suggest that the 'cholesterol' problem is really caused by dietary deficiencies of micronutrient vitamins and minerals required to properly metabolize cholesterol in our body. Researchers have shown that diets that are moderately high in cholesterol, which also include sufficient quantities of all vitamin and mineral micronutrients, keep blood cholesterol levels normal and prevent atherosclerosis.

Orthomolecular therapists lower high blood cholesterol levels simply by giving high doses of certain vitamins and minerals. Clinical evidence shows that atherosclerosis can be reversed by exercise, dietary manipulation, and a micronutrient supplement. Vitamins C and B_3 can lower a blood cholesterol level of 260 mg/dl by about 50 mg each. The minerals calcium, zinc, copper, and chromium are also helpful. Essential and other highly unsaturated fatty acids in their natural state can lower high cholesterol levels by up to 25%. Some types of dietary fiber also lower cholesterol levels by removing more from the body or inhibiting its production.[4]

Researchers at the Loma Linda School of Nutrition have explained the high incidence of atherosclerosis among meat eaters in a different way. They believe that man is by nature a vegetarian whose body does not know how to metabolize dietary cholesterol, much like his ancestors, the tropical primates. Strict vegetarians have less than one-quarter of the meat eaters' rates of death from cardiovascular disease (CVD), and people who include eggs and dairy products but exclude meat from their diets have only a slightly lower risk of death from CVD than meat eaters if they don't take nutritional supplements.

Resolution

Perhaps orthomolecular nutritionists and vegetarians are saying the same thing. A natural vegetarian diet is a richer source of vitamins, minerals, EFAs, and fiber than a non-vegetarian diet. Muscle meats (see Chapter 46, Meats) and dairy products (see Chapter 47, Mother's Milk and Dairy Products) contain fewer minerals and vitamins, less EFAs, more saturated fatty acids, and no fiber. Eggs are nutrient-dense but contain no fiber. Meat, eggs, and dairy products are poor sources of vitamin C and B_3, w3 fatty acids, and fiber, which are all important to cardiovas-

---

[4] Fiber from oats, apples, beans, peas, and flax lower cholesterol. Wheat bran does not.

cular health. When meat, eggs, and dairy products are augmented with the missing vitamin and mineral factors from vegetables, juices, or supplements, they present fewer cardiovascular problems.

Neither animal eaters nor plant consumers need fear CVD if they take their foods from unrefined natural sources, and especially if they supplement with C, B$_3$, w3, and fiber, and the rest of the substances long known to be essential for our health. Refined sugars, refined starches, hard fats, and refined, denatured oils from which vitamins, minerals, fiber, and protein have been removed should be expected to create problems. Sugar consumption and high serum triglycerides correlate with cardiovascular deaths at least as highly as do serum cholesterol levels.

The Dark Side of Cholesterol

Cholesterol has been given so much attention by the medical profession over the last 35 years that the word 'cholesterol' is automatically (and wrongly) equated with cardiovascular disease because it is often found deposited, along with fats, the protein fibrin, and calcium, in the inner lining (the intima) of human arteries, where it narrows them.

Theories. There are several theories about the causes of cardiovascular problems: one believable current theory suggests that arterial walls are first damaged by free radicals in our bloodstream, and that cholesterol deposition is part of a mechanism that attempts to repair this damage (see Chapter 21, Light, Free Radicals, and Oils). A second theory focuses on unnaturally rapid cell division (proliferation) in arterial walls. A third theory revolves around deficiency of micronutrient minerals and vitamins that destroy free radicals. A fourth theory blames oxidized cholesterol and triglycerides – produced when antioxidant (AO) levels in our blood are low – for causing arterial damage and thickening. A fifth theory blames increased consumption of refined, nutrient-poor sugars.

A Unifying Theory?

A unifying theory has been proposed by the team of Drs. Rath and Pauling – the latter is the only living winner of two unshared Nobel prizes (for Chemistry and Peace) and a humanitarian: "The purpose of my work is to minimize human suffering," he says. Rath and Pauling suggest that thickening arteries and cardiovascular disease revolve primarily around lack of vitamin C. Their theory turns orthodox cholesterol dogma on its head with its simplicity. Briefly, it goes like this.

Vitamin C functions. Vitamin C plays several key roles in the human body. It is *required for the synthesis of the 'glue' that surrounds our cells (mucopolysaccharides)*, makes them cohesive, and keeps our tissues from falling apart and landing on the floor in a pile of individual cells. In this role, vitamin C is important for tissue integrity and the prevention of invasion by foreign organisms and cancer cells.

Vitamin C is the *strongest antioxidant (reducing agent) normally present in our body*. In this function, it prevents oxygen and free radicals from damaging our cells and tissues. It also recharges other important AOs, notably oil-soluble vitamin E and water-soluble glutathione, allowing them to be reused many times. It also protects many B vitamins and other substances in our body from oxidative destruction. As such, vitamin C is 'king of the AOs'.

Vitamin C is *necessary for the production of the proteins collagen and elastin* (specifically, the hydroxylation of the amino acids lysine and proline), which keep our arteries, bones, teeth, cartilage, scar tissue, and other tissues strong. Lack of vitamin C results in weakened tissues. Tissue strength is particularly important in our arteries, since they are constantly under pressure. Lack of vitamin C (scurvy) results in weakened arteries and bleeding into tissue spaces.

Vitamin C, genes, and nature. Most animals can make vitamin C from glucose. They normally make several grams per 100 pounds of body weight, and can increase vitamin C production in response to infection, stress, or free radical-producing toxic influences.

Unlike most animals, human beings cannot make vitamin C from glucose. A genetic mutation in humanity's ancestors about 40 million years ago deprived us of that ability.

Vitamin C and health. To be healthy, we require the same large amounts of vitamin C as other organisms but, because our body cannot make it from glucose, we must get all this vitamin C from foods. Only a diet rich in fresh greens and fruits can provide the necessary amounts, and under certain situations of stress, no amount of such foods can provide enough vitamin C to equal what animals under stress normally produce.

But we do not eat a diet of fresh greens and fruits. Our diets have become deficient in vitamin C by storage and processing, and we have turned to other kinds of foods – meat, dairy, eggs, beans, grains – that are lower in vitamin C. As a result of vitamin C deficiency, our body develops a weakness of the connective tissues (scurvy) in our arteries. Scurvy must have killed many, many people in ice ages, when vitamin C was almost impossible to obtain in quantities sufficient for health.

Protection that kills. Under survival pressure, nature developed and selected for survival a way to protect us from early death due to scurvy – by thickening our arteries using an adhesive repair protein called apo(a) made in our liver. Apo(a) and its carrier vehicle in our bloodstream, lipoprotein(a) [Lp(a)], are stronger risk factors for cardiovascular disease than LDL which, if not associated with Lp(a), is only a weak risk factor. In cholesterol studies and measurements, the effect of the culprit Lp(a), which resembles LDL except for the apo(a) protein, have been mistakenly blamed on LDL.

Rath and Pauling suggest that in killing us by apo(a)-induced artery thickening, nature confers a survival advantage. For survival of the species, it is better to die from a heart attack or stroke after we have reproduced, than to die from scurvy before we have had a chance to reproduce.

Reversal. When ascorbate levels in our blood increase, apo(a) levels decrease, because less repair protein is necessary when there is enough vitamin C to keep the connective tissue in our arteries strong.

If Rath and Pauling's suggestion is correct, they lead the way to cure the most prolific killer disease in North America for a few pennies' worth of daily vitamin C (mineral ascorbate) supplements.

While it holds a major key to preventing and reversing cardiovascular disease, vitamin C is not the whole answer. Other keys are held by sulphur-containing amino acids, vitamin B_3, coenzyme Q_{10} and, for peripheral arterial disease, carnitine and lysine. W3 fatty acids keep platelets from becoming sticky, and have other beneficial effects on arteries. Ultimately, all essential substances must be present in optimum amounts for healthy cells, tissues, and organs.

Unification. Rath and Pauling's work combines the findings that led to the other theories. Lack of AOs leads to poor control of the free radicals normally produced by oxidation and other processes in our tissues, or produced by pollutants, drugs, pesticides, and synthetics from outside. These free radicals speed oxidization of cholesterol and triglycerides. Free radicals, and cholesterol and TGs (both oxidized) can damage arteries. Vitamin C-deficient, weakened, damaged arteries stimulate repair mechanisms including apo(a) synthesis and increased cell proliferation, which thicken and narrow arteries. Cholesterol and fats play a part in making platelets more sticky, which makes a clot blocking a narrowed artery more likely.

Politics. Rath and Pauling's article: "Solution to the Puzzle of Human Cardiovascular Disease," submitted to the prestigious journal: *Proceedings of the National Academy of Sciences (PNAS)*, was accepted for publication, and then later rejected. They subsequently published it in a tiny journal with a circulation of about 500. Pauling remarks that their explanation goes against established dogma and personal and economic interests of those who profit from cholesterol dogma and cardiovascular disease.

Those whose income depends on treating diseases of our heart and arteries by less effective or ineffective means, who profit from the fact that sickness is better business than health, and whose priorities place profit before truth, cure, care, and life stand to lose much from a solution to the puzzle of human cardiovascular disease (see Chapter 88, The Business and Politics of Health).

This political and economic controversy is part of an age-old battle between natural healer and drug pusher. A hundred years ago, the controversy involved the snake oil salesman who sold natural product and the patent medicine salesman (patented substances have to be synthetic; natural products cannot be patented), but the roots of the division go back to ancient Greece (see Chapter 56, Snake Oil and Patent Medicines).

In the end, cholesterol will be exonerated from its role as primary villain in cardiovascular disease. The accusing finger points at 'experts' who concocted the cholesterol theory to drum up business by spreading fear.

When the dust on the political-economic debate that parades as 'objective' scientific inquiry settles, and its heat dissipates, a nutritional solution that includes a full and balanced diet including all essential nutrients, the right kinds of fiber and digestive support (and perhaps several herbs) will make cardiovascular disease a non-threat for those who embrace the natural solution.

A Cautionary Note

Indiscriminately lowering cholesterol, as suggested by the National Cholesterol Education Program, statistically increases death rate from suicide and cancer.

Increased *suicide* may result from increased aggression, supported by the finding that low cholesterol levels reduce the number of receptors for serotonin on our brain cell membranes. Serotonin, a hormone and neurotransmitter, suppresses aggressive behavior. Lack of receptors might result in decreased suppression of aggression and violence.

Increased *cancer* may be due to lack of oil-soluble anti-cancer antioxidants: vitamins E and A, and carotene. These are transported to our cells by the same LDL transport vehicles that bring fats and cholesterol, and may become deficient when LDL levels in our blood decrease. Before embarking on a cholesterol-lowering program, one should first supplement with these antioxidant nutrients and vitamin C for two weeks. After all, it makes no sense to be saved from a heart attack only to be fed to cancer.

Essential Nutrients 13

To tell the complete story of nutrition, we must acknowledge *all* essential nutrients required by our body for health. Nutrients cannot work in isolation. All essential nutrients work as a team to build and support health, and to repair damage. *Absence* of any one of these essential nutrients is enough to destroy our physical health.

If we attempt to keep ourselves healthy by making sure that our fat intake is optimal without also making sure that optimum amounts of other essential nutrients are present in our diets, our attempts to attain, maintain, or regain health will inevitably fail.

Physical Components of Health

Essential factors. Physical components of health – the essential 'factors of physical health' – number about 50:

- 2 essential fatty acids (EFAs);
- 8 essential amino acids (10 for children, 11 for premature infants);

- 13 vitamins;
- 20 or 21 minerals (we're not sure yet about tin);
- a source of energy (carbohydrates are the cleanest source);
- water;
- oxygen; and
- light.

Out of these 50 factors, healthy bodies are built. A nutritional program designed to construct, defend, and rebuild health must contain peak (optimum) amounts of all essential nutrients. I have yet to meet a person whose health failed to improve from applying this approach.

In a healthy body, there is no room for disease. Disease results from an absence of health. In molecular terms, we need the presence of optimum amounts of the factors of physical health, and also absence of interfering (toxic) molecules in order to be healthy.

Not all essential factors need to be supplemented. Arsenic, for instance, is an essential mineral, but deficiency is unknown, and toxicity from excess can be fatal. Deficiencies of nickel and tin are unknown. Fluorine is not supplemented except through municipal water supplies and toothpaste. An excess of fluorine can be *very* toxic.

Accessory nutrients. In addition to 50 essential factors, there are accessory nutrients which, although not essential because the body can make them from other substances, may benefit health that is ailing due to infection, injury, obesity, suboptimal nutrition, degenerative disease, allergies, age, or a genetic constitution that interferes with biochemical conversions. We will list some of the accessory nutrients here but will not deal with them otherwise. They include orotic acid, pangamic acid, coenzyme Q_{10}, inosine, choline, inositol, lipoic acid, para amino benzoic acid (PABA), N-acetyl glucosamine (NAG), N-acetyl cysteine (NAC), carnitine, non-essential amino acids, hormones and neurotransmitters derived from amino acids, EFA derivatives, and bioflavonoids.

Digestive and intestinal help. Other factors necessary for health include fiber, friendly bacteria (acidophilus, bifidobacteria, streptofaecium, and others), hydrochloric acid, digestive enzymes, and adequate bile.

Herbs. Many herbs can help tone the human body to peak condition.

Deficiencies of Essential Nutrients

One might expect that diets in affluent industrial nations would also be nutritionally affluent, but this is not the case. Even though we have the necessary technology, money is not usually a problem, and we have both time and choices, over 60% (and rising) of North American people get less than the recommended amounts of one or more essential nutrients.

Let me list some statistics on North American nutrient status. Two government surveys, known as the Health and Nutrition Examination Survey (HANES,

1971-1974) and the Nationwide Food Consumption Survey (NFCS, 1977-1978), measured intake of 13 of about 45 essential nutrients in tens of thousands of people. Of the 13, only sodium was present in adequate amounts (actually, many people suffer toxic symptoms from an *excess* of sodium resulting from the overuse of table salt). They found the following percentages of people getting less than the government-set Recommended Daily Allowance (RDA), which was defined as the amount of an essential nutrient that is sufficient to keep most normal healthy adults from developing deficiency symptoms.

Nutrient	% who get less than RDA	Nutrient	% who get less than RDA
calcium	68%	vitamin B_1	45%
folacin	10+%	vitamin B_2	34%
iron	57%	vitamin B_3	33%
magnesium	75%	vitamin B_6	80%
phosphorus	27%	vitamin B_{12}	34%
vitamin A	50%	vitamin C	41%

The authors of these official surveys say that there is no cause for concern until intake of nutrients is down to seven-tenths of the RDA. This lower measure reduces the apparent incidence of deficiency, but those who think that optimums for health are far higher than the RDA strongly disagree. Statistics on food-related degenerative conditions also indicate that there is a high percentage of people that are deficient.

Clinicians observing smaller numbers of people 'unofficially' estimate the incidence of deficiency of other nutrients as:

Nutrient	% who get less than RDA	Nutrient	% who get less than RDA
biotin	10%	silicon	30%
chromium	90%	vitamin D	10%
copper	85-90%	vitamin E	20-40%
manganese	20-30%	vitamin K	15%
pantothenic acid	25%	w3s	95%
selenium	50-60%	zinc	35-60%

Deficiencies of essential nutrients may be due to many causes, including:
- poor food choices;
- poor digestion;
- poor absorption;

- food allergies;
- intestinal injuries;
- imbalances in bowel flora;
- drug interferences with metabolic processes;
- increased nutrient requirements for drug detoxification; and
- increased requirements due to genetic, congenital, life-style, athletic performance, and environmental conditions.

Deficiencies of the remaining essential nutrients are not likely to be widespread. However, deficiencies of some important non-essential substances necessary for health are widespread, in part due to deficiencies of essential nutrients necessary for their manufacture (hydrochloric acid, digestive enzymes), or because of a lack of fiber in refined diets, or due to use of drugs and poor bowel hygiene that destroy friendly bacteria.

Major Source of Deficiencies

Since deficiencies are widespread, we might well ask why this is so. Without going into a long explanation, let us examine what happens when whole wheat grain is turned into white flour. The following table shows the percentages of essential nutrients and fiber lost during processing. The figures are from work done by Henry A. Schroeder in the U.S. and by M.O. Bruker in Germany, both MDs.

Mineral	Loss (%)	Other Nutrients	Loss (%)
Calcium	60	Strontium	95
Chromium	40	Zinc	78
Cobalt	89	vitamins B_1, B_2, and B_3	72-81
Copper	68	vitamin B_6	72
Iron	76	pantothenic acid	50
Magnesium	85	folacin	67
Manganese	86	vitamin E	86
Molybdenum	48	linoleic acid	95
Phosphorus	71	alpha-linolenic acid	95
Potassium	77	protein	33
Selenium	16	fiber	95

Polished rice has lost between 26 and 83% of each mineral present in brown rice. Corn starch has lost between 31 and 100% of each mineral present in whole corn. Sugar has lost between 83 and 100% of each mineral present in raw sugar. Fat-free milk has lost all of its manganese and most of its selenium, as well as its vitamins A, D, and E.

Over half of the calories in normal American diets come from foods from which much of the mineral, vitamin, essential fatty acid, and fiber content has been removed – 17% from sugar, 20% from refined cereals, 3% from alcohol, 18% or more from refined fats (see Chapter 40, Why Calorie Counting Fails). This is the primary reason for deficiencies: the regular consumption of processed foods lacking essential nutrients.

Other affluent populations. Judging from the incidence of degenerative disease, the nutritional status of Europeans and affluent people around the world is about the same as ours. People in poorer nations are better nourished than the majority of the affluent. The former consume less food, but their foods are less processed and more nutrient-dense. Affluent populations have the luxury of choosing foods that undermine their health.

Reversal of Deficiencies

Impressive work is being done with vitamins, minerals and EFAs in the treatment of degenerative diseases. Much is being learned, and people are being relieved of degenerative afflictions that resist treatment with drugs, surgery, and radiation.

Gaps in knowledge. Although the basic essential components of human health are now known, the practice of healing through the use of essential nutrients is still poorly organized. This lack of organization keeps human health from being systematically learnable. The systematic study of biochemical nutrition is still young, and there are gaps in knowledge that need to be closed before we have *all* the information. Health, one of the key topics most vital to the well-being of every human, is not taught in schools, colleges, or universities. Nowhere in the world can a person earn a degree in a course of studies that explores the nature of human health. In our short-sighted, crisis-oriented approach, knowledge of health has lagged far behind knowledge of disease. The technology of food alteration is carried on without regard to its effects on human health, and has remained undefined and standardless.

Organization of the parameters of human health into a coherent discipline should be systematically and rigorously pursued. The benefits to health of such a teaching tool cannot be overestimated.

Essential Fatty Acids

Our body's content of EFAs fluctuates with the EFA content of our diet. An optimum dose of LA may be between 9 and 18 grams per day, and varies with body size, state of health, stress, season, and climate. Health effects of EFAs (especially w3s) have been studied less thoroughly than those of vitamins and minerals. Therapeutically, large amounts of w3 EFAs are being used to treat many degenerative diseases. Success requires that the other essential nutrient factors are also present in the amounts required for optimal cell functions. For successful therapy, junk foods and toxic substances must be removed from the food supply. Vitamin E is important to prevent rancidity of EFAs in our body. In some functions however, such as the treatment of malaria, short-term deficiency of vitamin E may make w3 fatty acids more effective killers of the malaria-causing protozoa. Table A2 gives an overview of EFAs.

Table A2. Essential fatty acids (EFAs).*

Name	Body Content (grams)	Daily Requirement (grams/day)	Estimated Optimum (grams/day)	Therapeutic Dose (grams/day)	Toxic Dose (grams/day)
Linoleic Acid (LA) 18:2w6	1000 or more	3	9	up to 60	none known**
Alpha-linolenic Acid (LNA) 18:3w3	200	2	6	up to 70	none known**

* oils used to improve health should be freshly made by mechanical (expeller) pressing while shielded from light and oxygen. They should remain unrefined, be stored in shelf-dated opaque containers, and used at temperatures below 160°C (320°F). Frozen solid while fresh, even the most sensitive oils can last a long time.

** provided that the natural antioxidants found in the seed are present, or vitamin E at the rate of 1:1500 is added to the oil.

EFA requirements vary with the total fat content of our diet, but should be about one-third of total fats consumed. A low-fat diet requires less EFAs, and a high-fat diet requires more. Traditional diets that maintained health without degenerative diseases contained 15 to 20% of calories as fats. Due to genetic differences, large variations in different individuals' optimums are to be expected.

Vitamins

Vitamins have been used successfully in therapy, with impressive clinical results, for many years now. The total body content for most vitamins is difficult to asses accurately, because vitamins (unlike minerals) degrade rapidly. They may also be meaningless, since concentrations of vitamins normally vary from tissue to tissue. Serum levels of vitamins and metabolites of vitamins in urine are measured therapeutically.

A few people do not absorb or metabolize vitamins well. These people may benefit from taking 'activated' forms of certain vitamins; for example:

- activated B_1 = thiamine pyrophosphate (TPP);
- activated B_6 = pyridoxine-5-phosphate (PSP);
- activated B_{12} = dibencozide.

If nutrients are not absorbed, they can be injected intramuscularly or intravenously. A three-hour intravenous drip of essential vitamins and minerals can give a person quite a lift in energy and disposition. Some nutrition-oriented doctors routinely administer them to people in their mid-40s or older. Table A3 gives an overview of vitamins.

Table A3. Vitamins.

Name	Body Contains (mg)	Daily Requirement (RDA) (mg/day)	Therapeutic Dose (mg/day)	Toxic Dose (mg/day)
Vitamin A (Carotene)*	500,000 IU (172 mg)	5,000 IU/day	50,000 to 500,000 IU/day short term	100,000 IU/day long term 18,500 IU/day long term (children)
Thiamine (B₁)	25	1.2	10 to 100	non-toxic
Riboflavin (B₂)		1.7	10 to 100	non-toxic
Niacin (B₃)		20	50 to 3,000	non-toxic (transient flush above 75)
Pantothenic Acid (B₅)		10	50 to 300	non-toxic
Pyridoxine (B₆)		2	50 to 500	over 500
Biotin (B₇)		0.3	up to 0.3	non-toxic
Folic Acid (B₉)		0.4	0.8 to 5	non-toxic
Cobalamin (B₁₂)	5	0.006	0.05 to 1.0	non-toxic
Vitamin C	1400	60	100 to 100,000 or more	non-toxic (diarrhea above bowel tolerance)**
Vitamin D		400 IU/day	500 to 1,000 IU/day	25,000 IU long term
Vitamin E		30 IU/day	50 to 1600 IU/day	non-toxic***
Vitamin K		not applicable****	up to 0.3	over 0.5

* Carotene is two vitamin A molecules hooked tail-to-tail. In this form, vitamin A is inactive, and therefore, carotene is non-toxic at all doses. As the body needs vitamin A, it splits carotene molecules to make active vitamin A.

** Bowel tolerance, above which diarrhea occurs, varies and must be individually determined.

*** People with rheumatic heart disease may need to limit dose to less than 200 IU.

**** Vitamin K is normally made in sufficient quantities by bowel bacteria.

Minerals

Mineral supplements are available in the form of inorganic salts, organic acid salts, and amino acid chelates.[1] All three forms have merit. Inorganic phosphates, sulfates, and chlorides are important for electrolyte balance; organic ascorbates, acetates, and citrates are natural and are more effectively absorbed by our digestive system than inorganic salts. Mineral amino acid chelates may be absorbed even better. The best formulations combine all three forms in appropriate ratios. Specific minerals chelate best with specific amino acids (e.g., magnesium with glycine or aspartic acid; copper with histidine, glutamine, or threonine; manganese with arginine; selenium with methionine; and iron with cysteine, to name a few). Table A4 gives an overview of minerals essential to human health.

Where no government RDA has been set for a mineral, parentheses indicate an RDA suggested by researchers in the field. So far no essential functions have been found for strontium and tin, although both are found in our body.

Essential Amino Acids

Traditionally, nutritionists were only concerned with whether or not proteins were 'complete' – containing all essential amino acids in the balance appropriate for the production of human proteins. Animal proteins were preferred because of this view. This attitude is slowly changing.

Vegetarian forms of protein are being given more attention, especially in terms of being able to feed about 20 times as many people by eating lower on the food chain, and in terms of balancing different plant proteins (e.g., beans and rice; or corn and beans) to improve their completeness. In addition, vegetable proteins may contain fewer toxic contaminants such as pesticides that are concentrated in animal tissues, fewer contaminants such as antibiotics, excess fat, and hormones, and fewer parasites that affect humans.

Individual amino acids are also being given more attention. They are beginning to be used for their therapeutic effects. Phenylalanine and tyrosine are used as anti-depressants, and for increasing assertiveness. Tryptophan is used as a sedative, but is now difficult to get because of regulatory interference. Arginine appears to decrease atherosclerosis and gallstones. Lysine is said to inhibit the growth of viruses, and is now being used to help in peripheral artery disease. The sulphur-containing cysteine[2] – and especially N-acetyl cysteine and reduced L-

---

[1] Our body must balance electrolytes, consisting of positively charged (cation) minerals with negatively charged (anion) groups in order to be healthy. Both food intake/absorption and loss (through stool and kidneys) are important regulators of electrolyte balance. Skin helps regulate electrolyte balance through sweating. In addition, carbon dioxide levels are regulated through our lungs. Increased carbon dioxide makes us more acidic; hyperventilation makes us more basic.

[2] Diabetics must exercise caution when using cysteine.

Table A4. Elements and minerals.

Name	Body Content (grams)	Daily Requirement (RDA) (mg/day)	Therapeutic Dose (mg/day)	Toxic Dose (mg/day)
Calcium (Ca)	1050	800-1200	800-2000	?
Phosphorus (P)	1000	800-1200	?	?
Potassium (K)	300	2000	up to 21,000 (not KCl)	25,000
Sulphur (S)	175	adequate protein		
Sodium (Na)	150	220		15,000
Chlorine (Cl)	140	220	?	15,000
Magnesium (Mg)	35	300-400	up to 2,000 (short term)	above 1000 long term
Silicon (Si)	30	?	200 to 1000	?
Iron (Fe)	4.2	18	up to 50 (short term)	5000
Fluorine (F)	2.6	(1)	1	above 2 long term
Zinc (Zn)	2.3	15	up to 100	over 300
Strontium (Sr)	.32	(1-3.2)	not used	?
Copper (Cu)	.125	(2)	up to 5	20
Vanadium (V)	.018	(1-3.2)	not used	?
Selenium (Se)	.013	(.05-.1)	0.2 to 0.8	0.9 (salt)
Manganese (Mn)	.012	(2.5-7)	10 to 100	?
Iodine (I)	.011	0.080-0.150	up to 0.5 (short term)	above 0.3 (long term)
Nickel (Ni)	.010	(less than 0.5)	not used	?
Molybdenum (Mo)	.009	(0.045-0.5)	0.5	?
Cobalt (Co)	.0015	(0.008)	not used	?
Chromium (Cr)	.0015	(0.090)	0.6	—

glutathione – is part of the body's nutritional antioxidant system. Several other non-essential amino acids are also used for special purposes. Amino acid therapy is a recent development in nutritional medicine, and a lot remains to be discovered. An excellent treatment of both essential and non-essential amino acids is found in Braverman and Pfeiffer's 1987 book: *The Healing Nutrients Within*. Table A5 (next page) gives an overview of essential amino acids.

Table A5. Essential amino acids.

Name	Body Content	Daily Requirement (RDA) (grams/day)	Therapeutic Dose (grams/day)	Toxic Dose (grams/day)
Protein	12% of total wt.	45-120		high protein diets
Isoleucine		1.1	10	
Leucine		1.0	10	
Lysine		0.84	1 to 8	140+
Methionine		0.65 to 1.3	1 to 3	25 for normal people over 5 for schizophrenics
Phenylalanine		1	1 to 8	toxic in PKU***
Threonine		0.35 to 0.7	food + 1 to 5	
Tryptophan		0.5	1 to 3	
Valine		0.85	1 to 5	
(Histidine)*			food + 1 to 5	
(Arginine)*			food + 6	40
Cysteine**				

* essential for children
** essential for premature infants
*** PKU is phenylketoneuria, a genetic condition in which dietary phenylalanine leads to brain damage.

Fat Cats in the Fats Lane

History, Oil Making,
Toxic Products, and Promotion

The oils you buy in a supermarket today are very different from those that people consumed 100 years ago. Oil processing methods have changed, and with them, oil molecules. In Section Two, we examined molecules as they are made by nature. In this section, we look at different kinds of processes used to make 'edible' oil products – past and present. While some of these processes provide fresh, natural oils, others can change these natural molecules into unnatural ones.

The molecular changes resulting from processing also change the way these molecules behave, and they can turn healing fats into killing fats. Unfortunately, they do not turn killing fats back into healing fats. We examine the nature of these changes and their effects on health. Again we see that diseases have their basis in the shapes and properties of molecules.

We examine scandals, controversies, and a few common advertising misrepresentations, and then go on to examine how oils should be, and are now beginning to be made, stored, distributed, and labeled if health is *really* the goal.

This information will enable you to make better oil choices for health.

Environmental Effects on Oils

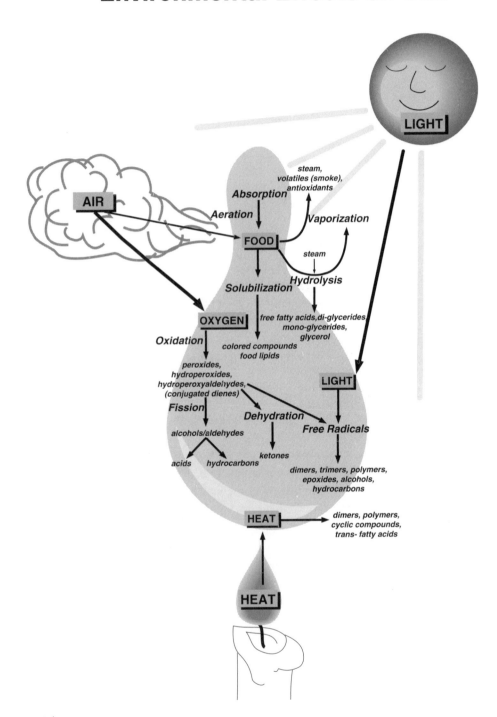

LIGHT

steam,
volatiles (smoke),
antioxidants

AIR

Absorption

Aeration

Vaporization

FOOD

steam

Hydrolysis

Solubilization

OXYGEN

free fatty acids, di-glycerides,
mono-glycerides,
glycerol

Oxidation

colored compounds
food lipids

peroxides,
hydroperoxides,
hydroperoxyaldehydes,
(conjugated dienes)

LIGHT

Fission

Dehydration

Free Radicals

alcohols/aldehydes

acids   hydrocarbons

ketones

dimers, trimers, polymers,
epoxides, alcohols,
hydrocarbons

HEAT

dimers, polymers,
cyclic compounds,
trans- fatty acids

HEAT

A Brief History of Oil Making 14

Changes in our food supply that have been made gradually, almost imperceptibly, over many years add up to major nutritional changes with major effects on our health. Oil production, too, has changed over the years, and has resulted in changes both in oil quality and in health.

In the Beginning

Traditionally in Europe, oil pressing was a cottage industry. Large estates, villages, and little towns had their own small oil press. Oil presses required parts that could withstand several tons of pressure per square inch, and they were difficult to clean and maintain; therefore they were (and are) too costly and complex for every home to have and maintain. Many older people who lived in Europe before the second world war remember how fresh oils were sold door to door like milk and eggs. Fresh flax oil was delivered once a week in small 100 mL transparent glass bottles. Since the oil was unprotected from light and air, it lasted only a few days.

Research showing the importance of protecting oils from destruction by light, oxygen, and heat had not yet been done, but people knew from experience that the best oils turn rancid quickly and then taste bad, so they had to be bought in small quantities and used fresh before they spoiled, just like fresh vegetables, milk, and eggs. Like fresh produce, unrefined oil was a staple in many homes.

Fresh oils are identifiable by their seed-specific characteristic odor and flavor. They are light and easy to digest. They sustain health and have therapeutic value because of the nutrients they contain. The most easily destroyed oils are also nutritionally the most valuable. All this was known over 50 years ago, before the advent of modern technology.

Bigger is Better

In the 1920s, the 'bigger is better' philosophy gradually took over the oil trade. Huge oil firms were constructed. Huge fields of oil seeds were planted. Huge continuous-feed, screw-type (expeller), heat-producing oil presses were built to replace small, slow, cold temperature batch presses in use prior to that time. The new presses were built to run around the clock, some pressing over 100 tons of seed per day. Automation made their operation highly efficient, and cut down labor costs. Figure 25 schematically illustrates batch and screw presses.

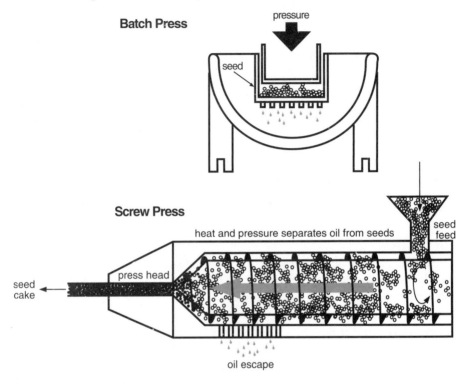

Figure 25. Schematic of batch and screw press.

Pesticides came into widespread use. Bigger crops resulted from not having to share the land and yield with weeds and insects.[1]

Technologies for seed preparation, oil extraction, refinement, bleaching, deodorization, and other processes were developed. Natural substances including carotene, vitamin E, lecithin, and others that keep oils from spoiling were removed because they were considered 'impurities', in the chemical sense of producing 'pure' oils. Synthetic antioxidants (AOs) were developed and added to the

---

[1] The pesticide advantage was short-lived, however. A recent report indicates that before we began using pesticides, 6% of crops were lost to pests. Today, the losses are up to 12%, in spite of pesticides. Pests have become resistant, and their natural predators have been killed off, making further reliance on less and less effective pesticides mandatory, unless we find a way to discontinue pesticides and help natural systems of pest control to re-establish themselves.

now refined oils whose natural AOs had been removed, to restabilize them and to extend their shelf life.

The cottage industry folded. It couldn't compete with the lower costs of mass production, afford the costs of mass media advertising, or match the clever and consistent ad-desk-inspired graphics that deceptively praised the 'new and improved' oil products. We got cheaper oil, greater confusion, and poorer health – and large companies profited.

Effects of the Mega Oil Industry on Nutrition

By the end of the second world war, flax oil, one of the more nutritious oils, had virtually disappeared from the market. Flax oil is highly unstable and spoils quickly because its so-called impurities include both essential fatty acids (EFAs): LA (18:2w6) at 20% and LNA (18:3w3) at 50%. The latter is the least stable of all essential nutrients, and flax oil is its richest source. More stable oils (poorer in the w3 essential fatty acid), with less chance of spoiling during transport and storage, replaced oils rich in w3s. The use of more stable oils of inferior nutritional value became commonplace, and helped upset the ratio of w6 to w3 EFAs that is important to our health. W6 consumption doubled, while w3 consumption decreased to one-sixth its 1850 level.

The paint industry continued to use flax. Boiled with lead to make linseed oil, it was, and still is, used as a 'drying' oil because it reacts chemically with oxygen from the air and dries rapidly in a thin film. In paints, this drying property is important.

Tasteless. Over the years, natural, unrefined oils were replaced by bland, refined oils without taste, and we have come to believe that oil *should* be tasteless. But fresh, natural seed oils have the delicate aromas and flavors of the seeds from which they are pressed.

De-vitalized. These tasteless, low-quality oils have had molecules with health benefits removed, altered, or destroyed. We lost fresh, natural, high-quality oils. We lost the complex, natural substances they contain, which help to digest and metabolize oils and have nutritional value of their own. These include: *phospholipids* including lecithin, with important fat-emulsifying and membrane functions (see Chapter 10, Phospholipids and Membranes); *phytosterols,* which block cholesterol absorption from our intestine; fat-soluble *vitamin E complex, carotene,* and their *precursors,* which protect oils against damage in storage and act as AOs in our body; *chlorophyll,* which is rich in magnesium; *aromatic* and *volatile compounds*; and *minerals.*

Toxic. Edible oils have become contaminated with pesticide residues that interfere with nerve functions and oxidation processes, and therefore lower our vitality. The invention of chemical extraction introduced gasoline-like chemical solvents (hexane, heptane) into our oils. These are lung irritants and nerve depressants. Very tiny (homeopathic) doses can have powerful detrimental effects on health. Non-natural AOs were added to edible oils. These improve oil shelf life, but may interfere with energy production, cell metabolism, and respiration, because they do not fit *precisely* into the precise molecular architecture of our enzyme systems and membranes. Over time, they may contribute to degenerative diseases and lack of vitality.

Chemically changed. The fatty acid composition of our diet was changed. Oils low in EFAs became the standard items on the shelves of our grocery stores.

We obtained oils altered by heat and chemicals. Natural nutrients in oils were converted into substances detrimental to health: *trans-* fatty acids, polymers, cyclic compounds, aldehydes, ketones, epoxides, hydroperoxides, and other compounds that have not yet been identified. Many of these are toxic and detrimental both to our body and our health even in small quantities (see Chapter 19, Other Toxic Products). The processes used to refine oils produce dozens of different new substances by random processes that cannot be controlled. Different batches of oil contain widely varying amounts and types of unnatural fat breakdown products.

Hydrogenation, a process introduced on a large scale in the 1930s[2] for making margarines and shortenings (cheaper substitutes for butter and lard, respectively), produces many altered fat substances in our diet. Just one of them – *trans-*fatty acids – brings twice as many food additives into our diet as all other food additives from all food sources combined (see Chapter 18, Margarines, Shortenings, and *Trans-* Fatty Acids).

With reduction in EFAs and increase in altered fatty acids in our diets, fatty degeneration rose to epidemic proportions.

'White' fats and oils. Refined fats and oils products – 'white' fats and 'white' oils – are nutritionally equivalent to refined white sugars and white flour in carbohydrate nutrition: protein-less, de-mineralized, de-vitaminized, fiberless, empty calories. They cannot be properly digested and metabolized, they rob our body of its stores of minerals and vitamins, and they lead to deficiency of essential nutrients and fatty degeneration.

In 1900, deaths from cardiovascular disease accounted for only 15% of deaths from all causes. Today, it kills 44% of the population, an increase of almost 300% in just 90 years, in spite of all of our amazing technological medical advances. Cancer in 1900 killed 3% of the population. Today, it kills 23% of us, and its incidence is rising. This is an increase of over 600% in 90 years. These two are the greatest killers in affluent nations. Other conditions of fatty degeneration: diabetes, multiple sclerosis, kidney degeneration, liver degeneration, and others, have also increased dramatically in the past 90 years.

Double-priced. Refined (but nutrient-impoverished) oils are sold both in

---

[2] The hydrogenation process was patented in 1903. The first commercial hydrogenated shortening, made by Procter & Gamble and called 'Crisco', went on sale in 1911.

supermarkets and natural (health) food stores. Lecithin, vitamin E, phytosterols, chlorophyll, and carotene have been sold to 'health nuts' as supplements in natural food stores for over 30 years. Consumers pay twice.

More recently, pharmacies and supermarkets have also begun to carry some of these natural products. 'Health food nuts' make up one of the fastest growing groups in the population, because we cannot escape – and *must* face – the fact that our body *is* made from foods. Supplements of nutrients benefit health, especially when the foods we normally eat – white bread, white sugar, and refined oils – are nutrient-poor. Research discovers and confirms this again and again. People are learning, trying, and benefiting. But, wouldn't it have been better just to leave the nutrients in our foods?

Bigger is Not Always Better

Slowly, we are beginning to get wise. Bigger is not always better. In Europe and America, fresh oils are making a comeback. Slowly, discriminating consumers are returning to eating habits of pre-processing days and regaining health. If the trend catches on, the incidence of degenerative diseases will decrease. In North America, a reversal appears to have been made – incidence of cardiovascular disease is now decreasing. Its decrease owes much to better eating and fitness habits, as well as the increased use of vitamin C and other nutrient supplements by 100 million (and increasing) Americans *against* the advice of many physicians. Expensive high-tech medicine being practiced on heart attack and stroke victims accounts for only a modest improvement in CVD statistics.

In North America, people are beginning to look for mechanically pressed, unrefined, natural oils. Slowly, the assumptions of the mega oil business are being examined, found to be false, and discarded.

A Fledgling Natural Oils Industry

Since the first publication of this book in 1986, under the title *Fats and Oils*, a fledgling natural oils business has been started. I was intimately involved with its development, setting the new guidelines for machinery design, packaging materials, shelf dating, and refrigeration – guidelines for making oils with human health in mind (see Chapter 28, Making Oils with Human Health in Mind). Poor industry practices and hidden agendas also had to be addressed.

Health or business? Business and health interests tend to move in opposite directions. In the short run, higher profits follow from cutting corners to minimize costs, but result in lower product quality and poorer health. If health is put first, short-term profits may be lower, because better health requires *more* care.

To manufacture products with health in mind requires a commitment to health that is rare in industry. Most manufacturers know little about the biology of human health. To them, the word 'health' is important in advertising copy, because *consumers* place value on health. Health-targeted advertising sells products. But most *manufacturers* place profit above health-sustaining product quality.

If a manufacturer does not know about or value health, how can he translate knowledge of health into products that support health?

15 The Business of Fats and Oils

Business interests are extremely powerful, and affect us all. When the conduct of business is not based on a clear commitment to the common good, it can become dangerous and destructive. The fats and oils business is no exception.

Just how large is the edible fats and oils business? One way to figure it out follows. Five billion people live on this planet. The average weight of a human being is about 150 pounds or 70 kg. The average human carries about 15% of his body weight (10 kg [22 pounds]) as fat.

According to these figures, human beings carry a total of 45 billion kilograms (99 billion pounds) of fat around with them in their bodies. That's a lot of fat. This body fat is constantly being used up in biological functions and then being replaced from food sources.

Fat Consumption

North Americans, Europeans, citizens of other industrialized nations, and wealthy people living in the poorer nations consume 40% or more of the daily calories (out of an average 2500 calories) as fats and oils. This is about 1000 calories, from just over 110 grams of fats per day (1 gram of fat produces 9 calories), amounting to just over 40 kg (88 pounds) per person each year. Actual fat consumption may be closer to 160 grams (about 1500 calories) per day, or 60 kg (132 pounds) per year (see Chapter 32, Fat Consumption and Daily Requirement).

For North America alone, human consumption of fats and oils adds up to 10 million tonnes each year. One source gives 25 kg (55 pounds) per person per year as the consumption of edible fats and oils worldwide, which adds up to 125 million tonnes.

Paint, chemical, soap, lubricant, and detergent industries gobble up a lot of fats and oils as well. Figure 26 gives a schematic view of how the mega oil industry processes oil seeds into processed consumer products.

Fats and Oils Sales

In 1975, the world market for edible fats and oils was over 41 million tonnes. The producers sold their products for almost 29 billion dollars. In 1981, they sold over

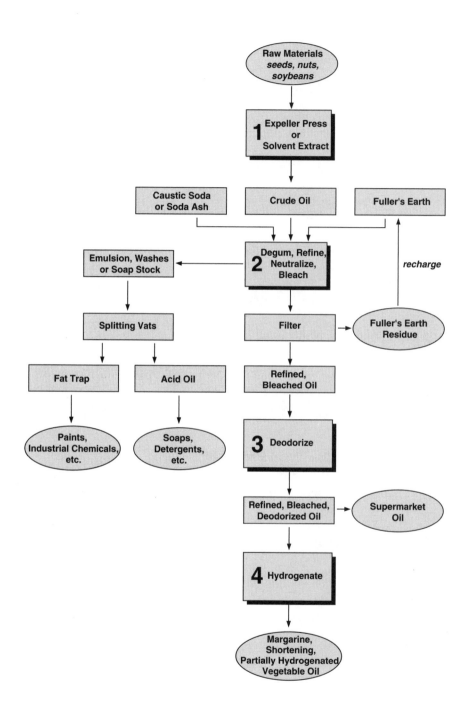

Figure 26. Schematic of the mega oil industry.

40 billion dollars' worth of fats and oils. In 1992, producers expected to sell 80 million tonnes, bringing in over 80 billion dollars.

Competition
From the size of the market involved, it is easy to see why the marketing arms of all sectors of the fats and oils industry – oil seed, meat, dairy, and egg – are engaged in fierce competition to sell their respective products. Each sector uses aggressive advertising campaigns, often short on facts and long on misleading half-truths and manipulative techniques, to capture the largest possible share of the attention, interest, and money of consumers. In these campaigns, health is not a major consideration, although some advertising campaigns make it appear to be the issue.

In the frenzy to create sales, consumers are 'educated' with misinformation. Armed with this misinformation, they change their buying and eating habits. Unhealthy fats and oils are over-consumed, and degenerative disease increases.

Lobbies
With huge volumes of products and profits at stake, the edible fats industry has developed powerful political and economic lobbies (now called government advocacies) to protect the sale of products for profits, even though the health value of some of these products is dubious. Modified oil products are used for various purposes in edible products, and some oils contain toxic fatty acids (see Chapter 19, Other Toxic Products).

Hydrogenated Oils in Food Products
About one-third of all edible oil produced is hydrogenated or partially hydrogenated. Hydrogenated oils end up in hardened 'edible' fat products, mainly margarines and shortenings. Hydrogenated oils are also used in baked goods, confections such as ice cream, chocolate, candy, and snack foods such as potato chips where the hydrogenated oils help to give the product crispness. Non-hydrogenated oils produce limp potato chips.

The market for limp potato chips is small, the health cost for crunchy ones is high. Why not eat whole potatoes? (see Chapter 17, From Oil to Margarine).

Conspiracy?
In private conversations, some researchers claim that the mega oil industry conspires to keep negative information about fats, oils, and health from the public in order to continue to profit from the sale of health-destroying products. They claim the industry doesn't want to make the costly changes in equipment, engineering, and methods that would be required to address new information about human health. Health-conscious methods would require greater care, and would make many of the industry's present methods obsolete.

One researcher, who prefers to remain nameless, even claims to know of secret meetings held specifically for the purpose of continuing to hoodwink consumers. Is this paranoia, or are these allegations true? It should not surprise us that one negative effect of industry's interest in profit is that it pays more attention to its bottom line than to our concern for health. Giant oil, food, drug, and medical industries are engaged in the pursuit of money. For all of them, health is a secondary concern. The blindly trusting consumer bears the consequences of the business bottom line with compromised health.

From Seed to Oil **16**

Commercial Oil Making Methods

A lot of strange things happen to super-nutritious seeds made by nature on the way to the tasteless oil we buy in a store. Changes made by processing have a bearing on our health. Processing turns fragrant seed and nut oils into bland tasting, colorless oils that cannot be distinguished from one another by our senses. The only oils that are not so treated are virgin olive oils (see Chapter 54, Virgin Olive Oils). In a commercial oil making facility, oil seeds and the natural oils they contain are subjected to many processes. Figure 27 summarizes oil processing steps.

Cleaning and Cooking
After being mechanically cleaned, seeds intended for mechanical pressing (see below) are cooked for up to 2 hours at varying temperatures, depending on the seed type used. They may be mashed before cooking to make this process easier. An average cooking temperature is 120°C (248°F). Cooking makes pressing or extraction easier by destroying the seed cells containing the oil, but it also cracks or breaks seeds and exposes their oils to air, beginning a process of deterioration (rancidity).

Mechanical (Expeller) Pressing
The cooked seeds are mechanically pressed in an expeller (or screw) press, a continually rotating spiral-shaped auger that moves seeds forward (like a home meat grinder or grain mill) and pushes them against a metal press head. The turning auger crushes the seeds and creates friction in the seed mass, which produces heat in the head of the press. The pressure generated in the head of an expeller press reaches several tons per square inch.

Heat and pressure squeeze oil out of the seeds, and the oil runs backward

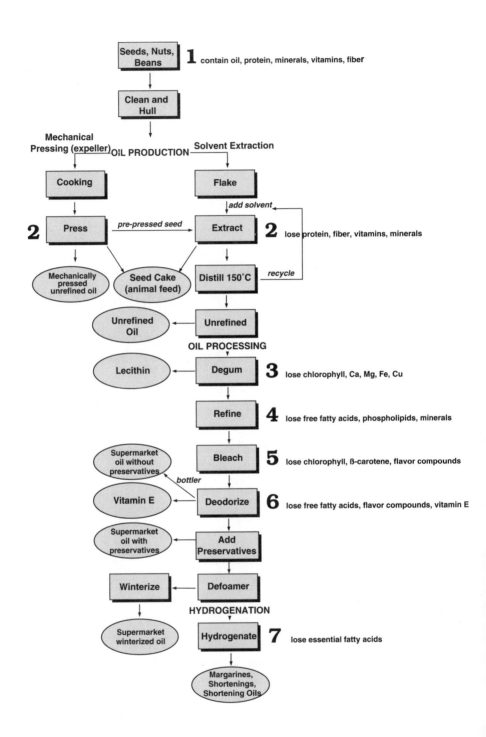

Figure 27. Summary of the steps involved in commercial oil making.

over the seeds and out through slots or holes in the side of the press head, while the oil cake – the solid remainder of the seed mash – is pushed out through slits at the end of the press head. The size of these slits, which is adjustable, determines the back pressure created in the press head, which in turn determines how hot the head and seed mash get, and how much of the oil contained in the seeds will be forced out of the seed mash. Higher temperatures and pressures produce better oil yields, and leave less oil remaining in the oil cake. In giant presses, the pressing process takes a few minutes, usually at temperatures around 85 to 95°C (185 to 203°F). At this temperature, oils react with oxygen more than 100 times faster than at room temperature. If the oil is not protected from exposure to air, much deterioration (rancidity) can take place in oils during pressing – at the front end – which must then be cleaned up at the back end by further processes that cause other problems.

Oil pressed in this way may be filtered, then bottled and sold in natural food stores and delicatessens as natural, unrefined ('crude') oil. In most operations, light and air are not excluded, and pressing temperature is high enough to damage essential fatty acids (EFAs). Until 1987, all unrefined oils commercially available in North America were in this state. That year, I (and others under my instructions) pioneered production methods for pressing oils protected from light and from air. This required us to custom-make modifications for existing presses. I bottle my protected and nitrogen-flushed balanced oil blend in amber glass, place the bottle in a completely opaque cardboard box to give the oil continued protection from damage by light and air (see Chapter 28, Making Oils with Human Health in Mind) and store the oil blend refrigerated or frozen solid. I have consulted regularly with manufacturers to develop innovative procedures for oils, and to develop nutrient-sparing procedures for making other nutritional products.

Mechanical pressing leaves about 9 to 18% residual oil in seed cake. This residual oil can react with oxygen and become rancid within the seed cake in a short time unless it is protected with the same care as the oil.

Solvent Extraction

A more *efficient,* but less healthy, method removes oil from seeds by dissolving it out of finely ground seed meal with a solvent such as hexane or heptane (gasoline) at 55 to 65°C (131 to 149°F), under constant agitation. These chemical solvents may also be used to increase oil yield by removing oil remaining in seed cake after mechanical pressing. The oil-less seed cake is usually fed to animals.

Once the oil-solvent mixture has been separated from the seed, the solvent is evaporated at a temperature of about 150°C (302°F), and reused. The solvents used for oil extraction are highly flammable. Occasionally, an oil factory blows up, with great damage and loss of lives.

Traces of solvent may remain in solvent-extracted oils. Some healers claim that even minute amounts of these solvents can have serious detrimental effects on health.

Oils from expeller pressing and solvent extraction may be mixed together and sold as 'unrefined' oils. More commonly, unrefined oils made by careless pressing or extraction procedures are processed by several further steps – degumming, refining, bleaching, and deodorizing – to produce refined oils. A description of these procedures follows.

Degumming

Degumming removes phospholipids, including lecithin. True gums (a kind of fiber), protein-like compounds, and complex carbohydrates (polysaccharides) are also taken out of the oil. Lecithin is isolated and sold separately as a supplement (*we* pay twice). Degumming also removes chlorophyll, calcium, magnesium, iron, and copper from unrefined oils. Degumming is carried out at about 60°C (140°F) with water and phosphoric acid.

Refining

During refining, oils are mixed with an extremely corrosive base, sodium hydroxide (NaOH, caustic soda, known under the trade name 'Drano'), or with a mixture of NaOH and sodium carbonate (Na_2CO_3). The mixture is agitated, then separated.

Refining removes free fatty acids from oils. Free fatty acids form soaps with NaOH, which dissolve in the watery part of the mixture. Phospholipids, protein-like substances, and minerals are also further removed during refining. Refining temperature is about 75°C (167°F). The oil still contains pigments, and is usually red or yellow at this stage.

Bleaching

Filters, 'Fuller's earth', and/or acid-treated activated clays bleach oils by removing pigments – chlorophyll and beta-carotene – as well as remaining traces of soap. Also, natural polycyclic and aromatic substances are removed. Bleaching takes place at 110°C (230°F), for 15 to 30 minutes.

During bleaching, toxic peroxides and conjugated fatty acids are formed from EFAs present in the oil. If air is excluded, peroxidation is prevented, but higher temperature must be used. This increases altered fatty acids produced by double bond shifts (positional isomers) occurring in unsaturated fatty acids.

Deodorizing

Deodorization is steam distillation under pressure and exclusion of air. It removes aromatic oils, free fatty acids, and molecules that impart pungent odors and unpleasant tastes that were not present in the natural oil before processing began.

Deodorization takes place at a destructively high temperature – 240 to

270°C (464 to 518°F) – for 30 to 60 minutes. When heated to temperatures above 150°C (302°F), unsaturated fatty acids become mutagenic, which means that they can damage our genes (and those of our offspring). Above 160°C (320°F), *trans-* fatty acids begin to form. Above 200°C (392°F), *trans-* fatty acids form in substantial quantities (see Chapter 18, Margarines, Shortenings, and *Trans-* Fatty Acids). Above 220°C, the rate of *trans-* fatty acid production increases exponentially.

Deodorization removes the peroxides produced during refining and bleaching. Tocopherols (vitamin E), phytosterols, and some pesticide residues and toxins are separated out. The oil is now (finally!) tasteless, and cannot be distinguished from oils derived from other seeds that have been similarly treated.

At the high temperatures necessary for deodorization, many unnatural isomers of unsaturated fatty acids form. These include molecules in which double bonds have moved to another part of the carbon chain (double-bond shifts); *trans-* fatty acids formed by twisting the molecule; cyclic compounds resulting from a fatty acid chain reacting with itself to form a ring; dimers and polymers formed when fatty acid molecules cross-link with one another to produce something similar to vulcanized rubber and plastics; and other altered fatty acid breakdown products. These changed molecules are not present in oils found in nature. Our body is not well equipped to handle them. They cause concern to biologists, nutritionists, and health professionals.

Oils resulting from these processes are vitamin and mineral deficient, the oil equivalents of white (refined) sugars, white (refined) flour, and 'pure' (refined) starch. Some clinical nutritionists call them 'nutrient robbers'.

After all of this heating, these oils can still be sold as 'cold-pressed', because there is no commonly accepted definition for that term. If no external heat was applied while the oil was being *pressed*, it qualifies as 'cold-pressed', according to one (ridiculous) manufacturer. Such oils are sold in supermarkets as well as in natural food stores alongside natural, unrefined oils. For health, it is important to know the difference.

Supermarket Step

To extend shelf life, refined oils sold in supermarkets may have synthetic antioxidants (AOs) added to them. The list of possibilities includes butylated hydroxytoluene (BHT), butylated hydroxyanisole (BHA), propyl gallate, tertiary butyhydroquinone (TBHQ), citric acid, and methylsilicone. In animal foods, the now controversial ethoxyquin is added as an AO to retard oil spoilage. These replace the natural AOs beta-carotene and vitamin E that were processed out of the oil. Defoamer is also added, and the oil is bottled and sold.

It may go through another step called winterization, where it is cooled and filtered one more time to prevent it from developing turbidity when cooled in the fridge.

Hydrogenation, an artificial saturation of fully refined oils to harden them into spreadable products, is so widely used and its health effects so widely unknown that the entire next chapter is devoted to this process. It is not, strictly speaking, part of oil making, but canola and soybean oils may be subjected to this process, and almost half of all refined edible oils are further processed using this destructive technique that was invented in the early part of this century.

Consumer Options

With one exception (see below), the oils available in **supermarkets, corner groceries,** and **convenience stores,** whether from safflower, walnut, sunflower, corn, grape seed, soybean, sesame, rice bran, canola, almond, peanut, avocado, other seed or nut sources, or oil blends – are fully refined and deodorized, and are either solvent-extracted or a mixture of expeller-pressed and solvent-extracted oils. The label does not advertise this fact, but trumpets less relevant selling information such as 'free of cholesterol' (all plant oils are cholesterol-free), 'low in saturates' (saturates in plant seed oils are, relatively speaking, always low), 'for frying, baking, and cooking' (no oil can *safely* be used to fry or cook [deep-fry]), and 'high in polyunsaturates' (such oils can lower cholesterol slightly but *increase* cancer). All of theses oils are colorless, odorless, and tasteless. The exception: virgin olive oils (see Chapter 54, Virgin Olive Oils), which are pressed without heat and remain unrefined.

Some suppliers in the **natural foods industry** sell only expeller-pressed oils. These may come from the giant commercial expeller operations, and may then be sold unrefined or be processed by the same methods that are used to produce supermarket oils.

In processed foods sold in the natural foods trade, solvent-extracted oils are often used because they are cheaper to buy.

Other suppliers to the natural foods industry sell only unrefined, unprocessed, expeller-pressed, fresh oils in dark containers. As long as they remain fresh, these oils taste like the seed from which they were pressed, and also have the color and aroma characteristics of their seed source.

Touring the Refinery

It is not easy to get permission to tour an oil-pressing facility. Most oil companies do not like the processes to be too well known. The average oil pressing facility is not a picture of care and cleanliness. If more people knew about how oils are made, what they contain, and what has been taken out, more people would complain, and fewer would buy these oils.

To be fair to oil processors, what is now known about oils and health was unknown when the huge oil pressing facilities were first developed. But important knowledge about the effects of processing artifacts on health has been around for 30 years now, much of it discovered under the stewardship of the oil industry itself, through work they did in their own labs or paid university laboratories to do.

There is great resistance in the industry to make the changes necessary to produce natural, unrefined oils. It takes effort to change mega oil industry momentum. In essence, the changes would make large presses obsolete. Fresh edible oils require a higher level of care.

The care required to make fresh, unheated, EFA-rich oils, with vitamins and minerals kept intact so our body can metabolize them properly, is not the present mandate of the mega oil industry; nor is a distribution system that gets fresh oils to consumers before they deteriorate from exposure to light and air high on their present list of priorities.

The Japanese claim that "the bigger the front, the bigger the back." In the case of commercial oil makers, there is a lot hidden behind the front.

From Seed to Oil

Let us briefly summarize what happens from a nutritional point of view when oils are made. We begin with a seed that is a rich source of essential minerals, essential vitamins, essential fatty acids, essential amino acids, fiber, lecithin, phytosterols, and health-promoting minor ingredients. Even in making a fresh, unrefined oil – the highest quality of oil there is – all of the protein and fiber present in the seed is lost, as well as some minerals and vitamins. It still contains essential fatty acids, oil-soluble vitamins, lecithin, phytosterols, minor ingredients and some minerals.

During processing, most of the remaining minerals and vitamins are removed. All of the protein and fiber is already gone. Lecithin, phytosterols, and minor components are also removed, and some EFAs are destroyed. In addition, processing introduces toxic molecules resulting from the breakdown and alteration of fatty acid molecules.

Fully processed oils are the equivalent of refined (white) sugars, and can therefore be called 'white' oils. Like sugar, they are nutrient-deficient sources of calories but in addition, they contain toxins that are not present in sugar.

17 *From Oil to Margarine*

Hydrogenation

Hydrogenation is the most common way of drastically changing natural oils. This process has major effects on health. Industry's reason for using the process is to provide cheap spreadable (plastic) products for (non-discriminating) consumers, or to provide shelf stability at the expense of nutritional value. It is important to know the effects of hydrogenation on oil molecules because they affect our health and, knowing these effects, we can make well-informed choices about whether or not to use hydrogenated products.

The Process

Hydrogenation changes the unsaturated and essential fatty acids present in a natural oil. In this process, oils are reacted under pressure with hydrogen gas at high temperature (120 to 210°C; [248 to 410°F]) in the presence of a metal catalyst (usually nickel, but sometimes platinum or even copper) for 6 to 8 hours. Figure 28 summarizes what happens to fatty acids during hydrogenation.

A 'nickel' catalyst often used in hydrogenation, called 'Raney's Nickel', is actually 50% nickel and 50% aluminum. Remnants of both metals remain in products containing hydrogenated or partially hydrogenated oils, and are eaten by people.

The presence of aluminum is particularly worrisome, because its presence in the human body is associated with Alzheimer's disease (mental senility), and osteoporosis, and may even facilitate the development of cancer.[1]

Complete Hydrogenation

If the process is brought to completion, all double bonds in an oil are saturated with hydrogen.[2] It contains no UFAs, no w6 polyunsaturated fatty acids (PUFAs), and no W3 superunsaturated fatty acids (SUFAs). A completely hydrogenated oil (which is now a very hard fat) has no essential fatty acid (EFA) activity whatsoever. Such a fat is 'safe' because it contains no *trans-* fatty acids to interfere with EFA activities in our body; and does not spoil, resulting in a a long shelf 'life' (if that

---

[1] Aluminum is also present in process cheese, canned soft drinks, acidic liquids in aluminum cans, antacids, underarm deodorants, flow agents in table salt and other powders, and some (acidic) water supplies.

[2] The completely saturated fat that results is neither *cis-* nor *trans-*, since *cis-* and *trans-* always apply to double bonds, and therefore only to *un*saturated fatty acids (UFAs).

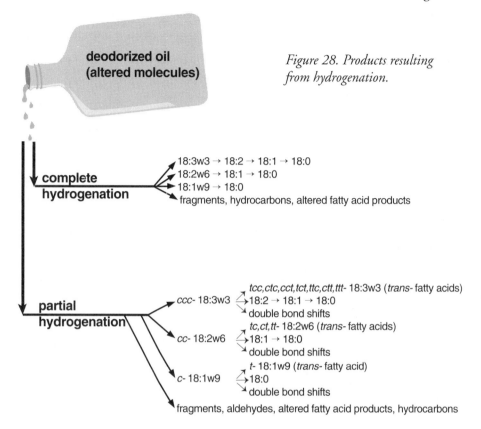

Figure 28. Products resulting from hydrogenation.

term can be applied to a dead substance). Completely hydrogenated oil (fat) can be heated without further damage: fried, baked, roasted, and boiled. Our body can store its saturated fatty acids (SaFAs) in triglycerides and membranes, or use them for energy.

Completely hydrogenated fat contains unnatural fatty acid fragments and other altered molecules derived from fatty acids, created during hydrogenation. Some of these may be toxic. It may also be contaminated by the metal catalyst used in hydrogenation. As stated above, aluminum is of special concern.

Except for the fact that our body does not need it and it contains some toxins, hydrogenated fat is a manufacturer's dream: an unspoilable substance that lasts forever.

Uses for Completely Hydrogenated Products

Completely hydrogenated oils, generally from coconut or palm, which are over 90% saturated to begin with, have commercial applications. Chemically inert, they can be used for frying without being made more toxic. They are used in products such as chocolate, which must be hard enough to stay solid in the package (except on scorcher days) yet soft enough to melt in our mouth. They can be used to extract oil-soluble substances, such as the flavors of onions or garlic, out of other plant tissues (see Chapter 64, Flax and Oil Blend Recipes), although non-hydrogenated coconut oil is preferable for this purpose. Completely hydrogenated coconut oil can be mixed with natural, EFA-containing liquid oils to make a 'vegetable spread' which is like margarine but is virtually free of *trans-* fatty acids.

Canola and cottonseed oils are also available completely hydrogenated, but contain more production artifacts. They are sometimes used as ingredients for making margarines, because they are hard (melt at 70°C [158°F]) and therefore only a small amount is needed to give plasticity to liquid oils used to make these into margarines.

Consumption of hydrogenated tropical fats appears to increase cholesterol levels, unlike the raw product from Malaysia, which apparently lowers cholesterol levels (see Chapter 52, Tropical Fats). Most affluent people consume too much saturated fat and too little w3s. Excess SaFAs crowd out EFAs from enzyme systems that insert double bonds into (desaturate) fatty acids, and EFA deficiency can result (see Chapter 8, The Healing Essential Fatty Acids). Saturated fatty acids can thereby upset the delicate balance of prostaglandins (see Chapter 58, Prostaglandins), with negative effects on health.

Partial Hydrogenation

When the process of hydrogenation is not brought to completion, a product containing many (dozens) of intermediate substances results. Double bonds may turn from *cis-* to *trans-* configuration. Double bonds may shift, producing conjugated fatty acids. Or, double bonds move along the molecule to produce positional double bond isomers. Fragments may also be produced. Figure 29 illustrates some of these chemical changes.

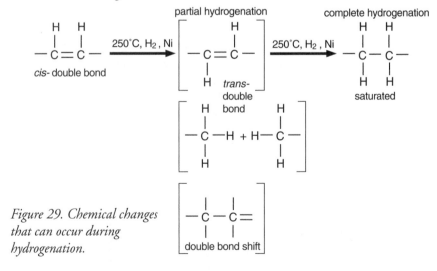

Figure 29. Chemical changes that can occur during hydrogenation.

So many different compounds can be made during partial hydrogenation that they stagger the imagination. Scientists have barely scratched the surface of studying changes induced in fats and oils by partial hydrogenation. Needless to say, the industry is hesitant to fund or publicize thorough and systematic studies on the kinds of chemicals produced and their effects on health. The industry is equally hesitant to publicize the information that already exists in research journals on this topic.

Hydrogenation randomly attacks double bonds within oils. It destroys w3s very rapidly, and w6s only slightly more slowly. It is impossible to control the chemical outcome of the process. We cannot predict the quantities of each different kind of altered substance that will be produced. We never know what any given batch of partially hydrogenated oil product contains.

It is possible, however, to stop the reaction when the desired degree of 'hardening' has been achieved, and this is one of the industry's major reasons for using the process. It allows cheap oils to be turned into semi-liquid, plastic, or solid fats with specific 'mouth feel', texture, spreadability, and shelf life.

Partial hydrogenation produces margarines, shortenings, shortening oils, and partially hydrogenated vegetable oils. These products contain large quantities of *trans-* fatty acids and other altered fat substances, some of which are known to be detrimental to health because they interfere with normal biochemical processes. Other altered substances have not been adequately studied regarding their effects on health. *Trans-* fatty acids have now been shown to increase cholesterol, decrease beneficial high-density lipoprotein (HDL), interfere with our liver's detoxification system, and interfere with EFA function (see Chapter 18, Margarines, Shortenings, and *Trans-* Fatty Acids).

Trans- fatty acids in partially hydrogenated products. Several research studies measured the content of *trans-* fatty acids[3] in commercial products. In some margarine samples from one such study, *trans-* fatty acid content of more than 60% was found, but virtually no EFAs (less than 5%).

Tables B1 and B2 show the pooled results of other studies.

Table B1. Average trans- fatty acid content of margarines, shortenings, and vegetable oils (numbers in parentheses show the range).

	Margarines	
Stick	Tub	Diet
31% (9.9-47.8%)	17% (4.4-43.4%)	(up to 17.9%)

Vegetable Oil Shortenings	Vegetable Salad Oils
20% (up to 37.3%)	(0-13.7%)

---

[3] *Trans-* fatty acids have received most of the attention of researchers, because they make up the largest part of the altered substances. They are not necessarily the most important altered fat products in terms of toxicity to biochemical processes and consumer health.

Table B2 Trans- fatty acid content of partially hydrogenated oils used in food products.

French Fries	Candies	Bakery Products
up to 37.4%	up to 38.6%	up to 33.5%

Margarines and shortenings contribute the bulk of the *trans-* fatty acids found in the human diet. We consume about 40 grams of margarines and shortenings daily, and they average 20% or more *trans-* fatty acids. The effects of these altered fatty acids on our body moved the Dutch government to ban the sale of margarines containing *trans-* fatty acids.[4]

Government concerns. A government committee in Canada in 1980 also expressed concern. It recommended that a minimum of 5% linoleic acid (LA, 18:2w6) should be required in all margarines and margarine-like products. This figure is too low, because 5% LA is neutralized and made ineffective by 95% of monounsaturated oleic acid and SaFAs (see Chapter 46, Meats), and therefore results in functional absence of LA (see Chapter 8, The Healing Essential Fatty Acids). According to the World Health Organization's recommendations, the *minimum* functional requirement of LA is 3% for an adult person, 4.5% during pregnancy, and 5 to 7% during lactation. A product should have 8% (5+3), 9.5% (5+4.5), and 10% (5+5) to 12% (5+7) LA, respectively to prevent functional EFA deficiency due to the presence of saturated and monounsaturated fatty acids, which can prevent EFAs from being able to function.[5] The presence of *trans-* fatty acids in products demands a higher content of LA to compensate for the inhibition of LA functions that *trans-* fatty acids are known to have.

The government committee was supposed to meet again in 1985, but has not yet done so.

Why Hydrogenate?

Hydrogenation allows manufacturers to start with cheap, low-quality oils, and to turn these into products that compete with butter in spreadability. They cannot compete in taste, because margarines often taste slightly rancid.

Butter too, can acquire a rancid taste when left out in summer, but this rancidity can be removed by heating it: short-chain free fatty acids, separated (hydrolyzed) from the glycerol molecule (see Chapter 9, Triglyceride Fats) and responsible for this taste, evaporate off. Margarine's rancidity is based on oxidation of long-chain UFAs that will not evaporate. Heating will not remove the rancid taste from margarine.

---

4 The Dutch, incidentally, enjoy the longest life expectancy among industrialized nations, 5 years more than Americans.
5 The calculation of these figures is described in more detail in Chapter 46.

The low cost of raw materials allows margarine to be sold at a much lower price than butter. Margarine sales generate good profits, with money left over to mount massive advertising campaigns. Shoppers who are more concerned with bargains and saving money than with health buy margarine. Advertising campaigns mislead uninformed people into thinking that margarine is better than butter, using health as an advertising tool without basis in fact, experimental proof, or even statistical or anecdotal evidence (see Chapter 24, Advertising and Jargon). Margarines sold in supermarkets and natural food stores usually contain the same junk fats, even when named after famous natural healers.

Alternatives

One alternative to partially hydrogenated margarines is *Becel* brand margarine which contains no *trans-* fatty acids, no hydrogenated fats, and no animal fats or cholesterol. It is made from *refined* sunflower oil and tropical fats. The latter increase cholesterol levels, but *Becel* may be acceptable in small quantities. It contains no w3s, but provides w6s from sunflower oil.

We can also dip our bread in fresh, unrefined olive, flax, or other fresh oils. The dipping custom of Mediterranean countries makes hydrogenation and processing to manufacture spreads completely unnecessary. It is therefore a step toward better health.

Expert Statements

Two statements sum up the story of hydrogenation and health. The first statement, made by G.J. Brisson, Professor of Nutrition at Laval University in Quebec, says that "It would be practically impossible to predict with accuracy either the nature or the content of these new molecules (produced in the process of hydrogenation). Between the parent vegetable oil, sometimes labeled 'pure', and the partially hydrogenated product . . . there is a world of chemistry that alters profoundly the composition and physicochemical properties of natural oils."[6]

The second statement was made by Herbert Dutton, one of the oldest and most knowledgeable oil chemists in North America. It goes like this: "If the hydrogenation process were discovered today, it probably could not be adopted by the oil industry." He adds, ". . . the basis for such comment lies in the recent awareness of our prior ignorance concerning the complexity of isomers formed during hydrogenation and their metabolic and physiological fate."[7] Translated into simple English, it means that we now know some of the ways in which fats are changed by hydrogenation. The body does not use these changed substances in the same way it uses normal fats and oils. Because of the known and unknown effects on health that the "complexity of isomers formed during hydrogenation"

---

6 Brisson, G. J., Lipids in Human Nutrition (New Jersey: Burgess, 1981), p. 39.
7 Brisson, G. J., Ibid. p. 39.

produces, government regulations passed to protect people's health would forbid the use of this process for making edible products if it were introduced today.

However, because partial hydrogenation has been used commercially on a large scale since the 1930s and now has a long tradition behind it, and because the oil industry has powerful lobbies in government, hydrogenation is allowed to continue to supply unnatural fat products to our foods.

From Seed to Oil to Margarine

Let us summarize what, nutritionally, we have done. In making the *oil* used in margarines and shortenings, we had already removed all proteins, all fiber, about 95 to 99% of all minerals, 65 to 100% of all vitamins, almost all of the lecithin, phytosterols, and other minor components (see Chapter 16, From Seed to Oil, and Chapter 54, Virgin Olive Oils). A small part of the EFAs has also been destroyed by processing. In addition, some toxic substances have been formed from fatty acids. The only essential nutrients left in this oil are some EFAs.

When we hydrogenate this oil to make margarines and shortenings, we systematically and preferentially destroy the only essential nutrients left in the oil. Hydrogenation attacks w3s more than w6s, and w6s more than monounsaturated fatty acids. In addition, hydrogenation produces many toxic substances.

We end up with a product that has had almost all of its essential nutrients deliberately removed or destroyed. The 60 grams (2 ounces) of margarines and shortenings we consume each day contains more than twice as many toxic 'food additives' than are found in the other 2640 grams of food that men consume each day, or the other 1740 grams of food consumed each day by women.

18 *Margarines, Shortenings, and Trans- Fatty Acids*

Although *trans-* fatty acids have been known for some time, only recently has public attention been focused on the negative effects of the *trans-* fatty acids that are present in margarines, shortenings, convenience foods, and even some oils.

Trans- fatty acids are produced by high temperatures and hydrogenation – discussed in the previous chapter – that turn refined oils into margarines, shortenings, shortening oils, and partially hydrogenated (stiffened) vegetable oils. Here, let us examine *trans-* fatty acids and their effects on health in more detail.

A very slight change – the rotation of the molecule around a double bond – twists a fatty acid from its natural *cis-* configuration into an unnatural *trans-* configuration, creating a *trans-* fatty acid. However, this slight change drastically changes its properties, its performance in our body, and its effects on our health. None of the atoms in the molecule has been changed: it still has the same number of carbon atoms and the same number of hydrogen atoms, and the bonds are still in the same place, but the molecule now has its "head on backwards".[1]

This rotation can occur at any one or more double bonds in the fatty acid, producing many different kinds of twisted molecules. I call them the 'twisted sisters' (old witches) of fatty acids.

Comparing Cis- and Trans-

Cis- double bonds have both hydrogen atoms on the carbons involved in double bonds on the same side of the molecule. The twist that occurs at high temperatures reached during frying, deep-frying, hydrogenation and, to a smaller extent, deodorization, flips the hydrogens on the carbons involved in double bonds onto opposite sides of the molecule. Figure 30 shows both *cis-* and *trans-* configurations of a fatty acid around a double bond.

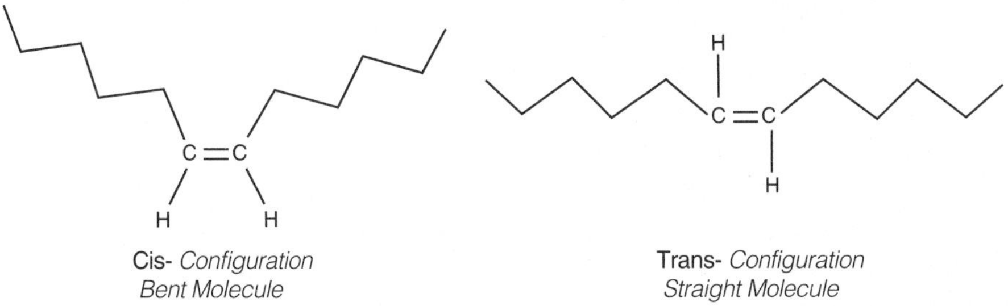

Cis- *Configuration*
Bent Molecule

Trans- *Configuration*
Straight Molecule

Figure 30. Cis- *and* trans- *configurations in a fatty acid.*

The results of this miniscule change are drastic. In a *cis-* double bond, hydrogens on the same side of the molecule repel each other in seeking space for themselves. Since the space on the other side of the molecule is unoccupied, the molecule bends to give each hydrogen more room. A *trans-* molecule remains almost straight because the hydrogen atoms are on opposite sides of the molecule. The difference in the shape of *cis-* and *trans-* molecules gives them different melting points, chemical activities, and enzyme fit.

Any double bond in a fatty acid molecule may be twisted into the *trans-* form. LA, with two double bonds, can produce 3 *trans-* forms of the molecule (one bond twisted, the other bond twisted, or both bonds twisted). LNA, with

---

[1] Imagine what kinds of problems you'd have if the top half of your body were back to front. You'd never know whether you were coming or going. On the molecular level, *trans-* fatty acids have this problem.

three double bonds, can form 7 different *trans-* forms. EPA, with five double bonds, could form 32 different *trans-* fatty acids. *Trans-* forms are biologically different from the parent molecule. During hydrogenation, the 2- and 3-times unsaturated EFAs LA (18:2w6) and LNA (18:3w3) are turned into SaFAs or twisted into different kinds of *trans-* fatty acid-containing monounsaturated or polyunsaturated fatty acid forms by the high temperatures (up to 250°C [482°F]) at which this process takes place (see Figure 28). Hydrogenation selectively and more rapidly destroys the biologically more valuable EFA molecules by *trans-* fatty acid production and saturation with hydrogen (see Chapter 17, From Oil to Margarine), because EFAs are more chemically active than fatty acids with only one double bond.

Properties and Functions of Trans- Fatty Acids

The simple change in shape from *cis-* to *trans-* has important effects on the physical properties and functions of the molecules. *Trans-* fatty acids are more stable than *cis-* configurations. This means that once a *cis-* fatty acid has been changed to a *trans-* fatty acid, it is unlikely to be changed back to a *cis-* fatty acid. The distance between carbon atoms (bond length) is shorter in *trans-* than in (natural) *cis-* fatty acids, which also changes the properties of the *trans-* fatty acids.

Misfits. The change in shape from the bent *cis-* form to the straight *trans-* form fits the molecules into body structures differently. In biological systems, the *trans-* form only half-fits into enzyme and membrane structures. It takes up the space and blocks out the *cis-* form, but cannot do the work that the *cis-* form can do.

Melting points. *Cis-* and *trans-* molecules pack differently, and therefore their melting points are different. For instance, each molecule of either *cis-* or *trans-* oleic acid (OA, 18:1w9) has one double bond. If this double bond is in its natural *cis-* configuration, a pot full of these molecules melts at 13°C (55°F). It is liquid at both room and body temperature. In its *trans-* configuration, a pot full of these molecules melts at 44°C (111°F) and is thus solid at both room and body temperatures. Non-sticky, liquid *cis-* form changes to sticky *trans-* form.

Dispersal. Natural *cis-* molecules are more dispersed. Unnatural *trans-* molecules are more sticky. They make platelets more sticky, increasing the likelihood of a clot in a small blood vessel causing strokes, heart attacks, or circulatory occlusions in other organs, such as lungs, extremities, and sense organs. *Trans-* fatty acids behave more like saturated (no double bonds) fatty acids than like their *cis-* fatty acid siblings: OA (18:1w9) melts at 13°C (55°F); *trans-* OA (t18:1w9) melts at 44°C (111°F); the saturated equivalent, stearic acid (18:0), melts at 70°C (158°F). While saturated fatty acids are even stickier than *trans-* fatty acids, they don't interfere with EFA functions.

Our body metabolizes *cis-* and *trans-* fatty acids differently. It prefers to use *trans-* fatty acids only as energy-creating fuel. It conserves *cis-* EFAs (see Chapter

8, The Healing Essential Fatty Acids) for use in cell membrane structure and prostaglandin (hormone-like regulator) formation.

Breakdown. The rate at which our enzymes break down *trans-* fatty acids is slower than the rate at which they break down *cis-* fatty acids. This is important for our heart, whose normal fuel is fatty acids. High *trans-* fatty acid consumption may lower its ability to perform. In a situation of increased activity, stress, or crisis, lowered heart performance could have fatal consequences.

Holes in membranes. *Trans-* fatty acids change the permeability of cell membranes. They impair the protective barrier around cells, which is vital for keeping cells alive and healthy. This means that some molecules that ordinarily would be kept out of our cells can now get in, while some molecules which would ordinarily remain in our cells can now get out. Cell vitality would then diminish. Also, allergic reactions may result, and immune function may be impaired.

Electrical short-circuits. The effect of *trans-* fatty acids that is most likely to generate negative effects on our well-being has received little research attention so far. It involves changes in electrical properties of *trans-* fatty acid molecules as a result of the twist and change in shape. EFAs and their highly unsaturated derivatives are involved, according to European research, in energy and electron exchange reactions that also involve sulphur-rich proteins, oxygen, and light. *Trans-* fatty acids are unable to take part in these vital reactions. Worse, they interfere because they almost fit, but not quite. This situation is comparable to what occurs when a spark plug has too wide a gap. The spark is unable to jump this gap. This fault, while tiny in comparison to the size of the car, prevents the car from functioning.

Energy flow. Life is energy. It flows in our body via electrons that move across molecules set up specifically for that purpose. Extremely precise structural and spatial arrangements of atoms and their electrons are required. When we change the molecular architecture of our body by introducing molecules with wrong shape, size, or properties, they do not fit, and throw the flow pattern of life's currents off course. Any molecule not normally part of our biological/biochemical construction could have such an effect, including altered fatty acid molecules, pesticides, synthetics, and drugs.

Life functions. Life energy currents are responsible for all life functions, including healthy heartbeat, nerve function, cell division, coordination, sensory function, mental balance, and vitality. To explain degenerative diseases on the molecular level, we must certainly look at altered molecules and their capacity to impair the natural flow of energy from molecule to molecule within our body.[2] *Trans-* fatty acids constitute a major class of these altered molecules.

Since the disruption that *trans-* fatty acids create may be primarily electrical

---

[2] Side effects of drugs and toxic effects of poisons can be also explained this way.

rather than molecular, it is difficult to lay conclusive blame on them. By the time degeneration becomes visible, the *trans-* fatty acids that started the electrical process that led to degeneration have been metabolized, and are gone.

EFA disruption. Finally, *trans-* fatty acids disrupt the vital functions of EFAs. They worsen EFA deficiency by interfering with the enzyme systems that transform fatty acids into highly unsaturated fatty acid derivatives found especially concentrated in our brain, sense organs, adrenals, and testes. *Trans-* fatty acids interfere with the production of prostaglandins (PGs) that regulate muscle tone in the walls of our arteries, and thereby interfere with PG functions that appropriately increase or decrease blood pressure; regulate platelet stickiness important in blood clotting; and regulate kidney function, inflammation response, and immune system competence. It is easy to see that whatever interferes with the production of PGs will also interfere with health.

Food Sources of Trans- Fatty Acids

How many *trans-* fatty acids do we get, and from where? Estimated average intake of *trans-* fatty acids is about 12 grams (0.43 ounces) per day in the U.S., and 9.1 grams (0.33 ounces) per day in Canada, of which 95% comes from partially hydrogenated vegetable oil products, and the rest from animal products, mainly beef and butter fat. This 12 grams is almost 10% of our total fat intake. Our annual consumption of *trans-* fatty acids is almost twice as much as our intake of all other unnatural food additives (and that is what *trans-* fatty acids are) put together.

The main products from which we get *trans-* fatty acids are margarines, shortenings, and shortening oils, all of which are made from partially hydrogenated vegetable oils. Margarine accounts for about 3.5 grams of *trans-* fatty acids per day, and shortening for about 4.6 grams per day. Salad oil accounts for around 0.5 grams, butter and milk add 0.25 grams each, and meat adds 0.12 grams.

How Our Body Deals With Trans- Fatty Acids

Just as a bricklayer can deal with defective bricks when building, our body has ways of dealing with *trans-* fatty acids in our diet. Some enzymes, luckily for us, recognize the difference in shape of *trans-* fatty acids from natural *cis-* fatty acids, and refuse to use *trans-* fatty acids in functions for which these changed molecules are not suited. Some tissues in our body also recognize and reject *trans-* fatty acids. Our brain is partially protected from them and the placenta does not let them pass through into the fetus completely, protecting the unborn child to some extent, but neither brain nor fetus is completely protected from *trans-* fatty acids.

A bricklayer may destroy defective bricks to prevent them from being used. Our body deals with *trans-* fatty acids in a similar way. It breaks them down as quickly as it can, metabolizing twisted *trans-* EFA molecules for energy, whereas it conserves natural *cis-* EFAs for more important functions. In this way, interfering *trans-* fatty acids are selectively removed, and their interference with EFA functions is kept to a minimum.

If too many bricks are defective, a bricklayer may have to use some of them in the structure. Our body's capacity to break down altered fatty acids is limited, although that limit has not yet been clearly determined by measurements. When our intake exceeds our limit, disease begins to manifest, because our body attempts to use altered molecules for vital structures and functions.

Trans- Fatty Acids and Disease

Atherosclerosis. *Trans-* fatty acids can increase blood cholesterol levels by up to 15% and blood fat (TG) levels by up to 47% very rapidly when partially hydrogenated vegetable oil containing 37% *trans-* fatty acids is ingested. High TG levels play a part in developing cardiovascular disease. If our diet contains cholesterol, the effect of *trans-* fatty acids is enhanced. *Trans-* fatty acids increase the size of atherosclerotic plaque in pig aortas in experimental situations. High levels of natural, highly unsaturated *cis-* fatty acids found in flax, hemp, and cold water fish oils reverse these effects of *trans-* fatty acids.

A large, well-controlled study published in the *New England Journal of Medicine* in 1990 shows conclusively that *trans-* fatty acids increase total cholesterol and 'bad' low-density lipoprotein (LDL), both of which are correlated with increased cardiovascular disease, disproving manufacturers' advertising claims that suggest that margarines can be good for the health of our heart.

Cancer. Many kinds of cancer are associated with diets high in fats. When this information is analyzed and compared to the increase in the incidence of deaths from cancer over the last 80 years (from 1 in 30 people in 1900 to 1 in 4 people in 1990), cancer increase parallels the increase in our consumption of fats of vegetable origin. Even closer correlation is found between cancer increase and increased consumption of *hydrogenated, trans-* fatty acid-containing vegetable oils. While statistical analysis is not *proof* that *trans-* fatty acids cause cancer, it should alert us to that possibility. The fact that *trans-* fatty acids interfere with vital functions of essential and other highly unsaturated fatty acids makes their involvement in cancer likely.

Research evidence shows that EFAs (especially w3s) inhibit cancer. The fact that at least some cancers appear to involve a functional deficiency in EFAs (see Chapter 70, Degenerative Diseases) lends further support to this theory.

Confirmations

A Silver Spring, Maryland researcher (Mary Enig, 1993) has researched, followed, and summarized others' research on the effects of *trans-* fatty acids for many years. Research from Harvard (Willett, 1994) and other institutions show that besides interfering with EFA functions, raising total cholesterol and lowering the 'good' HDL, inhibiting conversion of EFAs to their derivatives, and worsening essential fatty acid deficiency, *trans-* fatty acids also:

- raise Lp(a), a strong risk factor in human atherosclerosis;
- lower the efficiency of B cell response and increase proliferation of T cells (B and T cells are involved in immune function);
- decrease testosterone and increase abnormal sperm (in animals);
- interfere with pregnancy;
- correlate with low birth weight in humans;
- lower the quality of breast milk and decrease volume of cream;
- increase blood insulin in response to glucose;
- decrease insulin response (undesirable for diabetics);
- alter the activities of a liver enzyme system that metabolizes carcinogens and toxins (mixed function oxidase cytochromes P-448/450);
- alter membrane transport and fluidity;
- alter the size, number, and fatty acid composition of adipose (fat) cells;
- increase peroxisomal activity; and
- interact with fish oil and tissue w3s.

Since *trans-* fatty acids have detrimental effects on our cardiovascular system, immune system, reproductive system, energy metabolism, fat and essential fatty acid metabolism, liver function, and cell membranes, we should consider margarines, shortenings, shortening oils, and partially hydrogenated vegetable oils to be harmful to human health!

19 *Other Toxic Products*

Besides *trans-* fatty acids, which are treated separately in Chapter 18, we should know about several other toxic oil products.

Toxic Fatty Acids Found in Nature

Several oils contain toxic fatty acids, and are therefore not recommended for human consumption.

Cottonseed oil contains from 0.6 to 1.2% of a *cyclopropene fatty acid* with 19 carbon atoms, which has toxic effects on liver and gallbladder, and also slows down sexual maturity (at higher levels it causes female reproductive functions to stop, and at much higher levels, it kills rats within a few weeks). On the biochemical level, this fatty acid destroys enzymes (desaturases) that make highly unsaturated fatty acids, and therefore interferes with essential fatty acid (EFA) functions. It also enhances by many times the power of fungus-produced aflatoxins to cause cancer.

Cottonseed oil also contains *gossypol,* a complex substance containing benzene rings, which irritates the digestive tract and causes water retention in the lungs, shortness of breath, and paralysis.

Cottonseed oil contains high levels of pesticide residues. Cotton farmers must spray their crops in order to keep boll weevils and other cotton pests under control. Since many birds, the natural predators that once kept these pests in check, have been killed off by pesticides, the insects are now out of control, requiring more intensive pesticide application every year. Refining and deodorizing oils removes only part of the toxic fatty acids and pesticides.

Another fatty acid considered by some researchers to be toxic is *cetoleic acid,* a 22-carbon chain with a double bond between the eleventh and twelfth carbon atoms (22:1w11). **Herring** and **capelin oils** contain between 10 and 20% cetoleic acid; **menhaden** and **anchovetta oils** contain small amounts of this fatty acid. Most other fish oils do not contain cetoleic acid.

The hydroxy fatty acid *ricinoleic acid* which makes up 80% of the fatty acids in **castor oil**, stimulates the secretion of fluids in the intestine, and is therefore used as a purge, both during detoxification therapy and before medical intervention into gastro-intestinal problems. Aside from causing powerful intestinal contractions (the body gets rid of castor oil and everything else in the intestine as quickly as possible), this oil has no harmful effects. It is not absorbed into our body. Prolonged use leaches minerals and vitamins out of intestinal tissues, and is inadvisable unless enhanced nutrient support is provided.

Modified Oils

Heating oils to high temperatures (above 160°C [320°F]) produces many toxic substances besides *trans-* fatty acids. Many of these substances have not yet been identified.

So much of our food preparation involves **fried** and **deep-fried oils** that these constitute a major source of toxic fat substances in our diets. Oils heated in the absence of air form toxic cyclic monomers which are found in deep-frying oils. In experimental animals these cyclic monomers produce unnatural fat deposits in the liver (fatty liver). Fed to the young, they result in a high death rate. Oils heated in air form less cyclic monomers, but produce other substances equally toxic to animals. Heated either with or without air, deep-fried oils create a great health hazard for human beings.

Brominated oils rarely get attention. Made from olive, corn, sesame, cottonseed, and soybean oils, they are used to enhance cloud stability in bottled fruit drinks and to prevent ring formation on the necks of bottles; in other words, they serve purely cosmetic purposes.

Fresh juices have a natural, cloudy appearance. The solids in these natural juices settle out with time, and also dry on the bottle necks, forming (gasp! unsightly) rings. Brominated oils give a fresh look to old juices. They have been added to commercial fruit drinks for more than 50 years.

Brominated oils cause changes in heart tissue, thyroid enlargement, fatty liver, kidney damage, and withered testicles. They decrease the heart's ability to use saturated fats as fuel, and lower the liver's ability to metabolize pyruvic acid, a very common fuel for cells. They increase the levels of several enzymes that indicate imbalance or difficulty in important metabolic functions. They accumulate toxic bromine in the tissues of children. In Holland and Germany, brominated oils are not allowed in drinks.

Toxic oxidation products are formed from unsaturated fatty acids when oils become rancid. These include: *ozonides* and *peroxides,* which are toxic to lung tissues and can be fatal. *Hydroperoxides, polymers,* and *hydroperoxyaldehydes* are the most toxic oxidation products. All damage cell membranes. All impair liver and immune function.

Oils in number one grade, intact seeds usually have a peroxide value (PV) of less than 0.1 milli-equivalents per kilogram (meq/kg). Their oils have a taste characteristic of their seed source. Oil PVs vary, should always be less than 10, and can be kept below 0.5 for most oils under careful pressing and bottling conditions. Olive oil often measures in at a PV of 20. Corn oil in commercial trade may go up to 40, even 60. When its PV reaches 100, about 2 to 3% of the fatty acid molecules in an oil are oxidized (or rancid), and the oil is totally unpalatable. The PV at which the taste of an oil becomes unpalatable varies from oil to oil.

A substance called **phytanic acid,** found in milk and meat, is toxic for people suffering from a genetic defect called Refsum's disease. When phytanic acid-containing foods are omitted from the diets of people with Refsum's disease, their symptoms abate.

Toxic Products Due to Heat

We have already alluded to toxic products besides *trans-* fatty acids that are made during high temperatures used in deodorization (see Chapter 16, From Seed to Oil): *cyclic fatty acid derivatives* that result from fatty acid chains reacting with themselves, *cross-linked fatty acid chains, dimers,* and *polymers* of fatty acids, *cross-linked triglycerides, bond-shifted molecules,* and *molecular fragments.* While these kinds of altered molecules are produced only in small quantities, their toxicity may be substantial, and while some research with these molecules has been done and establishes their toxicity, no large-scale studies whose results can be directly applied to human populations have been carried out. Such studies are only available for *trans-* fatty acids, the largest (most obvious) group of altered molecules produced by heat. Studies comparing the toxicities of the various kinds of breakdown products are also waiting to be done. Such studies will likely show that many of the other breakdown products are even more toxic than *trans-* fatty acids.

Toxic Products Due to Frying and Deep-frying

Frying and deep-frying expose oils to the effects of the three major fatty acid-damaging influences – light, oxygen, and heat – simultaneously. Random free radical reactions due to light, oxidation-rancidity, and heat-twisting effects combine, interact, and synergize each other's destructiveness.

Besides producing atherosclerosis in the arteries of animals, fried and deep-fried oils can also impair cell respiration and other cell functions, inhibit immune functions, and lead to cancer. Over the next 10 or 20 years, research will verify the toxicity of fried and deep-fried oils.

Relative Toxicities

Exactly how toxic is each of the different kinds of altered fatty acids molecules? The research necessary to assign precise figures has not yet been done. Until these figures are available, we must console ourselves with a general discussion on relative toxicities.

The toxicity of molecules – the extent to which they can interfere with the biochemical reactions that underlie the biological functions necessary to keep our cells, tissues, and body alive – varies from substance to substance. We must consider three factors when assessing toxicity: *lethal dose* (a measure of toxicity), *speed of action* (a second measure of toxicity), and *frequency of exposure* (a measure of the concentration of the toxic substance). Lethal dose and speed of action depend on the precise way in which toxic molecules interact with biological molecules in our body, just how vital to life are the biological functions with which they interfere, and how well our body is able to detoxify them or find ways around their interfering effects. Frequency of exposure is an environmental issue.

Take cyanide, one of the most potent biological poisons known, for example. The *lethal dose* of cyanide for an average adult is tiny – about 50 mg – less than one-millionth (one ten-thousandth of one percent) of the adult body's weight. It blocks one of the most vulnerable steps in our cells' energy production. No energy production – no life. The *speed of action* is less than one-half hour, because it is absorbed and transported to all our cells very rapidly. The *frequency of exposure* to cyanide, however, is rare (cyanide poisoning is usually restricted to death row inmates, cult followers, and perhaps the occasional sloppy chemist).

In comparison to cyanide, altered fatty acid molecules are less toxic and far more slow-acting. It may take 5, 10, 20, or even 30 years of regular consumption of altered fatty acid molecules before their cumulative effects result in death. But we are exposed to these molecules far more frequently than to cyanide. As a result, many more people die from the effects of the less toxic altered fatty acid molecules than from the more toxic cyanide.

Among altered fatty acids, we are exposed to far greater quantities of *trans-*fatty acids than of other altered product. *Trans-* fatty acids are less toxic than some other altered fatty acid molecules that are present in processed oils and oil products in only small quantities. As a result, the small quantities of other, more toxic molecules continue to be largely overlooked, while *trans-* fatty acids are now getting much more attention.

Rating Toxic Molecules

Sugar, saturated fatty acids, oxidized fatty acids, oxidized cholesterol, *trans-* fatty acids, cyclic products of fatty acids, cross-linked fatty acids, fragments, and double-bond-shifted fatty acids can all have toxic effects. If we knew both the toxicity and the frequency of exposure, we could establish their relative toxicities. But, because we still don't have hard figures on human toxicity, we would have to guess, and the guess could be quite wrong.

The simple conclusion for health and well-being, supported by animal research evidence as well as clinical experience, is to avoid oil products that contain toxic substances. We make our best choices for health if we stick to fresh seeds and fresh, unrefined seed oils made carefully under protection from light and oxygen.

Since it is easy to avoid the effects of all the toxic molecules listed above by using fresh, natural foods (oils included) in our diet, we need neither to guess nor play Russian roulette with any of these poisons.

20 *Erucic Acid: Toxic or Beneficial?*

Rape and **mustard seed oils** contain *erucic acid,* a 22-carbon, once unsaturated fatty acid (22:1w9). In rats, these oils cause fatty degeneration of heart, kidney, adrenals, and thyroid. If a rat diet persistently contains erucic acid, the rat compensates for its presence by making enzymes that shorten the fatty acid chain from 22 carbons to 18 or less, but during the time that elapses before these enzymes become active, fatty deposits occur in the hearts of these animals. Although the fatty deposits are removed after some time, permanent scar tissue remains.

From 1956 to 1974, oils made from rape seed containing up to 40% erucic acid were marketed for human consumption in Canada. In response to government concerns about the results of the rat studies, geneticists bred new varieties of low erucic acid rapeseed (LEAR) containing less than 5% erucic acid. These are now known as canola (the Canadian Oil).

The Canadian government and industry spent $50 million to get the Canadian oil onto the U.S. Food and Drug Administration's 'Generally Recognized As Safe' (GRAS) list. They succeeded in this venture. The Canadian government outlawed the import of high erucic acid rape and mustard seed oils for human consumption. Taxpayers footed much of the bill.

Oops!

When researchers repeated the rape seed oil studies with rats, but used sunflower seed oil (which contains no erucic acid), the rats ended up having the same problems. It turns out that rats do not metabolize fats and oils well. Their natural diet is low-fat vegetables and grains.

Rat fat metabolism differs substantially from fat metabolism in humans. Contrary to the Canadian government's assumption in this case, humans are not rats, at least with regard to the complexities of fat metabolism. Human studies should have been done *before* the money was spent and the changes in the law were made.

Nevertheless, a huge new industry was created. Laws were enacted affecting international trade, commerce, and traditional diets. A new oil was invented and marketed, and a new lobby was created. All of this was based on an error of interpretation of research results from animal studies – the risky assumption that research results from animal studies can be generalized willy nilly to humans.

Vindication?

Erucic acid has been partially vindicated. It does not cause the same problems in the hearts of humans as it does in rat hearts, and is relatively harmless. In China and India, millions use high erucic acid mustard and rape seed oils (up to 40% or more erucic acid) as a staple, apparently without developing the problems that rats and governments have with these oils. They have used this oil traditionally for several thousand years now, without noting detrimental effects.

Chinese and Indians use high erucic acid oils in *unrefined* form. This may be an important consideration (see Chapter 54, Virgin Olive Oils).

Lorenzo's Oil

In fact, erucic acid may have some beneficial effects. In recent years, a preparation of 20% erucic and 80% oleic acids, called *Lorenzo's Oil* after the boy whose condition inspired its development, has been used to treat a rare, fatal degenerative genetic condition known as adrenoleukodystrophy (ALD), in which a buildup of very long-chain fatty acids (C22 to C28) destroys the white matter (myelin) in the brain. Erucic acid helps normalize the levels of these fatty acids, although it does not reverse damage already done to nerves and myelin.[1]

Thrombocytopenia. Recent research indicates that *Lorenzo's Oil* used in treating of ALD patients reduces the concentration of platelets in the bloodstream

---

[1] There is some evidence that W3 fatty acids may be helpful in ALD. Since most people's diets lack w3s, they should be incorporated into diets as a matter of course.

of many of them. This condition, known as thrombocytopenia (TCP), does not however appear to lead to impaired clotting of their blood after injury. The platelets seem to be fewer, but larger. TCP is reversed when the oil is withdrawn from the diet. It is not yet clear whether TCP results from erucic acid processing, the fatty acid combination, or some other factor.

The movie version of the story of Lorenzo Odone and his parents' fight to get erucic acid treatment for their son has been captured in the film *Lorenzo's Oil*. It chronicles the effort of two individuals – technically untrained, but highly motivated – to discover practical solutions for their son's genetic problem. It highlights the slowness of 'experts' to respond to real needs, and the interference with human and humanitarian issues caused by rules made by bureaucrats in institutions and organizations far removed from the needs of those living their lives in the more emotional arena of parents' pains, fears, and hopes.

It is worth noting that the U.S. Food And Drug Administration (FDA), the organization that gave GRAS status to Canada's canola (low erucic acid rape seed) oil has also made it difficult for parents of children with Lorenzo's condition (ALD) to obtain erucic acid. Lorenzo's oil is prepared in a laboratory in Europe and can be imported only 'for personal use'. It cannot be produced in North America, even though it appears to be relatively safe for humans, and may be helpful to the children who have ALD.

21 *Light, Free Radicals, and Oils*

In Chapter 8, The Healing Essential Fatty Acids, we introduced the fact that light produces free radicals in oils, and that free radicals can produce changes in molecules – changes that can drastically affect health. Free radicals serve vital, normal functions, but can also injure, age, degenerate, and kill our cells and tissues. And marketers can sell us products based on our fear of them. Since we will be hearing a lot about free radicals in the next few years, it is better that we know more about them.

Terrorists in Your Body?

Free radicals are almost perfect candidates for the honor of causal villain in the biochemical drama of degenerative diseases. Even the name 'free radical' has sinister overtones, great for a villain myth in the 1990s – hordes of evil-faced, mean-minded, scruffy terrorists loose inside our bodies!

Free radicals contain unpaired electrons, and electrons are very small and difficult to locate. A thousand of them can hide behind a hydrogen atom, and there are so many atoms in our body that the number is incomprehensible. Electrons are even smaller, and their numbers even more staggering, more than 4 times 10 to the power or 28, or 4 followed by 28 zeroes! They are impossible to catch or pin down, because they are constantly flitting from place to place at the speed of light (300,000 km or 186,000 miles per second), and can change from a particle to a wave and back again in a fraction of a second. When you stop, out of breath from chasing them, you can almost hear them laughing at you.

The free radical theory explains the ultimate cause of degenerative conditions such as cancer, aging, and cardiovascular disease. All are widespread and all, so far, have eluded attempts to cure and control them, except with nutrients that prevent or slow down aging and damage caused by free radicals.

But free radical theory also lends itself to enormous misuse. As a story about invisible terrorists within us, this theory can be used as a tool to advertise any number of substances that promise to destroy, remove, capture, scavenge, neutralize, trap, or otherwise immobilize these terrorists in our systems. If we can be terrorized by hucksters to believe that any one of the 4 times 10 to the power of 28 electrons in our system will damage us unless we buy their product, a market is created for endless 'anti-terrorist' health products, and great profit. An understanding of the nature of free radicals will enable us to separate fact from market fiction.

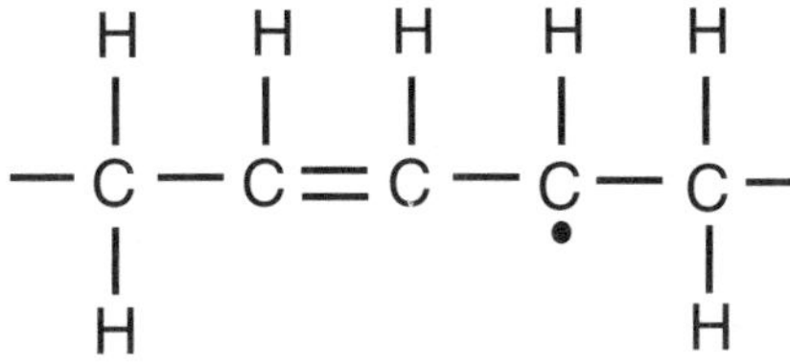

Figure 31. Molecular fragment with an unpaired (free radical) electron.

A free radical is a molecular fragment or element with an unpaired electron. Figure 31 illustrates a molecule with a free radical electron.

A free radical electron is very active,[1] because it is not tied up in a bond or an electron shell with another electron. It is looking for a partner, because electrons, like humans, hate to be alone and like to be paired. It will therefore draw an electron from wherever it can, including another electron pair. So a free radical

---

[1] By forming the bonds between atoms that create molecules, electrons provide the basis of chemical activity. The *strength* of the bond that an unpaired electron from one atom forms with an unpaired electron from another atom expresses the *intensity* of their need to be paired. The number of unpaired electrons found around an atom is constant for each element, and determines the number of bonds that an atom of that element will form. A hydrogen atom always has 1, an oxygen 2, a nitrogen 3, and a carbon, 4 unpaired electrons. These elements, therefore, always form 1, 2, 3, and 4 bonds, respectively, when they share electrons with other atoms to form the bonds that hold these atoms together in molecules.

might be described as a sub-atomic, free-wheeling, loose-living electron bachelor playing the field for a mate to settle down with, and willing to break up other pairs to find that mate.

Free radicals are intermediates in thousands of normal chemical reactions taking place in our body, including oxidation reactions that are absolutely necessary for producing the energy our cells require to live, and we require to be active. Between 2 and 5% of the free radicals involved in oxidation escape from molecular confinement, and it is these escapees that can damage molecules in cells and tissues. Lots of free radicals are produced every second, and our body uses antioxidants (AO) nutrients like vitamins C, B_3, and E, carotene, cysteine, selenium, bioflavonoids, and coenzyme Q_{10}, as well as several enzymes containing zinc, manganese, and copper to neutralize them. During AO deficiency, free radical chain reactions can occur, leading to biologically unsuitable biochemical reactions, abnormal and toxic substances, and disease.

Free Radical Chain Reactions
Let's take a closer look at free radical chain reactions that can occur in oils. If we expose a bucket of oil to light, a ray (photon) of light may be caught by an electron on a carbon next to the double bond carbon in a molecule of unsaturated fatty acid[2] (see Chapter 3, Fatty Acids Overview). The electron now carries more energy than it did before, and it is in an excited state. It takes off with a hydrogen nucleus, leaving behind a lone electron desperate for a partner. This in turn will grab a partner from wherever it can, leaving another electron unpaired and desperate, which then repeats the process in a chain reaction, until the original excited electron returns home to pair with the other lone electron (whoever and wherever it may be by this time), or until a special AO molecule traps the loose electron. A typical chain reaction of this kind may go through 30,000 cycles before it is stopped, and another single ray of sunlight can start another chain reaction. Because chemical bonds are made up of electron pairs, it is easy to see that when light starts electrons bouncing in chain reactions, bonds break and change, and when bonds change, new and different molecules form from the fatty acids with which we started in our bucket of oil. Billions of photons are present even on a cloudy day. Each photon can alter, denature, and destroy oil molecules exposed to light, especially if the oil was processed, and the natural AOs – vitamin E and carotene – were removed. Figure 32 illustrates a few possible light-induced free radical reactions.

Oxygen destroys oils in a similar way. Light first activates oxygen to a form containing an unpaired electron, a singlet oxygen radical. Its unpaired electron then pairs with an electron stolen from a fatty acid, starting the chain reaction.

---

[2] Saturated fatty acids(SaFAs) do not catch photons as readily as do unsaturated fatty acids, because SaFA electrons are less active, more stable in their pairing.

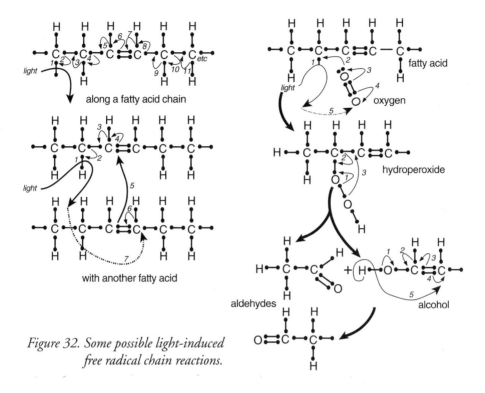

along a fatty acid chain

with another fatty acid

Figure 32. Some possible light-induced free radical chain reactions.

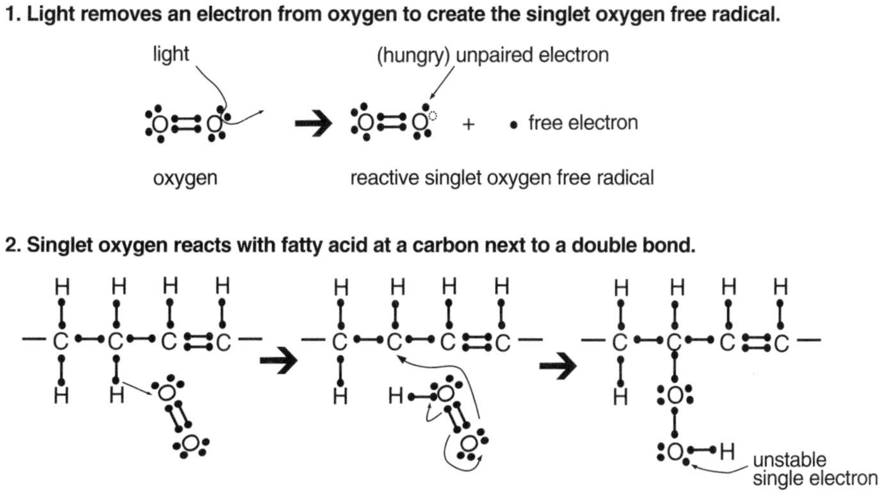

fatty acid

oxygen

hydroperoxide

aldehydes

alcohol

1. Light removes an electron from oxygen to create the singlet oxygen free radical.

light

(hungry) unpaired electron

oxygen

reactive singlet oxygen free radical

+ • free electron

2. Singlet oxygen reacts with fatty acid at a carbon next to a double bond.

unstable single electron

Figure 33. Oxygen-induced free radical reactions.

Figure 33 shows how this happens. Light-induced oxidation spoils oils 1000 times faster than oxidation in the dark, because light produces 1000 oxygen free radicals for every oxygen free radical produced spontaneously in the absence of light.

In an unrefined oil, natural AO molecules such as vitamin E (Figure 34) and others trap loose free radical electrons. Carotene (Figure 35) and others 'quench' oxygen free radicals. Vitamin C reactivates used-up glutathione (cysteine) and vita-

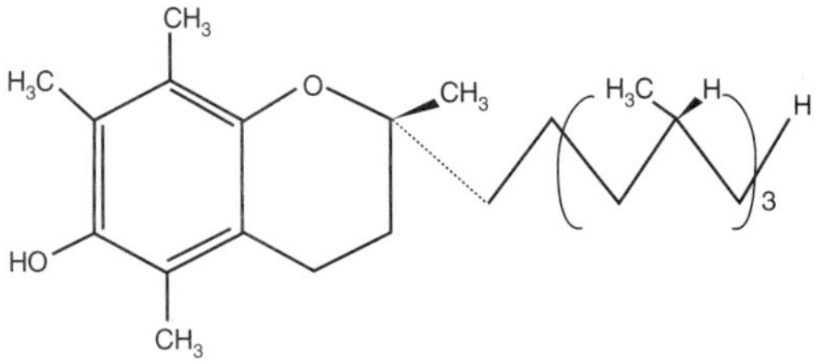

Figure 34. Vitamin E.

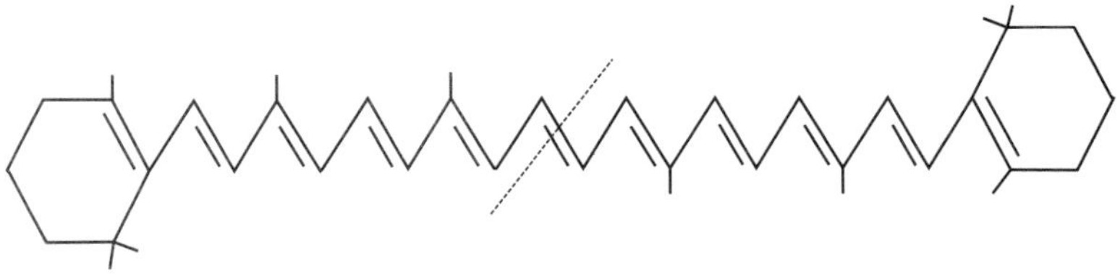

Figure 35. Carotene.

min E, which in turn reactivates carotene and other antioxidants. Hence vitamin C plays a key role in AO functions that prevent free radical chain reactions.

On the other hand, chlorophyll and finely divided 'pro-oxidant' metals such as iron and copper encourage free radical reactions. They help light to destroy oils even more rapidly. When oils are refined, vitamin E and carotene, as well as chlorophyll and most metals, are removed. Cheap artificial AOs such as BHT and BHA, which trap free radicals and slow down light-induced destruction of oil, may be added to replace the natural AOs that were removed.

Protection From Free Radicals

In our body, vitamins E and C, carotene, bioflavonoids, and other AOs protect essential and other highly unsaturated fatty acids from free radical chain reactions.

The three-dimensional architecture of the enzymes responsible for facilitating our body's biological reactions keeps most free radicals that are normal intermediates in biological reactions confined so they cannot escape and cause destruction. When reactions in which they are involved are completed, these free electrons reunite with the other lone partner. Free radical electrons that escape the architectural confines are snaffled by AOs. The latter do not fit into enzyme architecture, and thus cannot interfere with the natural free radical-involving biochemical reaction taking place.

The most likely place for free radical chain reactions from fatty acids is in cell membranes. Here is where vitamin E and carotene are found, protecting against that possibility. The watery parts of our body are protected against damage from free radicals by vitamin C, sulphur-containing amino acids (cysteine and sulphur-rich proteins), the metal selenium, bioflavonoids, and naturally occurring cyclic (phenolic) compounds found in foods. Our body also makes enzymes to protect us against free radical damage, including catalases and superoxide dismutases containing zinc, copper, and manganese. With these nutrients and cell-made molecules, our body can prevent, reverse, and repair free radical damage very efficiently (but not forever, which is why we age).

Free Radicals and Nutrition

Some nutrition writers, knowing that highly unsaturated fatty acids form free radicals easily, suggest that people should minimize their intake of polyunsaturated (w6 and presumably also w3) fatty acids. This suggestion is ill advised for three reasons.

First, because two highly unsaturated essential fatty acids (EFAs) and oxygen, all of them free radical formers, are absolutely necessary for life and health, and most modern diets are already deficient in one of them (w3). It is as ludicrous to remove EFAs from our diet because they can form free radicals as it would be to strangle ourselves because oxygen can form free radicals in our body. Both are essential to life. The ability to form free radicals is important for normal biochemical functions of life.

Second, a healthy body contains a large quantity (about 1 kg [2.2 pounds]) of essential linoleic acid (LA, 18:2w6). Some people less prone than average to degenerative disease – strict vegetarians, Japanese fishermen, and traditional Inuit – have even higher tissue content of highly unsaturated fatty acids. People suffering from degenerative diseases – obesity, cancer, cardiovascular disease, diabetes, and liver degeneration – usually have lower EFA tissue content.[3]

Third, highly unsaturated fatty acids are used successfully in nutritional treatments of degenerative diseases. EFAs help bring oxygen into our system. Lack of oxygen is a key factor in degenerative diseases like cancer, aging, and cardiovascular disease. Since these diseases are often associated with deficiency or function-

---

[3] The human body also requires more LA daily than any other essential substance. Nature had a reason for arranging it this way.

al deficiency of essential fatty acids, the supply of EFAs should not be compromised. But it must be accompanied by optimum intake of the necessary vitamins, minerals, amino acids, and antioxidants.

Free radicals become dangerous only when they get out of control. In a diet deficient in AO factors that keep free radicals in check, it might seem to make sense to decrease EFA intake, but it makes even more sense to bring the intake of essential AOs up to optimum levels.

Fire and Sparks

Our life is like a fire. For health and vitality, we need a strong, bright fire, produced by clean-burning fuel (carbohydrates) in the presence of a good supply of oxygen. Highly unsaturated fatty acids are like fire starter. They help to build a strong fire of life by their chemical reactivity, producing free radicals and increasing oxidation rate.

At the same time, a strong fire scatters more sparks than a weak one. The sparks generated by the fire of life are free radicals. To protect the living room carpet from being damaged by these sparks, we use a screen. Antioxidants screen the free radical sparks that the fire of life produces.

During the last 20 years, the role of antioxidants in health has been given a lot of well-deserved attention, but oxidants have been neglected. Both are important to health. Our health is a delicate balance between two factors: *oxidation* of foods to produce energy (fire) by means of free radical reactions; and *antioxidants,* which keep free radicals (sparks) from doing damage to our cells. (see Chapter 39, Antioxidants and the Fire That is Life).

History of Free Radicals

Free radicals are not a new creation of nature. They have been around for millions of years, along with minerals, EFAs, vitamins, and protective natural AOs found in foods. Oils high in EFAs from seeds such as flax, hemp, sunflower, and sesame have been pressed and enjoyed for their health-supporting properties for at least a few thousand years. Degenerative diseases on a large scale are recent in origin. What are the reasons for the epidemic increase in their occurrence during the last 100 years?

First is the rising deficiency in modern refined food diets of essential nutrient (vitamin and mineral) factors required to metabolize fatty acids properly, and lack of antioxidants that protect us from free radical chain reactions. Better eating habits, fresh juices, special super-foods resulting in nutrient enrichment, or good multi-vitamin, multi-mineral supplements can take care of this deficiency.

A second reason for widespread degeneration is deficiency of w3s, as well as imbalance in the ratio between w3 and w6 fatty acids.

Third is the increasing presence of synthetic and toxic substances – drugs, *trans-* fatty acids, pesticides, heavy metals, additives, etc. – in our foods, due to industrial practices that remove nutrients, alter natural molecules into unnatural (toxic) ones, add synthetic toxic molecules such as additives, preservatives, colors, and flavors, and increase pollutants in our environment, as well as medical practices that invade our body with drugs and other toxic molecules out of line with our biology.

Synthetic substances, which can mimic some effects of natural substances in our body but are in other ways quite different from natural substances, are likely to 'misfit' our body's enzyme architecture – monkey wrenches into our body's natural works. They might produce more free radicals, be more likely to start damaging free radical chain reactions, use up more of our body's antioxidant nutrient defenses (increasing our requirement for these nutrients), do even more damage when our processed foods lack antioxidants, and lead to degenerative diseases. The 'side effects' of many prescription drugs, and the toxic effects of many pesticides and poisons can be explained by free radical chain reactions initiated by these substances.

Common sense suggests better ways to heal our aches and pains. Improved diets and greater care in the way we live are more likely to bring lasting relief from degenerative conditions than swallowing unnatural substances that mask symptoms while producing further damage and no cure. When our diets become natural, and the levels of all essential nutrients including antioxidants become optimal, free radicals cease to be major concerns to health.

Frying and Deep-Frying 22

Frying and deep-frying are two of the most popular methods of (fast) food preparation, but they are also the two most damaging to health. Having looked at the chemical changes that occur in oils unprotected from the damage done to them by light, air, and heat, let's focus on what happens when we fry and deep-fry oils in restaurants and home food preparation.

The dangers to health of frying and deep-frying result from rapid oxidation and other chemical changes that take place when oils are subjected to high temperature in the presence of light and oxygen. First, antioxidants in the oil (vitamin E and carotene) are used up. Then, frying and deep-frying produce free radicals that start chain reactions in oil molecules (see Chapter 21, Light, Free Radicals, and Oils). Under these conditions, many chemical changes take place in oils. Frying and deep-frying produce some *trans-* fatty acids (see Chapter 18, Margarines, Shortenings, and *Trans-* Fatty Acids). These are the least harmful of the altered molecules produced by these processes. Other oxidation products are far more toxic than *trans-* fatty acids. Scores of unnatural breakdown, dimer, and polymer products with unknown effects on health are produced by frying and deep-frying.

Frying with oils once will not kill us, and so seems harmless. Our body copes with toxic substances. But over 10, 20, or 30 years, our cells accumulate altered and toxic products for which they have not evolved efficient detoxifying mechanisms. The altered and toxic substances interfere with our body's life chemistry, our 'bio-chemistry'. Cells then degenerate, and these degenerative processes manifest as degenerative diseases.

'Safe' Frying

Frying is not recommended, because safe frying is a contradiction in terms. Frying temperatures are too high. When foods turn brown, they have been burned. The nutrients in the browned material have been destroyed. Proteins turn into carcinogenic acrolein. Starches and sugars are browned (caramelized) through molecular destruction. Fats and oils are turned to smoke by destruction of fatty acids and glycerol.

Minimizing damage. Although frying cannot be recommended for health, some oils and some frying methods are safer than others. Knowing them can be helpful to those who will not give up this destructive practice.

Changes due to high temperature, oxygen, and light present in frying and deep-frying take place rapidly in unsaturated fatty acids, and even more rapidly in essential fatty acids (EFAs). Saturated fatty acids are less valuable to our health than EFAs but, being more stable in the presence of light, heat, and air, stand up better to high-heat uses. Whenever a fat is needed for frying, one which is mostly saturated and/or monounsaturated is preferable. Most oils in bottles are unacceptable for frying, because they are too rich in EFAs. Frying turns EFAs into toxic products which damage health. Saturated fatty acids (SaFAs) are destroyed only minimally.

EFA-poor, saturated fatty acid-rich fats. The least damaging frying fats include *coconut, palm, palm kernel, cocoa butter,* and *butter* – in small quantities. But high heat turns SaFAs, too, into smoke, which is obviously made of destroyed fatty acids. Smoke damages health in many ways, and increases cancer incidence.

EFA-poor tropical oils, such as coconut oil contain mostly saturated fatty acids 10 to 16 carbons in length, and contain only about 3% EFAs. Other oils must supply the essential w3 and w6 fatty acids.

Usually, tropical 'oils' are hydrogenated, which means that the double bonds in their EFAs, and their carotenes, vitamin E (tocopherols), and tocotrienols have been saturated. In this state, they raise cholesterol levels. In their natural state however, tropical oils have been shown to lower cholesterol levels. What a difference a chemical process makes! On the other hand, hydrogenated tropical oils have little left in them to be destroyed by light, air, and heat during frying.

Butter contains SaFAs between 4 and 18 carbons in length, plus 18-carbon monounsaturates, and 5% EFAs. About 3 to 6% of its fatty acids are easily digested vaccenic acid, an 18-carbon *trans-* monounsaturate. Its short-chain fatty acids are easier to digest than longer chains. Its 16- and 18-carbon SaFA chains can interfere with EFA metabolism.

Used in moderation, fried butter and tropical fats create fewer health problems than fried oils. But, since they fail to supply EFAs, they are nutritionally deficient. They provide only fat calories our body must burn for energy or store as fat.

Lard, traditionally used for frying, has largely been replaced by shortenings and margarines. These cheap 'funny fats' are not recommended for frying, because they contain too many altered molecules to begin with, and frying makes them worse (see Chapter 18, Margarines, Shortenings, and *Trans-* Fatty Acids).

EFA-poor, monounsaturated fatty acid-rich fats. Monounsaturated oils such as *olive* (unrefined) are acceptable for low temperature frying. *Refined peanut* and *avocado* oils withstand heat relatively well. *High oleic sunflower* and *high oleic safflower* oils are also quite stable, but are more difficult to find. Low-LA, high monounsaturated fatty acid strains of safflower and sunflower seeds (called high 'mono' saff and sun by oil traders) were created by genetic engineering from 'regular' safflower and sunflower seeds, which are not suitable for high temperature frying because they are EFA-rich.

Frying with EFA-Containing Oils

There *is* a way of frying with oils that contain EFAs that is less damaging than common frying practices, but this way of frying requires more care on our part than we ordinarily take in our frying operations.

Traditional Chinese cooks first put water in their wok, not oil (North American Chinese cooks have largely abandoned this wise practice). Water keeps the temperature down to 100°C (212°F), a non-destructive temperature. In European gourmet cooking, vegetables placed in the frying pan *before* oil is added protect the oil from overheating and oxidation. The food tastes less burned, retains more of its natural flavors and nutrients and, most important, supports our health better.

It requires care to fry foods in this way, because we cannot be away doing something else at the same time. It would be best to not fry at all, and to eat our fresh oils on salads or get them from eating seeds. We are creatures of habit, but a small change in the way we fry with oils pays large dividends in health and well-being.

No-No's

The following oils should not be used for frying at all. Fresh, unrefined, mechanically pressed, light- and oxygen-protected EFA-rich seed oils can support and improve health. *Flax oil* is rich in alpha-linolenic acid (LNA), the w3 EFA. Use it to reverse dietary w3 deficiency and in the natural therapy of cancer, inflammation, and weight loss. *Hemp seed oil* is one of nature's reasonably balanced oils. It contains a 3:1 ratio of w6s to w3s for long-term use, and provides the w6 derivative gamma-linolenic acid (GLA). *Sunflower* and *sesame seed oils* are rich in the w6 EFA, but contain no w3s. These and other unrefined oils smoke at lower temperatures than refined oils. Natural substances they contain do not stand up well to heat (from this point of view, refined oils are preferable to unrefined oils for frying).

Unrefined EFA-rich oils should be fresh, mechanically pressed from organically grown seeds, and stored in dark containers. Some stores carry acceptable oils, but not all oils even in natural food stores are acceptable. I prefer an arrangement in which fresh oil is shipped by a manufacturer directly to retailer or consumer, arriving less than a week after pressing. Healers, patients, health-conscious retailers, and consumers who want super-fresh oil can call to set up this kind of quick delivery system.

Slower methods of oil delivery can result in old, bad-tasting oil, which is bad for health. Even people who *need* the oil for health will not comply to taking bad-tasting oil for long.

Refined oils in transparent bottles have lost many protective natural nutrients – lecithin, carotene, tocopherols, phytosterols, and others. They may have been degraded by light, and have lost some of their EFAs during refining processes. They are often made from cheap, inferior, pesticide-sprayed oil plants (cottonseed oil is especially contaminated).

More No-No's. In frying, our usual custom is to pour oil into an empty frying pan, and to let it heat, shimmy, and smoke before adding the foods we want to fry. During this time, the oil is being destroyed. The temperature is too high. Light-catalyzed free radical oxidation reactions occur extremely rapidly. Oil kept at 215°C (419°F) for 15 minutes or more consistently produces atherosclerosis when fed to experimental animals. In commercial deep-frying operations, the same batch of oil is often kept at a high temperature constantly for days. Many altered substances have been isolated from such oils. Some are known to be toxic; the effects of many others are not known; and we can be fairly confident that none of them will improve health. What keeps the level of these altered and toxic substances from getting too high is the fresh oil added to replace the oil that stuck to the fish and chips, onion rings, or whatever was deep-fried – and that we ate.

Boiling and Baking

Boiling is less destructive of oils than frying because the temperature goes only to 100°C (212°F). Even the most sensitive, EFA-rich oils can be used in cooked grains and steamed vegetables without deterioration.

Baking fits between safe boiling with water and unsafe frying. The temperature of baking pan and crust gets very high, damaging (browning) molecules of oils, starches, and proteins. Butter or tropical fat should be used to line baking pans and to brush the top of what you are baking. The temperature inside the bread being baked goes up to only just above boiling – perhaps 116°C (240°F) – and the inside of bread is also protected from air and from light.

The inside of 'baked' bread is actually steamed at an acceptable temperature for even the more sensitive oils. Only the crust is actually baked (meaning 'burned'). The oils in the brown (or black) crust are destroyed.

Summary

If you insist on frying and/or deep-frying, it bears repeating that the less oils are heated, the less they are destroyed, and the better they are for us.

Frying and deep-frying destroy *all* oils and cannot be recommended for health. But some oils are damaged less by frying than others. If you *must* fry, use *refined* oils that contain the *lowest amount of EFAs* and the *greatest amounts of SaFAs and MUFAs*, and use sulphur-rich *garlic* and *onions* in frying to minimize free radical damage.

Oils least damaged by high temperatures and oxygen include:
- medium chain triglycerides (MCTs) (in small quantities only, less than 1 tablespoon;
  - butter;
  - tropical fats;
  - high oleic sunflower (not regular sunflower) oil;
  - high oleic safflower (not regular safflower) oil;
  - peanut oil;
  - sesame oil; and
  - olive oil;

in that order of preference. These oils are EFA-poor, and produce the lowest amount of toxic molecules when heated. The EFAs required for health must come from other sources.

Frying and deep-frying are completely prohibited if optimum health is what you are after, or if you are attempting to reverse cancer or any other degenerative condition using natural means.

Fractionation and Transesterification 23

What kinds of processes are these? Can we eat fractionated and transesterified products without harm to our health?

These processes are more recent in origin than refining and deodorizing. Neither process *adds* to the nutritive value of an oil. Both serve industry. They make oils easier to work with, confer properties that natural oils don't have, or help replace products such as tropical oils that now have a bad reputation. The starting materials for these processes are always fully refined, deodorized, bland oils (see Chapter 16, From Seed to Oil). The 'minor' natural ingredients present in unrefined oils – carotene, chlorophyll, phytosterols, and others – would interfere with these processes.

Fractionation (FR)

Oils are triglycerides (TGs) with three free swinging fatty acid molecules hooked to a molecule of glycerol (see Chapter 9, Triglyceride Fats). As illustrated in Figure 18, the fatty acids in TGs can vary widely. By mechanical means, we can separate TGs with different fatty acid composition (and therefore different properties) from any oil. This is *fractionation:* separating an oil into two or more different TG 'fractions' due to their having different physical properties based in differing fatty acid compositions.

For instance, coconut oil can be fractionated into a harder, more saturated fraction with a higher melting point and a softer, more unsaturated, more liquid fraction with a lower melting point. It can also be fractionated into a harder, an intermediate, and a softer fraction, or into even more fractions. The intended use determines which fraction we want and into how many fractions the oil will be separated.

In chocolates, for example, coconut oil was commonly used in the past, because coconut oil stays solid at room temperature and most climactic temperatures, but melts at mouth temperature. If a liquid oil were used, chocolate would remain a liquid pudding. If it stayed hard in our mouth, it would not be chocolate.

Then along came the 'tropical oils scare' of 1988. The world was told that tropical oils (such as coconut, palm, and palm kernel) increase cholesterol, and high cholesterol causes heart attacks. Chocolate sales went down. "Not good," said chocolateers, "Is there something besides tropical oil that we can use?" "Yes," said chemists. "We can isolate from other oils the fraction with the same properties as coconut oil." No sooner said than done. Such fractions can be isolated from cotton, avocado, peanut, soybean, and other oils.

The downside of this change in source materials is that the fraction that goes into chocolates has the same as properties as coconut oil, and has the same effects on health. In this application, the industry has simply avoided the negative effects of the 'tropical oils scare' on sales, without actually providing a product with different properties. The ploy works until the public finds out what fractionated oils in chocolates consist of. The point is, to get the melting properties required in chocolates, an oil with the properties of coconut oil *must* be used. Only hard oils (tropical or animal) or hydrogenated oils fit this bill. In making chocolates and confections, the use of 'fractionated' oils is a marketing gimmick. It gives the appearance of real changes toward using better oils having been made without actually having made those changes. Only the name has been changed. Fooled again.

Fractionation can also be used with better motives. One could isolate EFA-rich fractions from EFA-poor oils. For industrial purposes, one could isolate fractions with superior lubrication properties. Being a simple mechanical separation, FR does no further great damage to the refined, deodorized oils used, and could have useful applications. Hoodwinking consumers is not one of them.

Transesterification (TE)[1]

If we mix two oils with different physical properties, (e.g., coconut and corn oil – heaven only knows why anyone would do that, but someone will come up with a reason to do so sooner or later – they will tend to separate (fractionate) naturally on cooling. If the mixture was used in a spreadable product or an oil-water emulsion, this could be a problem. The product might have inconsistent texture, form coarse crystals, and have an unpleasant mouth feel – important marketing considerations.

To avoid this problem, we can clip the fatty acids off all TG molecules of both the coconut and the corn oils and then reattach the fatty acids randomly to the glycerol molecules. The random reattachment process results in a product in which fatty acids from both oils end up on the same glycerol molecule, forming 'hybrid' TGs with fatty acid compositions unlike those of the two separate oils from which they were derived.

The term 'transesterification' consists of two parts. 'Trans' means 'across', and refers to the fact that fatty acids from coconut TGs move 'across' to positions on corn oil TGs, and vice versa. 'Esterification' refers to the kind of bonds, known as 'ester' bonds, by which each of a TG's three fatty acid molecules is hooked to a glycerol carbon. Each TG molecule has three free-swinging fatty acid molecules 'esterified' to glycerol, one to each of glycerol's three carbons.

To remove (hydrolyze) fatty acids from glycerol molecules, our body uses enzymes called lipases. In industry, hydrolysis of fatty acids from glycerol is brought about by adding water in the presence of acid. In our body, enzymes also attach (esterify) fatty acids to glycerol to make TGs. In industry, sodium anhydride is commonly used to reattach fatty acids to glycerol. Enzymes are more precise and specific. Industrial methods are more random. In TE, randomness is preferred, producing a uniform end product.

The effects of transesterified fats and oils on our health has not been well researched. The body may rearrange fatty acids yet again in keeping with its biological preference for EFAs on the middle carbon and saturated fatty acids on outside carbons. Other than product contamination by reagents that are used and the

---

[1] The term transesterification is sometimes used interchangeably with the term interesterification.

fact that the oils used for TE are fully refined and deodorized, TE probably creates no major health hazards.

Hydrolysis, Fractionation, Re-esterification

Products such as medium-chain triglycerides (MCTs) (see Chapter 65, Medium-Chain Triglycerides) are made by removing (hydrolyzing) fatty acids from tropical oils, separating (fractionating) the fatty acids into glycerol and short-, medium-, and long-chain fatty acid fractions, and reesterifying the medium-chain fatty acids to glycerol, using sodium anhydride. The separation of fatty acids allows a product to be made that is 'purer' (in the chemical sense) than natural products. MCTs are used by athletes as a source of energy during workouts. They do not produce body fat, unlike long-chain saturated fatty acids. In medicine, MCTs are used as a source of energy for patients with liver damage because, unlike long-chain fatty acids, they require little liver involvement for their metabolism. During digestion, they are absorbed directly into the bloodstream rather than into lymphatics, and go directly to our cells rather than first to our liver.

The above combination of processes can be used to make chemically 'pure' TGs that contain only SaFAs, only EFAs, or only monounsaturated fatty acids. These processes could have many industrial applications.

Why we would want to apply these technologies across-the-board to human health is less clear. In some genetic and metabolic health disorders, 'pure' products have valuable applications, but for most people, the way nature designed our foods over the course of millions of years of evolution is likely to be most conducive to health. Why mess with it?

24 *Advertising and Jargon*

A close link exists between molecular, biological, biochemical facts – the truths of nature – and health. Good research attempts to explore, discover, and explain these facts without bias. Advertising, on the other hand, is about sales. If truth were told about mediocre products, that would be bad advertising. For their protection, consumers need to know the difference.

Winners don't need much advertising. They radiate success on their own merit, by what they are and what they do. Their reputation spreads by word of mouth, based on their performance. Quality speaks for itself.

Losers require cosmetic jobs and a lot of advertising noise to succeed. They have no track record, because they don't perform. To support a loser, you have to be informed by urgency techniques, sold with fancy talk and pleasant imagery, and develop a habit based on hype rather than results. The same is true for foods.

Advertising Foods

Nutritious natural foods don't need a lot of advertising. A fresh, crisp apple looks good, smells good, and tastes good. It doesn't cause upset stomach, varicose veins, or illness. Fresh fruit, fresh vegetables, fresh juices, whole grains, nuts, and seeds need little advertising (the human body likes nutritious, whole foods, even though our tongue may have been miseducated to prefer junk). Particular brands of whole foods are advertised, but we know them generally from our personal experience since childhood. Our body recognizes their health value on the molecular level, and a recognition of their virtues has even been programmed into our genes.

Refined, denatured, nutrient-impoverished foods require much hype, much flash, much dress-up. The worse the product is, the more enticing and insistent the ad must be. Pleasant results must be implied from the use of the product to get buyers motivated: to buy unnourishing products, consume them, and develop a consumption habit. Cigarettes, alcohol, ice cream, boxed instant breakfast foods, soft drinks, chocolates, processed convenience foods and sugary snacks, powdered soups, candy, canned foods, and children's junk foods belong in this category. If these products were not constantly advertised, we would not buy them. While they may have been doctored to taste good, they cannot keep us healthy.

Body Language

Advertising for inferior products, therefore, has to be vigorous enough to override our body's subtle (or not so subtle) signals, which flash: "Deficient!"

When food products are new to a particular market, they may need initial advertising exposure to let people know they exist. Beyond that, they advertise themselves in our mouth, our stomach, our intestines, our colon, and throughout our entire body. Our body lets us know. It talks to us in feelings. Feelings of vitality, positive and stable moods, clarity of thought, and stamina in action are associated with health. Lethargy, emotional instability, bad moods, foggy thinking, and physical fatigue accompany deterioration of health. The changes from one to the other may be gradual, but they are perceptible if we practice self-awareness.

It is important in self-care to become sensitive to what our body tells us, learn what symptoms mean, and learn enough about health to know what to do to respond to its messages.

The feeling of health is subtle, and deserves more attention than it usually gets. When we are healthy, we tend to focus on and get involved with other things. Only as the feeling of health and well-being is replaced by discomfort or pain is our focus drawn to it, and we become motivated to find out how to make ourselves feel good again.

When room temperature is just right, we tend not to notice. When it gets too hot or too cold, we perk up from our diversions, adjust windows or thermostat to make it so we can forget about the room temperature again, then shift our focus to other matters again. Health too is like that.

Exposing Advertising Claims

There are laws against false advertising. But words are flexible, and can be used creatively to get around legal restrictions. Words can simply say something that is true about the product, but imply to the customer something desirable that is not actually true of the product. Here are examples from the world of oils.

"From 100% Corn Oil!" Margarine marketed as made "from 100% corn oil" makes a correct statement, but implies to the consumer that it must therefore be good margarine. Why? Because corn oil is high in polyunsaturated fatty acids (PUFAs) and the public associates PUFAs with good health. Corn oil in its natural state contains about 60% w6 PUFAs.[1]

The ad leaves out the fact that the corn oil used to make margarine is refined, missing some natural substances that protect it from chemical deterioration during storage and in our body; it contains chemically altered breakdown products made from essential fatty acids (EFAs), and other unnatural or toxic products (see Chapter 16, From Seed to Oil).

And here is the kicker. To make margarine, corn oil is partly hydrogenated (see Chapter 17, From Oil to Margarine). EFA molecules are saturated, and/or broken or twisted. The "100% corn oil" margarine contains (advertisers leave out this important information) an average of 25% *trans-* fatty acids, both mono- and polyunsaturated (See Chapter 18, Margarine, Shortenings, and *Trans-* Fatty Acids), which can interfere with EFA functions and do other kinds of damage in our body. If we are lucky, we end up with 25% LA (more likely to be about 10%) remaining in the margarine out of the 60% we started with. One writer puts it this way: "Hydrogenated corn oil is similar to hydrogenated soybean, or canola oil, and offers no advantages over it, [except] the promotional claim: 'contains 100% corn oil'"[2]

'Polyunsaturated'. We think that 'polyunsaturated' means 'healthful' or 'EFA-containing'. Both essential fatty acids, LA (18:2w6) and LNA (18:3w3), are polyunsaturated fatty acids (PUFAs), but most PUFA oils contain no LNA. Our body makes about 8 other natural and valuable PUFAs from LA and LNA, or it can get them from foods. This is a total of 10.

But dozens of unnatural PUFAs, some harmful, may be present in refined and hydrogenated oils. These PUFAs hurt health, but are included with the natural, health-enhancing PUFAs (see Chapter 25, Polyunsaturates and Superunsaturates). Advertisers use our ignorance to hoodwink us.

'High in Polyunsaturates'. How high is high? Compared to zero, 2% polyunsaturates in an oil is high. But 2% is low in terms of body needs and

---

[1] But corn oil contains no alpha-linolenic acid (18:3w3), which is also essential.

[2] Weiss, T. J., *Food Oils and Their Uses*, 2nd Ed. (Connecticut, Avi Publishing, 1983) p.40

health. A product 'high in polyunsaturates' may be devoid of w3s (and therefore poorly balanced), may contain unnatural PUFAs, or may decrease cholesterol levels while increasing cancer. All these possibilities are left out of the advertising statement.

'Contains lecithin'. How much? Even a tiny amount of lecithin in a product allows the term to be put on a label. We know that lecithin is nutritious, so we like to see that on the label, but there may be less lecithin than a cat (or even a mouse) could carry away on its tail. And, while the label 'lecithin' might make bells ring in our heads, the lecithin might make no bells ring in our bodies, if it is low in EFAs (see Chapter 11, Lecithin).

'For cooking, frying, and baking'. Heat destroys the EFAs, and oxidation and light reactions occur far faster at high temperatures, making oils toxic. This recommendation encourages sales ("use our oil for everything!"), but has little to do with science, correct product use or health. Any oil can be used for boiling, but no oil is good for cooking, frying, and baking (see Chapter 22, Frying and Deep-Frying).

'No preservatives'. The oil may contain pesticide residues, toxic fatty acids (cottonseed), solvents, residues of soap, *trans-* fatty acids, and toxic fatty acid breakdown products. Refined oils lack natural protective vitamins and minerals. They deteriorate more rapidly if light or oxygen come in contact with the oil. *Natural* preservatives would help the oil last longer. Keeping an oil free of natural preservatives (vitamin E and carotene) is like the famous last words: "Look Ma, no hands!" before the crash. It is not a service to the customer's health.

'No cholesterol'. This is true for all products of plant origin. The claim cashes in on our fear of cardiovascular disease, for which cholesterol is not even primarily responsible (see Chapter 12, Cholesterol). The claim can be used to sell refined oils, tropical fats, margarines, shortenings, partially hydrogenated vegetable oils, etc., which, although free of cholesterol, may kill you by means of other toxic ingredients far more rapidly than would the feared cholesterol.

'For the good of your heart' or 'For health'. Scientific evidence fails to back up claims that margarine is good for our heart, or that it has other health benefits. Heart disease and cancer deaths have increased at a rate parallel to increased sales of margarines and other hydrogenated and partially hydrogenated products. The claim, based on the fact that EFAs are necessary for health and that the vegetable oils from which they were made contained EFAs, avoids mentioning that hydrogenation and partial hydrogenation systematically destroy EFAs and produce many toxic substances detrimental to health. Not a shred of evidence for health benefits! In fact, scientific evidence points in the opposite direction.

'Low in fat (or saturated fat)'. Some products advertised as low in fat still contain over 50% of their calories as fat. Milk, for example, contains only 3.5% fat but, because milk is mostly water, the fat makes up about 51% of its calories.

'Light (or lite)'. Light foods contain less fats than their non-light equivalents, but may still contain substantial amounts of it. Advertisers like to invent marketing terms for which no rules exist, but which can be used to give the impression of health concern. Having worked in advertising, I can assure you that health is a minor concern, and that marketing advantage is the primary goal of advertising departments.

These are examples of how advertisers of inferior products tell only part of the story. We get taken in as long as we don't know the facts. Advertisers count on us to remain ignorant, or at least confused.

Advertising and Media

Advertising makes use of a field of research that studies how people's buying responses are affected by factors such as color, shape, imagery, music, movement, setting, background, context, and other considerations. Advertisements are aired by media (TV, radio, newspaper), not because they are true, but because they bring in revenue. When we turn on the tube, we program ourselves with the information sellers use to motivate us to buy. Advertising works – we buy.

Businesses are created to profit their owners. Unscrupulous owners do whatever is necessary to get us to buy. Advertising is business putting its best foot forward while hiding its defects.

If we want quality, we must first *know* quality. That's not easy in a world of high-tech smoke and mirrors, unless we educate ourselves or stick to what is simple and natural. If we know *and* insist on quality, we will get quality.

25 Polyunsaturates and Superunsaturates

The extent to which the term 'polyunsaturated' is misused in advertising products defies description. We think we are getting health-supporting products, when actually they may be health-destroying. Read on to find out why, and what to do about it.

By definition, polyunsaturated fatty acids (PUFAs) are all fatty acids with more than one double bond in their carbon chains (see Chapter 3, Fatty Acids Overview). We equate the term with health-enhancing oils, because EFAs – which *are* PUFAs – are necessary for health. But, while EFA PUFAs are necessary for health, other PUFAs are unnecessary, and still others are detrimental to health.

The value to health of oils and oil-based products can be estimated by knowing their content of the EFA PUFAs present in their natural, unaltered state.

In practice, the term 'polyunsaturates' is used to refer to the w6 EFA linoleic acid (LA, 18:2w6) and its natural derivatives. The w3 EFA alpha-linolenic acid (LNA, 18:3w3) and its derivatives are sometimes referred to as 'superunsaturates' to distinguish between w6s and w3s – a useful distinction, because w6s and w3s have certain opposing functions in our body.

Natural Polyunsaturated and Superunsaturated Fatty Acids

Polyunsaturates (PUFAs). From the w6 EFA, linoleic acid (LA, 18:2w6), most healthy human bodies can make all other natural w6 PUFAs they need. These other natural PUFAs can also come from foods. From LA, our body makes: gamma-linolenic acid (GLA, 18:3w6) which is also found in hemp oil, evening primrose oil, borage oil, and black currant oil; arachidonic acid (AA, 20:4w6) also present in meats, eggs, and dairy products; and docosapentaenoic acid (DPA, 22:5w6) which is found in the oils of cold-water fish and marine mammals.

 Superunsaturates (SUFAs). From the w3 EFA, alpha-linolenic acid (LNA, 18:3w3), most healthy bodies can make all other natural w3 SUFAs they need. These can also come from foods. From LNA, our body makes stearidonic acid (SDA, 18:4w3) found in the seed oils of black currants and several wild plants; and eicosapentaenoic acid (EPA, 20:5w3); and docosahexaenoic acid (DHA, 22:6w3), which are found in the oils of cold-water fish and marine animals (such as trout, salmon, sardine, albacore tuna, mackerel, eel, seal, and whale).

 All of the above PUFAs and SUFAs are in the natural, all *cis*- configuration, are methylene interrupted, and are vital for health. We want both EFAs in their natural state in the products we buy, since they provide the basis for making the other natural PUFAs and SUFAs important for health. For special health needs, therapeutic oils are available (see Chapter 57, Evening Primrose, Borage, and Black Currant Oils; Chapter 60, Hemp; Chapter 59, Flax; and Chapter 55, Oils from Fish and Seafoods).

Unnatural PUFAs and SUFAs

Many fatty acids are neither natural nor beneficial, although they *are* polyunsaturated or superunsaturated. These are usually generated by destructive processes used to make oils, and by frying. In this group we find: *conjugated fatty acids,* in which one or more of the double bonds has moved closer (2 carbons apart) to another double bond than methylene interrupted (3 carbons apart); fatty acids with one or more double bond in a position further away (4 or more carbons apart) from the other double bond(s); *trans- fatty acids,* in which the molecule has been twisted at the location of one of the double bonds (see Chapter 18, Margarines, Shortenings, and *Trans*- Fatty Acids); or combinations of the above.

 Margarines and shortenings. *Trans-* fatty acids constitute a major deception in advertising PUFAs. In one study of margarines on the Canadian market, some samples were found to contain up to 20% *trans*- PUFAs. Shortenings contain similar quantities of *trans*- PUFAs. The manufacturer is allowed to advertise this product as 'high in polyunsaturates', which is technically true and therefore legally permissible, but entirely misleading, because not only are *trans-* PUFAs unable to support health, but they also antagonize the health-building EFAs. *Trans-* PUFAs compete for enzymes, produce biologically non-functional derivatives, and interfere with the work of EFAs in our body. Because we associate the term 'polyunsaturates' with health, we get fooled into thinking that we are buying a health-enhancing product. In reality, we may be getting a product that is health-destroying.

Not all margarines and shortenings have 20% of their PUFAs in the detrimental *trans-* form, but it is not possible for the average consumer (or biochemist, for that matter) to easily determine whether a sample of margarine in the supermarket is high, medium, or low in these unnatural PUFAs, or even free of them. What we do know is that they will not cause problems if we avoid them.

Partially hydrogenated vegetable oils also contain *trans-* PUFAs and SUFAs. Small amounts of *trans-* PUFAs may also be found in refined oils and products made from EFA-containing oils that have been heated to high temperatures during processing.

Manufacturers are not presently required to give information on unnatural PUFAs and SUFAs present in their products. They do not have this information because hydrogenation (see Chapter 17, From Oil to Margarine) is a random, uncontrollable process. Different batches of the same brand of margarine or shortening show widely fluctuating amounts of *trans-* PUFAs.

Procedures to identify and quantify each of dozens of unnatural substances found in hydrogenated products are expensive and time-consuming. They would have to be performed for each new batch of product. This time and expense cannot be justified commercially, and so they are simply not done at all.

Manufacturers motivated primarily by profit take molecules supplied by nature, subject them to often destructive processes, package them for convenience, and sell us less nutrition for a higher price. Where business interests to maximize profit take precedence over health – so far, that's generally the way of our 'modern' world – consumers have to be doubly careful. If labels on the products we buy were required to separately list their content of EFAs and of non-natural PUFAs, consumers would be in a better position to make health-oriented food choices.

Polyunsaturate/Saturate (P/S) Ratio

Oils are often rated for health value by the P/S ratio, which is the amount of PUFAs over the amount of saturated fatty acids (SaFAs) present in the oil. A P/S ratio of 2 or higher – meaning that PUFAs outnumber SaFAs by at least two to one – is considered desirable.

Correcting the P/S Ratio. Our biological consideration of the polyunsaturates makes it clear that the P part of the P/S ratio should include only natural PUFAs, which are EFAs. In addition to SaFAs, the less desirable S part of the P/S ratio should include all *trans-* fatty acids, since they act like SaFAs in the body and worse, have anti-EFA activity that worsens EFA deficiency.

If we use this biological perspective to compute *true P/S ratio,* we discover that this ratio for some oil products touted as valuable decreases from just less than 4, which is excellent, to a true P/S ratio of 0.05, which is 70 times lower, and unmasks the product as exceptionally poor. Margarines and shortenings perform badly when true P/S ratios are determined in keeping with our body's biological requirements. They generally contain large quantities of non-natural *trans-* fatty acids. Only small quantities of the natural PUFAs – EFAs – remain when the processes that create them are completed.

In a study of Canadian margarines, only 1 out of 100 different samples had a true P/S ratio of 2. The rest were lower. The true P/S ratio of the oils from which these margarines were made ranged from 3.8 to 6.5 in their natural, unprocessed states. Making margarine thus appears to be a way of ruining a perfectly good oil for the sake of imitating butter's spreadability.

Other failings of the P/S ratio. The P/S ratio fails to take into account our body's need for w3s. It also ignores the importance of the balance between w3 SUFAs and w6 PUFAs. A too simplistic formula, the P/S ratio has limited value as a tool for determining which oil products are health-promoting.

Vitamin E and Polyunsaturates 26

We have been warned that increased intake of polyunsaturates requires an increased intake of vitamin E. Some poorly informed writers have suggested decreasing our intake of polyunsaturated fatty acid (PUFA)-containing oils, so that the intake of vitamin E does not have to be increased. Where is the truth?

Natural Oils

In nature, vitamin E and other natural antioxidants (AOs) are *always* found in fresh oil-bearing seeds and nuts. Generally, the more essential fatty acids (EFAs) an oil contains, the richer in AOs it is, in keeping with the need to protect oils from destruction by light and oxygen both in the seed and in our body. We suffer no problem of lack of vitamin E (and other AOs) if we rely on fresh nuts and seeds to fill our requirement for oils and EFAs.

When oils are pressed, vitamin E and other oil-soluble AOs remain in the oil. If we consume *fresh* seed and nut oils mechanically pressed under protection from light and air, there is still no problem of lack of AOs. Fresh, protected oils will not go rancid in our body.

Vitamin E and other natural AOs in foods protect our molecules, cells, and tissues from free radical damage.[1] They prevent abnormal clotting of blood, protecting us from heart attacks and strokes. They also help protect us from cancer by inactivating free radicals that might otherwise get out of control and start free radical chain reactions (see Chapter 21, Light, Free Radicals, and Oils).

As long as AOs are present, oils are protected from destruction by light and air. During exposure to light and oxygen, AOs in an oil are used up rapidly (within a few hours or days). Only then can the process of rancidity proceed.

Processed Oils

When oils are degummed, refined, bleached, and deodorized after pressing, AOs, including vitamin E, are removed from them. The oil-refining industry does not throw away the vitamin E. They collect the sludge from deodorization, separate and concentrate the vitamin E, and sell it at a profit (vitamin E is one of the more expensive vitamins).

When we use refined, deodorized oils, we may end up short of vitamin E. Without vitamin E, EFAs and other highly unsaturated fatty acids including PUFAs in our body are unprotected from free radical damage. If our diet consists mainly of nutrient-deficient refined foods, uncontrolled free radical chain reactions will occur in our body, causing degeneration and aging (see Chapter 21, Light, Free Radicals, and Oils).

Refined oils in transparent bottles exposed to light are subject to light-induced damage. Refined oils that have been fried have been exposed to the destructive influences of light, oxygen, and heat, and are especially bad. Consuming these vitamin E-deficient oils eventually produces brown spots on the skin, especially prominent on the head, face, and back of hands of older people.[2] These spots, descriptively called 'fleurs de cemetière' ('cemetery flower'), are a sign of fatty degeneration. They indicate deficiency of the AOs vitamin E and seleni-

---

[1.] Plants produce hundreds of natural antioxidants besides vitamin E. Sesame oil contains an antioxidant called sesamol; many kitchen spices including rosemary, celery, sage, oregano, cumin and cloves, as well as the exotic herbs myrrh and frankincense contain their own specific potent antioxidants; vanilla contains antioxidants. In addition, there are the familiar antioxidant vitamins A, C, B1, B3, and B6, the minerals selenium, zinc, manganese, and copper, the bioflavonoids, the amino acids cysteine, N-acetyl cysteine, and tyrosine, the tri-peptide glutathione, and various proteins made by our body. Every kind of food, including potatoes, cabbage, broccoli cauliflower, brussels sprouts, bananas, red grapes, and other fruits contains antioxidants that protect their (and our) life.

[2] In 1988, I visited with the president of the American Heart Association in Pennsylvania. The backs of his hands were almost completely covered with big brown spots, more than I had ever seen before. Like the association as whose figurehead he served, he did not believe in nutrient enrichment or supplementation.

um. 'Cemetery flowers' contain denatured oils and protein (lipofuscin). They are also found in the cells of heart muscle and brain of older people, where with time, they may take up more and more of the cell's space, and may reach 60% of the cell's total volume. Soon thereafter, they choke the cell, killing it.

Getting Enough

It is good to take vitamin E supplements to prevent the deterioration of oils in our body. Many people do, and books have been written on the health benefits of this wonderful vitamin. We benefit from decreased consumption of refined, denatured, calorie-rich but nutrient-poor oils because they have been altered through processes invented by man out of touch with nature. It makes sense to switch to fresh, unrefined oils, and to eat fresh nuts and seeds that contain the full palette of vitamins, minerals, proteins, fats, fiber, and AOs – the way nature made them for us, the way our body can best use them to keep vital and healthy.

It is nonsense to lower an already low intake of PUFAs because of fear of free radicals. It does make sense to increase the levels of the AOs present in our body, which protects the PUFAs we consume from free radical damage.

'Cold-Pressed': A Meaningless Term 27

Most people are surprised to hear that oils labeled 'cold-pressed' are not cold-pressed at all. "But the label says so," I am told by misinformed people.

Store owners and customers alike believe that when oil is labeled cold-pressed (wrongly implying that the oil remained cold while being pressed), it is nutritionally superior; and they also believe (rightly, in part) that heat destroys oils. What does 'cold-pressed' actually mean?

History of Cold-Pressed

'Cold-pressed' is a term searching for a meaning. Since neither industry nor government has an agreed-upon definition, anyone is free to invent one that suits their particular purpose.

The term was into advertising by a distributor of mass-market oils, strictly for advertising mileage. Spokespeople for other oil companies, when asked point-blank what 'cold-pressed' means, say: "Nothing."

One company calls oils that have been heated to very high temperatures during deodorization (see Chapter 16, From Seed to Oil) 'cold-pressed' because "no external heat was applied to seeds while they were being *pressed.*" This definition belies the fact that *external* heat is *never* necessary in modern presses, because the pressing itself produces heat due to pressure and rotational friction. It also belies the heat applied before and after pressing, including deodorization temperatures of over 200°C (400°F) for up to an hour.

'Cold-pressed' is a translation of the German words 'kalt geschlagen', which literally mean 'cold pummeled'. A hundred years ago in Germany, oil was produced at home in very slow, mallet-hammered, manually-operated wedge presses. Seeds were poured into a wedge-shaped container, and a wooden wedge was driven into it. Every hour or so, the housewife would hit the wedge with a wooden mallet, and the oil would drip for an hour. Then she would give it another whack and the oil would drip again. She would carry this on all day, to produce the oil needed for her household. 'Kalt geschlagen' meant that no heat was applied to either seed or oil, and referred to a completely natural, unrefined crude, fresh, high-quality oil.

The term is still used in Germany today for oils made more by more modern methods. It gives the sense of the quality of the old method without actually employing that method. In North America also, the term is widely used for oils that are made by heat-producing methods.

In fact, it is almost impossible today to find oils commercially pressed without heat. **Note:** Virgin olive oils are one exception; the other exception is a brand of peanut oil available in the natural foods trade, which is made by the old hydraulic pressing method that produces no heat.

Seeds were cooked to increase oil yield even when hydraulic presses were being used 80 years ago. Screw (mechanical, expeller) presses generate heat by friction as seeds and crushed material are simultaneously compressed and rotated into a squeeze. Heat makes oils run out of seed meals faster. The higher the heat, the less oil remains in the pressed seed cake, the more efficient the operation, the better the price and profit, and the less waste.

The lowest temperature at which it is possible to expeller press oils in small presses is around 50°C (122°F), although the temperature inside the press head gets higher than that. Inside, small presses heat up to between 54 and 72°C (130 to 160°F); the next size up, 65 to 85°C (150 to 180°F). Huge presses run even higher temperatures. It is customary in the industry to measure the lower temperature of the oil dripping out of the press and call that its pressing temperature, although it would be better to call that the 'dripping' temperature.

In Switzerland, 'cold-pressed' is defined to mean that oils have reached temperatures not exceeding 50°C (122°F) during their entire journey from seed to bottle. In North America, there is no such agreed-upon definition, so anything goes. The usual temperature of oil that drips out of huge presses may be between 85 and 95°C (185 to 203°F). Inside the press, the temperature is somewhat higher, and some presses generate so much heat under the tremendous pressure and friction at which they operate that the oil dripping out of the machine has a slightly burned taste. Some people prefer this taste, and some oils on the market contain added burned flavoring to cater to this taste preference.

Pressing Oil with Minimum Heat

Oils should be pressed with minimum heat for two reasons.

First, as temperature increases, chemical reactions speed up. For every 10°C (18°F), the speed of chemical reactions more than doubles. The higher the temperature of the oil, the faster it is destroyed by light, oxygen, and other chemical reactions. This can be minimized by excluding light and air from the pressing process. Pressing facilities usually run without this protection.

Second, internal changes take place in oil molecules at high temperatures. Unsaturated fatty acids may twist into unnatural *trans-* configurations (see Chapter 18, Margarines, Shortenings, and *Trans-* Fatty Acids), or fatty acids may cross-link, oxidize, dimerize, or polymerize, changing the shape and properties of the fatty acid molecules, destroying their nutritional and biological value, and making them toxic.

These processes begin to take place measurably when oil temperature reaches about 160°C (320°F), and become really serious above 200°C (392°F). Oil pressing temperatures rarely exceed 100°C (212°F). Thus, the heat produced during *pressing* is not a major problem if light and air are excluded from contact with oils. 'Cold-pressing', in this sense, is based on fiction and ignorance. It offers no quality advantage.

The term is meaningless. Its use by manufacturers is unethical, to cater to uninformed consumers who still believe that 'cold-pressed' means high quality. For quality, it is more important that the oil was *protected* from light and oxygen during pressing, and was also *sheltered* during bottling, storage, and shipping.

Too Hot

Deodorization, carried out for about an hour at high temperature (245°C, 473°F), destroys the nutritive value of the oils, and produces *trans-* fatty acids and chemical changes (see Chapter 16, From Seed to Oil).

Hydrogenation, used to turn liquid oils into semi-solid or solid fats, is carried out at a temperature of 250°C (482°F) for several hours. Hydrogenation purposely creates *trans-* fatty acids, because *trans-* fatty acids have higher melting points and are more solid than *cis-* fatty acids, and give products made from oils (such as margarines and shortenings) body, consistency, texture, and shelf life.

Frying and *deep-frying* with oils, especially if the oil is allowed to sizzle or boil for hours or even days, occurs at temperatures between 160 and 220°C (320 to 428°F), depending on the kind of oil used, and produces *trans-* fatty acids, as well as light-, oxygen-, and heat-induced chemical destruction of fatty acids.

While the pressing temperature should be kept as low as possible, the major heat problem in oil manufacture is not the pressing temperature if we exclude light and air from the oil, but temperatures reached during deodorizing, hydrogenating (see Chapter 16, From Seed to Oil; and Chapter 17, From Oil to Margarine), and frying (see Chapter 22, Frying and Deep-Frying).

The term 'cold-pressed' is based on misunderstanding, and has no value whatsoever as a term denoting oil quality.

Terms with Meaning

We need new terms for high-quality oils, and a precise definition of the meaning of those new terms. We need to look for *unrefined* oils that have been *mechanically* pressed rather than chemically extracted, that have been *completely protected from light and air during pressing*, that have been *completely sheltered from light and oxygen* during filling, storage, and transport, that have been *stored frozen*, and that *taste fresh* like the seed from which they came. As consumers we need to make sure that we do not destroy these quality oils during food preparation.

28 *Making Oils with Human Health in Mind*

If health rather than shelf life and convenience is our primary concern, we must make oils in a more careful way than is the present practice of large oil processors. Let me acquaint you with new methods that I pioneered for making such oils, beginning in 1983. When health-conscious, educated consumers demand such oils and refuse inferior oils, the oil industry will more widely develop and adopt such methods.

Destructive Factors

Of the factors that destroy oils while they're being made, light is most damaging; oxygen from air is next; and heat speeds up the destruction by both light and oxygen. High temperatures, such as those attained during frying, deodorizing, and hydrogenating, cause damage even in the absence of light and oxygen. Water, certain minerals, and some pigments also damage oils, especially in the presence of light.

This knowledge leads one to certain conclusions regarding oil production. The way to make *health-sustaining* oils is to prevent damage to oils at the front end by treating them with care, instead of following industry practice of pressing them without care, allowing deterioration to take place, and then cleaning up the damage done by these sloppy practices, with high-tech, high-temperature industrial methods that damage oil molecules in other ways.

I worked with others who expressed a willingness to make oils with human health in mind. We chose to use organic seeds because non-organic seeds may contain a greater amount of poisonous pesticide residues. Their removal from oils requires deodorization which only takes out about half the pesticides, and at the same time produces other toxic substances (see Chapter 16, From Seed to Oil).

Custom Design

To treat oil with care at the front end, we custom-designed and custom-made parts for existing presses to prevent any contact of the oil with light and air while being pressed. Such parts do not come standard with oil presses. Machine modifications had to be made of special metals, especially avoiding copper, brass, and iron,[1] which catalyze oil breakdown. These metals could not be used in lines and tanks, either.

Containers to store freshly pressed oils had to be opaque and oxygen-free. We settled the oil by gravity rather than using filter presses. Use of the latter introduces an unnecessary step during which contamination and oil breakdown can take place. All containers, lines, and space inside presses were flushed with inert gas to clear them of oil-damaging oxygen (easier said than done): either nitrogen or argon, or a mixture of inert gases.

We chose black polyethylene (PE) as our bottle material and had it thickened to make it *completely opaque* to light and ultraviolet (UV) rays, to completely protect the oil from its most destructive influence. PE is lighter and more durable than ceramic and glass. It is also cheaper. We rejected tin and soldered cans, because metals tend to speed oil deterioration and solder contains lead.

Brown glass bottles are necessary for people with allergies or sensitivities to synthetic materials. In fact, further research has convinced me that oils do better in glass than in plastic. I've had to change my mind on this issue and now recommend oils only in amber glass bottles. To counter the negative effects of light, I suggest using cardboard packaging around the glass bottle. I developed an EFA-rich oil blend for seeking a convenient product which contains everything they need, but nothing they should avoid from oils. The box excludes all light as well as UV.

Cold Store, Shelf Date, and Quick-Ship

We pioneered refrigerated storage and shipping for fresh oils. No one in the mainstream oil industry refrigerates oils. They choose convenience over product freshness and human health. We shelf-dated our oils, because even refrigerated fresh oils (especially sensitive therapeutic oils such as flax) spoil within a short time.

---

[1] When one of the partners decided to use brass fittings (to save money!), the oil was spoiled and one person got diarrhea from using the 'brass-made' oil. When the wrong kinds of material were used to coat the press head, they too ended up in the oil. These and other sloppy practices resulted in my separation from the people with whom I originally developed flax oil.

Frozen solid at a low enough temperature, however, oils last a long time. The manufacturers of the new oils still think that freezing is going too far with care but, being stubborn about health issues, I continue to advocate frozen oils.

Distribution methods for sensitive fresh oils require attention too. Many distribution systems are too slow. Fresh oils should go directly from manufacturers to retail stores or, in cases where consumers have serious health concerns, directly from manufacturers to consumers.

Education

Touring the North American continent, I have educated consumers about the fats that heal and the fats that kill. About five million people have been exposed to my message about fats, oils, cholesterol, and human health through lectures, seminars, and media.

As a result of these efforts, several companies now make and sell oils made by the methods that I pioneered. Not all of them make oil with the recommended care. Not all of them distribute oils as quickly as possible. Over the next few years, methods for making, storing, and distributing oils will continue to be improved. Steps in that direction continue to be taken.

29 Packaging and Storing Oils

If oils are not packaged and stored properly, they spoil, and when they do, they spoil our health. Here is some insight into what must be done to keep oils safe for human health.

Exclusion of Light and Air

Just as oil seeds should be pressed in a dark, oxygen-free environment, so bottling and storage should exclude light and oxygen. Light catalyzes oxidative destruction of oil, speeding it up 1000 times over destruction by oxygen in the absence of light. Refrigeration slows down this deterioration – to about half the rate at room temperature.

Oil in clear glass is subject to light-induced deterioration, and may contain altered fatty acid derivatives. The longer oil is exposed to full spectrum light while standing on the shelf, the worse deterioration is likely to be. Cardboard shipping cartons are opaque, and protect oils from light as long as they stay in the box. But deterioration begins to take place as soon as an oil is exposed to light, and each ray (photon) of light can begin a free radical chain reaction that destroys or alters many molecules in an average of 30,000 reactions before it stops (see Chapter 21, Light, Free Radicals, and Oils). Each second that an oil is exposed to full spectrum light, thousands of photons strike it. The best protection is *no* exposure to light – from the time the oil is enclosed in light- and oxygen-excluding seeds until the time it ends up in the darkness of our stomach.

Black bottles are best, then brown (which block all but a fraction of the long, weak, non-destructive wavelengths), green, and clear, in that order. A cardboard box enclosure for oils completely blocks exposure to light.

For complete protection, oils should be filled into and stored completely opaque, and packed under inert gas (nitrogen, argon, or inert gas mixtures) to exclude oxygen. If everything has been done right, oils may keep for years without spoiling.

Refrigeration and Rapid Use After Opening

Opened bottles of oils should be kept in the fridge and used up rapidly (3 to 6 weeks for flax, 6 to 12 weeks for hemp, longer for less sensitive oils) because they start to go rancid (oxidize) on contact with air. Keeping the lid on tightly between uses does not prevent damage because air enters the bottle as soon as we open it (gas molecules move extremely fast, only a bit slower than the speed of light). Each oxygen molecule inside the container can induce many cycles of free radical chain reactions without being used up. Only a little oxygen is needed to create a lot of damage.[1]

Reactions of oils in which oxygen is used up to produce stable fatty acid epoxides proceed much slower than reactions in which unstable peroxides are formed. Peroxides can start free radical chain reactions and release oxygen to start another round of chain reactions. Figure 36 illustrates both types of reaction.

Quantities of Sealed Product to Purchase

In order not to waste oil due to spoilage, it should be bought in small quantities: 250 mL for flax oil with its high alpha-linolenic acid (LNA, 18:3w3) content; 500 mL for safflower, sunflower, and other oils high in linoleic acid (LA, 18:2w6); and 1000 mL for olive oil, which is high in oleic acid (OA, 18:1w9).

The difference in quantities has to do with the speed at which the three unsaturated fatty acids react. Triply unsaturated LNA (18:3w3) is most chemically reactive, and spoils most rapidly. It reacts with oxygen about 5 times faster than doubly unsaturated LA (18:2w6), and LA reacts 2.5 times faster than monounsaturated OA (18:1w9).

Because of these differences in reactivity, properly made flax oil keeps about 3 months while in a cool and sealed container; my oil blend keeps 6 months refriger-

---

[1] One cubic centimeter (about 1/15 cubic inch) of air in the space at the top of an 8-ounce bottle contains roughly 6 quintillion (6, followed by 18 zeroes) oxygen molecules, each of which can become an EFA-destroying free radical.

[2] The protein impurities in fats can also spoil. Butter will spoil if left out in hot weather. If it is 'clarified' to remove protein and other 'impurities', leaving 100% butter fat (ghee), it will keep quite well. Butter clarification is practiced by cultures living in hot climates without access to refrigeration.

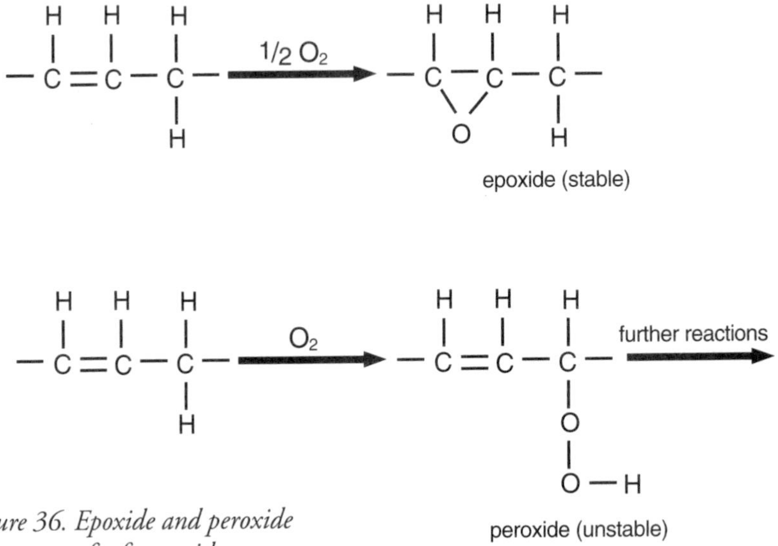

epoxide (stable)

*Figure 36. Epoxide and peroxide
of a fatty acid.*

peroxide (unstable)

ated and 3 to 5 years frozen solid; safflower, sunflower, sesame, and pumpkin seed oils keep 9 to 12 months when cool and sealed; and olive oil will keep up to 2 years when cool and sealed. Walnut and soybean oils are less sensitive than flax oil because they contain less LNA, but are more sensitive than oils containing only LA. Fats that contain mostly saturated fatty acids are much more stable, and spoil only slowly. [2]

Healers versus Manufacturers

Healers and manufacturers head in opposite directions regarding oils. Manufacturers want oils that won't spoil, which are low in essential nutrients. Healers want oils that are good for us because they are EFA-rich, but these oils spoil easily.

There is a saying among nutritional therapists and healers using natural medicine. They tell us to: "Eat things that spoil, but eat them before they do." Whoever coined that saying was probably thinking of fresh vegetables, but the saying is equally valid for fresh, EFA-rich edible oils.

30 Labeling Oil Products

We are now aware of some of the destructive processes to which oils may be subjected on their journey from nature to our stomach. To conclude this section, we will look at how oils are presently labeled and how, in the best of all possible worlds, fats and oil products *should* be labeled to help consumers make informed choices in their purchases of these food items.

Labeling Conventions

In present labeling practice, most of the information that you need to know about an oil (relevant to health) is left off the label. In purchasing oils, therefore, it is as important to know what a label leaves out as it is to know what the label says. Manufacturers are not required to state on the label when an oil has been degummed, refined, bleached, deodorized, or even partially hydrogenated, and they therefore do not give this information.

If an oil is *unrefined* (in its natural state – not degummed, not refined, not bleached, not deodorized, not partially hydrogenated) the word 'unrefined' will appear on the label. If the label does not carry this word, it is degummed, refined, bleached, and deodorized (for canola and soybean oils perhaps even partially hydrogenated), and is an oil from which natural ingredients important to health have been removed, and in which fatty acids altered by heat, light, oxygen, and processing – and detrimental to health – are present.

If an olive oil is virgin (unrefined) quality, the word 'virgin' will be printed on the label, perhaps in combination with other words such as 'extra virgin'. If the word 'virgin' is not on the label, the oil is non-virgin, which means: refined, bleached, deodorized – an oil that has lost all the virgin virtues of olive oil for health (see Chapter 54, Virgin Olive Oils). But the words 'non-virgin, refined, bleached, deodorized' will *not* be found on the label.

In the best of all possible worlds, what should the label tell us?

Essential Fatty Acid (EFA) Content and Balance

Since EFAs – LA and LNA – hold key importance in maintaining our health, labels of all edible oils and products containing them should list the amounts of all *cis-* LA and all *cis-* LNA in the finished product in grams per 100 grams of oil. A product containing less LA than 5 grams per 100 grams of oil is useless, and a product containing less LA than 8 grams per 100 grams is nutritionally deficient in LA. A good product has at least 25 grams of LA per 100 grams (33% or more LA is recommended).

LNA content should be stated separately from LA content (see Chapter 8, The Healing Essential Fatty Acids). A balance of w6 to w3 fatty acids should ideally be between 3:1 and 1:2 for the long term. For the short term (6 months) to make up for w3 deficiency, and in therapeutic situations involving cancer, cardiovascular disease, inflammatory, and other degenerative conditions, w3 supplementation with flax oil, which contains 4 times as much w3 as w6, is recommended.

Trans- Fatty Acids and Other Altered Fat Products

Since *trans-* fatty acids act against EFAs, interfere with EFA functions and make EFA deficiency more severe, an edible product should list the amount of *trans-* fatty acid isomers present in grams per 100 grams of product. Health-conscious consumers know to buy only products containing no *trans-* fatty acids (see Chapter 18, Margarines, Shortenings, and *Trans-* Fatty Acids). Other altered fat molecules, such as positional isomers, dimers, and polymers of fatty acids, and breakdown products of fatty acids such as aldehydes, ketones, epoxides, and alcohols are also dangerous, and it would be a good idea to list the total amount of altered fat substances on the label, in grams per 100 grams.

Exclusion of Light and Air, and Maximum Temperature Reached

Whether light and air were excluded during the whole processing, filling, and storage of the product should be known. We can then choose between natural and deteriorated products. Oils in transparent bottles are exposed to destruction by light (see Chapter 29, Packaging and Storing Oils).

New terms should be coined and defined for fresh oils that have been pressed and packaged under exclusion of light and air, and stored and transported either refrigerated or frozen (see Chapter 27, 'Cold-Pressed': A Meaningless Term).

The highest temperature to which the seed and oil have been subjected during post-pressing processing procedures used to manufacture finished products should be on the label. We can then choose products that have been processed at non-destructive temperatures.

Pressing Date

Pressing (or expiry) date should be printed on the label. By the age of the product, we would know how fresh the product is, and could avoid age-deteriorated products. Depending on what kind of oil it is, EFA-containing oils might stay edible for 3 to 12 months in unopened containers, and from 3 weeks to 3 months once opened. Skin preparations containing EFAs deteriorate within 6 months.

Pressing date should not be confused with processing date or other gimmicks that make older oils sound fresher.

Mechanically Pressed or Chemically Extracted

The label should state whether the oil was mechanically pressed or chemically extracted. We know that mechanically pressed oils contain no traces of chemical solvents (see Chapter 16, From Seed to Oil).

Crude or Refined

The label should state whether the oil was degummed, bleached, deodorized or otherwise refined. We know that completely unrefined (crude) oils still contain nutrient co-factors required to metabolize the oil, as well as antioxidants, and therefore do not rob the body of essential nutrients (see Chapter 16, From Seed to Oil).

Hydrogenation

Whether or not the oil was hydrogenated is important to keep on the label. We know that hydrogenated oils and fats contain *trans-* fatty acids and other altered molecules. If health is our concern, hydrogenated products are unacceptable.

Organic or Non-Organic

Whether or not the seeds were organically grown should be stated on the label. We know that oils from organic seeds are likely to contain fewer pesticides (nothing anywhere is *completely* free of them anymore). Many pesticides are oil-soluble, and can be kept out of foods only if pesticides are not used during seed production, transport, or storage.

In a free market economy, manufacturers are free to offer for sale to the public many kinds and qualities of products. The public is free to buy or to refuse any product available. If the above information were present on the label of the oil products, we would know what kinds and qualities of products we are being offered. With this information, we could take greater responsibility for our choices and our health. To make responsible choices, we need that information.

In the best of all possible worlds, we would be given that information. In this one, we must fight to get it.

Fats and Figures

Fats in the Human Body

Having looked at natural fats and how processing changes them, we turn our attention to body fat which, although it has a bad reputation, serves important functions in health. We look at our requirement for lipids, examine how our body digests and metabolizes them, and discuss other essential nutrients that our body requires in order to properly metabolize lipids.

Then we shift gears to talk about the uniqueness of each individual in terms of nutritional requirements, the use of natural substances normally present in the body to improve health and treat disease, the nature of stress and how to overcome it, and the importance of balance between fuel foods that increase energy and protector substances that prevent us from burning out.

I have included a chapter on the futility of calorie counting, and suggest a simpler, more effective method for weight control. You'll also find a note on liposuction, stomach stapling, partial removal of intestine, and other high-tech methods of weight control.

The section ends with a chapter on cholesterol. It introduces revolutionary new information about cholesterol and heart disease that throws a completely new light on cardiovascular disease (CVD), the number one killer of this century – and shows simple, practical ways in which you can prevent and reverse CVD.

The Fire Inside Each Cell

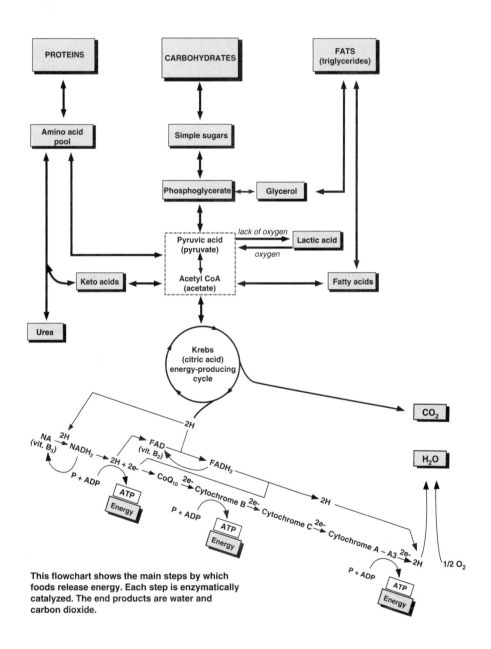

This flowchart shows the main steps by which foods release energy. Each step is enzymatically catalyzed. The end products are water and carbon dioxide.

Body Fat **31**

Next to water, which makes up about 70% of the total weight of a human adult, and 84% of that of a newborn infant, fat is the most abundant substance found in our body. We may not like that, but there it is.

The exact amount of fat present in the body is influenced by diet, exercise, age, gender, and genetic disposition, and can vary from 5% to over 60%, with an average of 15 to 22%. Degenerative diseases are associated with both overweight and underweight.

Diet. Concentrated high-calorie foods – those rich in refined sugars, starches, proteins, and saturated fats, and low in fiber and water – increase fat deposition. When we gain weight, the extra 'weight' is plain old fat unless we gain muscle through strenuous physical activity. Bulky foods rich in water and fiber, such as leafy vegetables, tend to keep us slim.

Exercise. Athletes need to be more slim and trim than average. Extra fat during competition means that their muscles must do more work, which could cost them the medals they aim to win. Male swimmers trim down to 12% fat, runners down to 8%. Women athletes usually trim down to around 15%. World class body builders carry 12% fat between competitions, and go down to 6% body fat during competition, for better cut and definition of muscle profile. Although it is possible for women to lose most of their fat, this may not be desirable from a health point of view, as low body fat may affect female hormonal balance. Olympic and other female athletes often lose their menstrual cycles. Loss of the menstrual cycle is also one diagnostic sign of the eating disorder *anorexia nervosa.*

The best way to lose excess fat is to build muscle. Losing fat through the use of self-imposed starvation diets is self-defeating in terms of health and, in the long run, even for weight loss. Liposuction – the high-tech, expert-administered alternative – is safer than starvation, but undermines personal initiative and responsibility.

Exercise, good food choices, and thinking (or visualizing) 'slim' are the three keys to successful slimming. During exercise, our muscles consume fat to produce energy. Fat deposits around our entire body are rearranged and reduced when we exercise. Since muscle weighs more than fat, exercising may actually increase weight rather than decrease it, but an exercised body looks slimmer and feels better. Our bathroom scales are therefore less reliable than mirror, eyes, and feelings.

Age. Our body's fat content tends to increase with age, although this is not inevitable. Old natives of South Sea Islands are as slim as their young, and as active and child-like. Their use of unrefined foods, active life-style, simplicity, and sunny disposition help them remain slim into old age.

Gender differences. On the average, fat accounts for about 15% of the total weight of males, and about 22% of the weight of females. The tendency for women to carry more fat than men evolved during ice ages or even more primitive times, when a primary female role was to produce offspring under living conditions characterized by fluctuating food supplies. It was important for them to store in their body the energy (fat) necessary to complete fetal growth even if the food ran out. Now that food supplies are more stable, the climate warmer, and procreation no longer their main purpose, women still carry the genes and hormones adapted for survival in ice ages, perhaps in preparation for future chills.

Female hormones, responsible for the extra fat that women carry, also protect women from the deleterious cardiovascular effects of fats.[1] Women suffer heart attacks and strokes only one-third as often as men, until their hormones fade at menopause. Within 6 to 10 years after menopause, women become as prone as men to cardiovascular disease. The edge of obesity is considered to be 23% of body weight as fat for men, and 32% of body weight as fat for women.

Genes. Some people have excessive fat deposition because of inherited genetic traits. Such mutations are rare, occurring in less than 5 per 1000 in the population. Most of us cannot hide behind our genes on this one. About 300 per 1000 of adult North Americans and Europeans are overweight, largely due to calorie-rich, nutrient-poor diets and inadequate exercise.

Comparisons. Compared to fluctuating fat levels, proteins constitute a fairly constant 12% of the weights of both genders, less than fat on the average. Excess proteins are converted into stored fat. Carbohydrates – glucose in our blood, and glycogen stored in tissues, muscles, and liver – make up only 0.5% of body weight. Carbohydrates above this low level are turned into fat. Minerals make up about 3.5% of body weight.

On average then, fat is the most abundant body component next to water. Nature chose wisely to store energy reserves in this efficient way. Each gram of fat stores more than twice as much energy as the same weight of protein or carbohydrates. Furthermore, while most cells contain about 70% water, our fat cells contain up to 70% fat and very little water. Thus fat and fat cells store energy for future use in an extremely economic and efficient way.

---

[1] This hormonal protection is thought by some researchers to be due to decreased iron (a strong pro-oxidant that can damage fats which then damage arteries and start the process of narrowing them) from women's monthly blood loss, and not a *direct* effect of estrogen hormones.

Fat tissues store more cholesterol than other tissues except our brain, whose cholesterol content is even higher than that of fat tissues.

Fatty Acid Content of Body Fat

The fatty acids profile of body fat can vary greatly as a direct consequence of differing contents of saturated, monounsaturated, and essential fatty acids (EFAs) in different diets. Table C1 gives the percentages of linoleic acid (LA, 18:2w6) and alpha-linolenic acid (LNA, 18:3w3) found in fat tissues of various groups of people.

Table C1. Essential fatty acids in human body fat.

	% 18:2w6	% 18:3w3	
New Zealand Maoris	2.6	0.93	
Hottentot	5.9	0.6	
obese American	8.7	1.1	
normal American	10.2	0.58	
American students	17.3	2.0	
Israeli students	22.1	2.4	
Japanese (surgery patients)	14.8	1.2	} +2% w3 long-
Japanese	16.5	0.97	chain fatty acids
Leipzig normal	7.9	1.5	
British omnivores	11.0	2.1	
British vegans	25.4	2.4	

Three interesting points emerge from this information.

1. In both tissue samples from people living in hot, sunny, dry climates (New Zealand, Africa), low-fat tissue levels of LA and LNA are found, in keeping with low LA and LNA content in their food supply. Neither Maoris nor Hottentots are especially prone to degenerative diseases (see Chapter 67, Oils and Sunshine) but, on the other hand, neither are known for longevity, either.

2. In temperate areas, obese people have levels of less than 10% LA in their adipose tissue, and 'normal' adult Americans (remember that 68% of these 'normal' people die from degenerative conditions) generally have only about 10% LA in their fat tissues.

3. People in temperate regions with the lowest incidence of degenerative diseases (Japanese, British vegans) have higher than average levels of LA and LNA in their fatty tissues.

The evidence does not support the opinion of writers who warn against high levels of polyunsaturates (PUFAs) because of fear of cancer. If the PUFAs are fried, oxidized by light or air, hydrogenated, or processed at high temperatures – in other words, if EFAs in the oils are altered – they may indeed increase cancer incidence. If antioxidants (vitamin E and carotene) are removed from PUFA (w6) oils by refining, these oils also increase cancer incidence. If the diet also lacks vitamin C, selenium, and sulphur, PUFAs that peroxidize within our tissues may cause damage and increase cancer. It is important to distinguish between health-destroying kinds of PUFAs and EFA-containing oils in their natural (unrefined) state, which are health-enhancing (see Chapter 25, Polyunsaturates and Superunsaturates).

Changing the Body Fat Picture

How can we change the fat content of our body? To increase the amount of w3 EFAs in our fat tissue, which is desirable for both beauty (they make skin soft and velvety) and health (they decrease our risk of degenerative diseases), we must replace excess calories (refined sugars, refined starches, refined oils, and saturated, hard, sticky fats) with whole foods including seeds such as flax and hemp, or their fresh oils. W6 (but not w3) EFAs are found in sunflower and sesame seeds. Hemp seeds are a balanced source of both.

To decrease body fat, we must replace some of our concentrated, calorie-rich foods with bulky, calorie-poor foods. Bulky foods spend less time in our intestines and contain fewer calories. Our efficient digestive mechanisms therefore absorb less unnecessary calories.

Proportions. When I start to get fat (which is easy for me), I don't cut out the foods I like, but simply change proportions: less cheese, meat, bread, sugar, and pasta, and more salads and vegetables. Instead of using the sprig of parsley to garnish the meat, I use a little meat to garnish the salad: more natural, fiber-rich foods, and less processed, concentrated foods.

Lean (fiber-rich) foods. It is impossible to gain weight on a diet of vegetables. To get 2000 calories, the amount needed to maintain constant body weight, we must eat:

- 6 kg (13 pounds) of broccoli;
- 4.75 kg (10 pounds) of carrots;
- 7.7 kg (16 pounds) of spinach;
- 14 kg (30 pounds) of lettuce;
- 7.4 kg (16 pounds) of cauliflower; or
- 13 kg (28 pounds) of cucumbers.

It is impossible to eat this much food. Eating less food than this means fewer calories. Also, fresh vegetables are rich in minerals and vitamins, which help metabolize our foods properly.

Concentrated (protein, fat, and starch) foods. But 2000 calories are supplied by amounts of concentrated foods that one can easily consume, namely:

- 0.571 kg (1.25 pounds) of cheese;
- 0.378 kg (0.83 pounds) of chocolate chip cookies;
- 0.476 kg (1.05 pounds) of beef;
- 0.606 kg (1.34 pounds) of wheat;
- 0.371 kg (0.81 pounds) of pork;

- 0.588 kg (1.3 pounds) of beans, peas or lentils;
- 0.497 kg (1.1 pounds) of soybeans; or
- 0.355 kg (0.78 pounds) of peanuts.

One can easily gain weight from eating too much of these foods.

Finding the balance. An average adult U.S. *male* eats about 2.7 kg (5.9 pounds) of food per day. Less than 1000 calories, which usually result in weight loss, are contained in 2.7 kg of broccoli but over 10,800 calories, which must result in weight gain, are contained in 2.7 kg of soybeans.

An average U.S. *female* eats about 1.8 kg (4 pounds) of food each day. Only 600 calories, too few to maintain weight, are contained in 1.8 kg of broccoli but 7200 calories – too many, leading to weight gain – are contained in 1.8 kg of soybeans. We must combine lean foods and concentrated foods in such a way that we maintain normal body weight between the extremes of anorexia and obesity.

When we gain weight, we must eat more lean foods like salads, green leafy and flower vegetables, and root vegetables like carrots and beets. Fiber added to foods also cuts down calories. Also, eating our main meal early in the day helps to ensure that calories are used for activity instead of being stored as fat, because we are physically inactive late in the evening and at night.

When we get *too* skinny, we can gain weight by eating more concentrated foods like meats, cheese, and eggs, and starchy vegetables like grains, corn, and potatoes. Eating a main meal late in the day may help put on extra pounds of fat, but only strenuous exercise will build a more muscular and more attractive body.

EFAs. Since EFAs increase our metabolic rate, they are preferable to saturated fats that slow down metabolic rate, deposit more fat, and make us feel lazy and lethargic (unenergetic). A balanced supplement of vitamins and minerals can also help increase metabolism and vitality.

Exercise. Activity burns off calories, speeds up metabolic rate, and invigorates. It is easier to be active if we feel like it, but this should be easy if our foods are nutrient-rich and balanced. Diet and activity go hand in hand, building each other. Active people eat better. Good eating gives us energy to act.

Overweight is associated with every kind of degenerative disease. Too little body fat also makes us prone to disease, because our reserves run out sooner in times of stress. The middle road leads to health.

32 Fat Consumption and Daily Requirement

According to 1979 figures, the average U.S. citizen consumed 135 pounds (61 kg) of fats that year, about 168 grams per day. The consumed fat was made up of 34% saturated, 40% monounsaturated, and 15% polyunsaturated (w6) fatty acids. The information did not distinguish essential fatty acids (EFAs) from non-essential, altered, denatured, and toxic polyunsaturates (see Chapter 25, Polyunsaturates and Superunsaturates). W3 intake was completely ignored. The amount of EFAs left in their natural state after hydrogenation, exposure to destruction by light and air, and food preparation (both commercially and in the home) will be lower, and some of this may be unavailable to our body because saturated and monounsaturated long-chain fatty acids, *trans-* fatty acids, and sugars present in the diet interfere with EFA functions. Fat consumption has been increasing by about 1 pound per person per year for the last 10 years.

According to *Nutrition Reviews* (1984), fat calories make up about 42% of all calories consumed by Westerners, but 168 grams per day is closer to 56% of the average daily calories (168 grams fat, multiplied by 9 calories per gram is 1512 calories, which is over half of 2500 calories consumed daily by an average adult). High-fat diets speed growth, sexual maturity (from 17 years old at first menstruation, on average, in the 17th century, to 13 years old now), aging, and death.

Nutrition Reviews also states that only 15 to 25 grams of fat (5 to 8% of total calories) are required daily if it is the right kind of fat. The author does not specify what is the right kind of fat.

In countries such as Thailand (27 grams per day), the Philippines (30 grams per day), Japan (40 grams per day), and Taiwan (45 grams per day), fat consumption is much lower than in Western countries such as Denmark (160 grams per day), New Zealand (155 grams per day), the United Kingdom (142 grams per day), the United States (168 grams per day), and Canada (142 grams per day). People in the nations consuming a low-fat diet have a low incidence of fatty degeneration, and people in the high-fat nations have a high incidence of fatty degeneration.

Recommendations

Official. Several official bodies in the U.S., including the National Academy of Sciences, Senate Select Committee on Health and Nutrition, American Heart Association, and National Research Council have recommended decreasing our consumption of fats in order to improve health. Their general recommendation is that only 30% of our calories should come from fats, with 10% each made up by saturated, monounsaturated, and essential fatty acids. This change will improve

160

the health of people of Western nations. But people in nations like Japan with a low incidence of fatty degeneration consume only about 15% of their calories as fat, indicating that 30% of calories as fat is still too high.

Seventh Day Adventists. Researchers at Loma Linda School of Nutrition, who are less bound to the fats and oils industry and inclined toward vegetarianism by Seventh Day Adventist beliefs, have studied diets of vegetarians and other groups of people around the globe. They conclude that 15 to 20% of total calories as fats is optimum, and should be made up of no more than 4% saturated fatty acids, around 6% linoleic acid (LA, 18:2w6), and 5 to 10% monounsaturated fatty acids. They give no figures for alpha-linolenic acid (LNA, 18:3w3), which is also essential.

Some researchers recommend that as much as 20% of total calories should be LA (18:2w6). This is far too high in the long term. In the short term, people with severe cardiovascular problems stemming from atherosclerosis appear to be helped by high intake of LA. But highly unsaturated w3 fatty acids including LNA (18:3w3), EPA (20:5w3), and DHA (22:6w3) appear more effective for this purpose. Optimum mineral and vitamin intake is more important for cardiovascular health than high levels of LA (see Chapter 12, Cholesterol).

Pritikin. Nathan Pritikin, an engineer who founded, and until his death in his sixties directed the Centre for Longevity in California, recommended 10% of calories from fats as the absolute maximum. Beyond 10%, he considered all fats poison. People with obesity and cardiovascular problems use his diet (which contains only 7% of calories as fat) to reverse these conditions but, to maintain long-term health, this diet is too low in fats[1], w3s, and vitamin E (he did not use supplements). Many of his patients cheat. Also their skin becomes dry and their energy levels eventually take a nose-dive. Pritikin's program of diet (80% complex carbohydrates, 10% protein, 10% fat) and exercise (a lot of walking) is calorie-restricted. It lowers blood cholesterol levels by 25%. But his diet contains only 10 units of vitamin E, even less than the minimum daily requirement of 15 units set by government. Vitamin E is required to protect highly unsaturated fatty acids and cholesterol from oxidation; and lack of vitamin E promotes cancer. Pritikin wrongly claimed that since lettuce contains 7% fats, getting enough fats cannot be a problem (common sense tells us that few foods contain less fat than lettuce!).[2]

Pritikin's diet is clearly too low in fats. Research shows that fat consumption of 5% or less of total calories compromises the absorption of fat-soluble vitamins A, D, E, and K and leads to increased occurrence of blindness and cancer, both

---

[1] Slightly defective nutrient absorption, common with age, could bring fat absorption to the critical level (5%) below which fat-soluble vitamin absorption is impaired and cancer increases.

[2] Fats provide 7% of the *calories* in lettuce, but only 0.2% of the *weight* of lettuce. To obtain the minimum daily fat requirement of 15 to 25 grams, one would have to eat 7.5 to 12.5 kg (16.5 to 27.5 pounds) of this herbivores' green delight each day.

probably due to lack of vitamin A and possibly also vitamin E.

According to the U.S. Department of Agriculture's *Handbook on the Composition of Foods,* lettuce contains between 0.1 and 0.3% fats, depending on the variety. To get our *minimum* daily requirement of fats (15 to 25 grams per day) from lettuce, we'd have to eat 15 to 25 kg (33 to 55 pounds) of this vegetable. Only a cow could do that.

World Health Organization. Other research reported in scientific journals and adopted by the World Health Organization sets the requirement for LA at 3% of calories for children and adults, at 4.5% of calories during pregnancy, and at 6% of calories during lactation, but makes no recommendation about saturated and monounsaturated fatty acid intakes, or about w3 intake.

No one encourages us to increase our consumption of fats, except manufacturers of fat-containing products. Of course, our health is not their motive.

Overweight, which is almost always fat (Arnold Schwarzenegger is overweight, but *his* type of overweight is muscle), is a major risk factor for cardiovascular disease, cancer, and diabetes.

A healthy perspective. Some of the above recommendations are extreme, and none recognize the importance of getting enough w3 EFAs, the balance between w3 and w6 EFAs, and the balance between EFAs and non-essential fatty acids. However, it is clear that we need to decrease our consumption of fats and calories from sugars, starches, and concentrated foods in order to come down to our ideal weight and to enjoy ideal health. Consuming 15 to 20% of calories as fats, with one-third of this as LA and LNA in the appropriate ratio, and not more than one-third as saturated fatty acids, is a strong step in that direction.

Remember also that 20% of *calories* as fats is less than 10% of the weight of our *food* as fat, since fats store more than twice as many calories as an equal weight of protein or carbohydrates.

We also need to decrease our consumption of (saturated) fats from land animal sources because saturated fatty acids make platelets more sticky. Also, fat tissue contains more cholesterol than lean body tissue and can therefore increase the cholesterol load carried in the low-density lipoprotein (LDL) fraction in the blood of those 30% of the population whose serum cholesterol levels are sensitive to dietary cholesterol.

Our body's capacity for metabolizing LDL appears to be limited, and by present-day nutritional standards, it requires 2.5 days after a meal to remove this cholesterol from our bloodstream. This suggests that unless other aspects of our diet (such as vitamin and mineral intake) change, sensitive people should eat cholesterol-containing foods only about every 3 days, to give their body time to metabolize it completely and to avoid a buildup of cholesterol in their blood.

Requirement for Essential Fatty Acids

LA (18:2w6). About 1% of daily calories (about 3 grams in a 2500-calorie diet)

as LA is enough to relieve the symptoms of LA deficiency, and therefore constitutes a minimum daily requirement for LA. But this is not the optimum dose,
which is probably between 3 and 6% (or 9 to 18 grams per day).

LNA (18:3w3). The daily requirement for LNA is less well known. LNA
deficiency described in journals include a 6-year-old girl who required 0.54% of
daily calories as LNA in order to reverse symptoms of LNA deficiency, and older
people who required somewhat less. The optimum for LNA is unknown, but can
be estimated. Inuit (Eskimos) consumed 4.1% or more of their daily calories as
EPA (20:5w3) and DHA (22:6w3), both of which are made from LNA. Several
other traditional diets associated with good health contain around 2 to 2.5% of
calories as LNA. This figure may be an optimum.

People using fresh, unrefined flax oil in the treatment of terminal cancer
may consume up to 100 grams of the oil (mixed with skim milk yogurt or baker's
cheese containing 40 to 50 grams protein) daily until the tumor dissolves. This
much flax oil contains about 60 grams of LNA, or about 20% of daily calories.
No side effects are seen at this dosage in the short term if whole foods rich in
minerals, vitamins, and fiber are eaten. As health is reestablished, the amount of
flax oil is decreased to 1 or 2 tablespoons per day. (1 tablespoon per day of flax oil
supplies about 2% of calories as w3s).

Other factors. A well-balanced diet containing vitamin C, carotene, selenium, vitamin E, N-acetyl cysteine, and other antioxidants keeps LA and LNA
from oxidizing. Optimum amounts of all 50 essential nutrients are necessary for
building health.

Digestion of Fats, Oils, and Cholesterol 33

Our body's processing of dietary fats and oils begins with digestion. When problems arise in our body's ability to digest, or when we exceed its capacity to digest,
our health deteriorates.

Mouth and stomach. Nothing much except mixing happens to fats, oils, or
cholesterol in our mouth. Our stomach produces an enzyme that can split fats
into their components, but the enzyme is inactive under normal stomach acid
conditions.

Our small intestine can digest a maximum of about 10 grams of food fats
every hour. Figure 37 shows where digestion and absorption of fats take place
in the human digestive system.

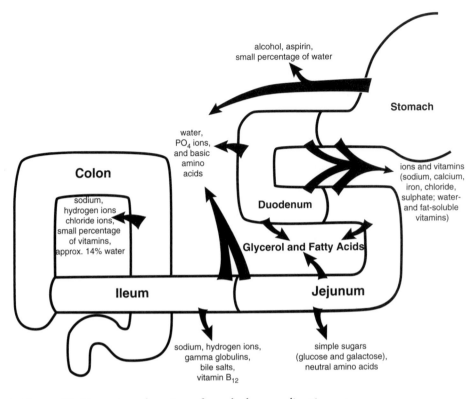

Figure 37. Absorption of nutrients from the human digestive system.

Bile

The churning action of our intestines mixes fatty food material with bile that our liver produced from cholesterol and stored and concentrated in our gallbladder.[1] Bile contains lecithin, which emulsifies fatty material, breaking it into tiny droplets. This increases the surface area of fat exposed to fat-digesting enzymes, and speeds up the rate at which fatty material can be digested by these enzymes. Fat-digesting enzymes are made by our pancreas and released into the food mixture in the first part of our small intestine (duodenum). Digestion and absorption of fats continues to take place as food passes through our small intestine. Figure 38 shows a cross-section through the intestinal wall.

Enzymes

Different enzymes contained in the alkaline pancreatic juice digest triglycerides,

---

[1] Bile actually consists of bile salts, phospholipids (lecithin), and cholesterol in a ratio of 12:2.5:1.

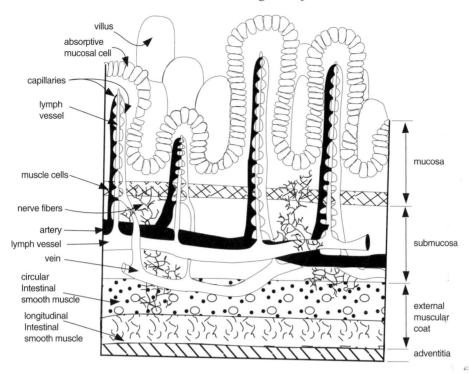

Figure 38. Cross-section through the intestinal wall.

phospholipids, and cholesterol esters present in food fats.[2] These enzymes split fatty acids from the outside carbon positions of the glycerol molecules in triglycerides and phospholipids, and remove fatty acids attached to cholesterol. The components are absorbed separately into cells lining our intestinal tract (mucosal cells), where they are put back together.

Free fatty acids may also be hooked up with albumin protein, and taken directly to the liver for further metabolism. Figure 39 summarizes the steps by which fats are digested, absorbed, reassembled, and carried into lymph and blood fluids.

Why digest? It might seem pointless to take apart foods just to put them back together, but it is really quite clever. By breaking down the molecules, our body makes sure that the complex chemical substances[3] (proteins) that make up tissues of other species of animals or plants don't get into our blood. If this were to happen, an alarm reaction would be set off, and several different kinds of white blood cells (leukocytes) – the soldiers among our blood cells – would mobilize,

---

[2] Pancreatic juice also contains enzymes that to digest starches and proteins.

[3] Allergy-producing substances are usually proteins, but sometimes complex fatty, hydrocarbon, or carbohydrate substances may also cause allergic reactions.

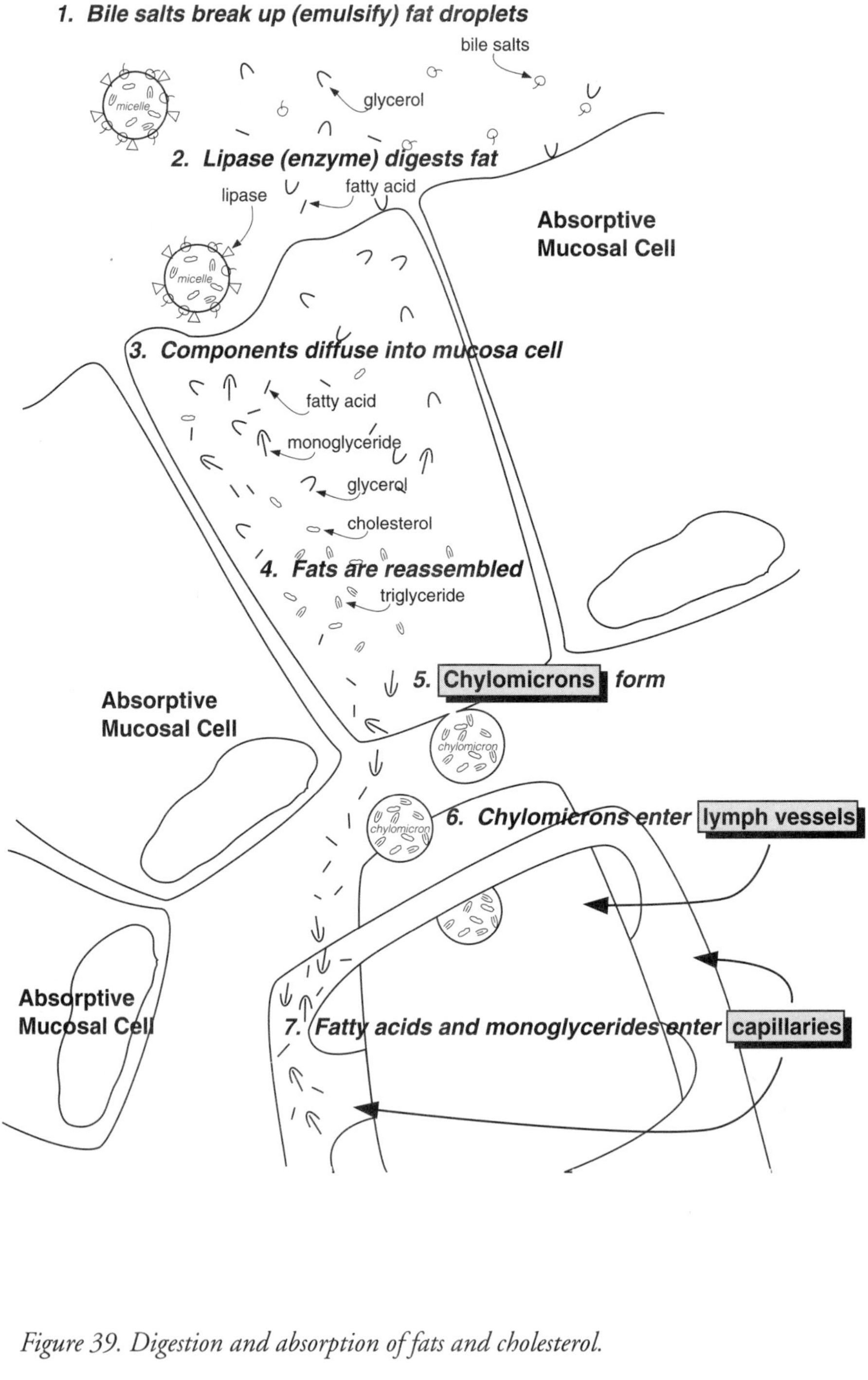

Figure 39. Digestion and absorption of fats and cholesterol.

declare war, and destroy the 'intruder' molecules. The disassembly (digestion) of molecules into component parts makes it unnecessary for our body to wage such molecular wars which, like all wars, are extremely stressful, wasteful, and costly to its molecular economy, harmony, and integrity – its health.

When, due to mechanical or biochemical injury or biochemical (nutritional) deficiency, foreign substances *do* get into our body, our immune system builds a standing army of antibodies against future intrusions by the same foreign substance. The result is food allergy. When we eat the food in question, we might manifest a long range of possible physical and mental symptoms of molecular wars or, in extreme cases, suffer anaphylactic shock which can be fatal.

Transport

Our mucosal cells build transport vehicles for fats. Out of proteins and phospholipids, they make a membrane bag, and stuff the reconstituted food fats into this bag. The loaded bags (chylomicrons) are dumped into our lymph vessels,[4] which ship them to a large vein close to our heart (left subclavian vein), where they merge into our bloodstream. The heart pumps the blood containing chylomicrons to all parts of our body.

Lipoproteins. Chylomicrons never reach our cells. They transfer their fats to high-density lipoproteins (HDL) circulating in our blood, and both HDL and empty chylomicron remnants are taken to our liver. Our liver also makes transport vehicles called very low-density lipoproteins (VLDL).

VLDL exchange material with HDL or are transformed into other vehicles called low-density lipoproteins (LDL and Lp[a]), which also exchange material with HDL (see Chapter 41, Blood Cholesterol). Our blood carries VLDL- and LDL-containing fats and cholesterol to our cells. Figure 40 illustrates the relationships between transport vehicles.

Loading docks. Each of our body's 100 trillion cells has on its membrane several 'docks' for receiving and unloading VLDL and LDL, drawing from them the fats and cholesterol our cells require for their functions.

When the requirement is filled, the docks are shut down. Excess fats and cholesterol from foods continue to circulate in our blood (high blood triglyceride and cholesterol levels are the measurable result) until they are metabolized by our liver or taken to fat cells for storage.

Fatty acids serve as fuel for our cells' energy-producing factories (mitochondria); membrane phospholipids and cholesterol are incorporated into membranes according to need; triglycerides are kept as fat reserve in our cells, and excess fats not needed by our cells are transported to fat depots around our organs or body, and stored there for later use.

---

[4] After a fatty meal, the lymph fluid turns a milky white color due to the presence of millions of fat-filled chylomicrons being transported in that fluid.

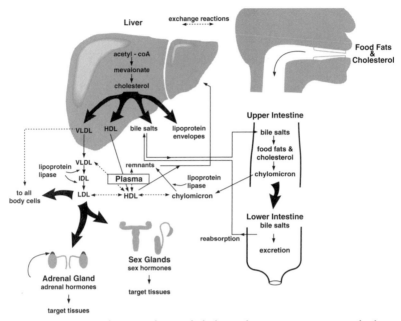

Figure 40. Interactions between fat- and cholesterol-carrying transport vehicles.

Fats that HDL pick up from the other transport vehicles are taken to the liver and further metabolized. Standard medical dogma considers HDL to be 'good', and LDL to be 'bad', but both play important roles in cardiovascular health and disease (see Chapter 41, Blood Cholesterol).

Regulation and Control. This extremely complex lipoprotein system ensures that fats are digested, absorbed into our body, and transported to all cells to supply them with the needed fats. It also ensures that excess fats don't build up in our blood. This system also moves excess cholesterol from our cells to our liver, which converts cholesterol into bile salts, pours these salts into our intestine to aid in fat digestion, and gets rid of excess cholesterol (as bile) through our stool.

Many points of regulation and control ensure proper functioning of the lipoprotein system. It is sensitive to our body's changing needs for fats and cholesterol, and balances its needs against fluctuating food intake of these two substances.

Our body does not digest or absorb castor and mineral oils. Rancid oils have toxic effects, from which our body only partially protects us: by unpalatability; by irritation of the delicate lining of our intestines, perhaps leading to diarrhea as well; and by decreased digestion and absorption.

Lipoproteins work effectively when we eat foods as nature makes them. Marvelously efficient, the system that digests, absorbs, and transports fats can cause problems when we eat over-rich, over-fat, over-sweetened, and over-processed foods. If we eat foods short of antioxidant minerals and vitamins needed to process fat, sugar, and cholesterol, we inhibit lipoprotein function, weaken and damage arteries, and oxidize cholesterol and fats, which do further damage. Toxic substances including drugs can create additional damage and disruption.

Realistically, we cannot blame our digestive system for what goes wrong. It deals with whatever we put into our mouth. Digestion is, after all, its purpose. If we are dissatisfied with the results of the work or our digestive system, then we, as its employer, can change what we give it to work with.

Lp(a) and Vitamin C

Accepted cardiovascular dogma – the link between 'bad' LDL and cardiovascular disease (CVD) – is weakening. Some people with high LDL are free of CVD. Others with low LDL suffer from CVD. There has to be an explanation.

Recently, this and other observations have led Drs. Matthias Rath and Linus Pauling to propose a solution to the puzzle of CVD. A third lipoprotein, called Lp(a), often confused with LDL in measurements, is a strong risk factor for CVD. As the levels of vitamin C – the strongest antioxidant normally present in our body – decrease, Lp(a) levels increase. Lp(a) contains an adhesive protein that thickens our arteries to protect them from damage due to vitamin C deficiency (scurvy). When the levels of vitamin C in our blood increase, the levels of this adhesive protein decrease.

Vitamin C and other antioxidants prevent oxidation of LDL cholesterol and triglycerides, minimize arterial damage by free radicals, and keep our arteries strong. Vitamin C, therefore, helps prevent and reverse CVD by at least two different mechanisms (see Chapter 71, Is the Cholesterol Theory Wrong?).

Metabolism of Fats and Oils 34

Metabolism includes all of the chemical changes that molecules undergo as they function in our body – in energy production, growth, maintenance, repair of body structures, and removal of wastes and toxic materials.

A discussion of *fat* metabolism includes how fats and oils are made, broken down for energy, transformed into other substances, used up, and/or destroyed and discarded. Thus the study of fat metabolism concerns itself with the birth, life, death, and disintegration of fat molecules in our body.

The components of fats: glycerol, saturated fatty acids, monounsaturated fatty acids (MUFAs), and essential fatty acids (EFAs) each play different roles in our body. We will consider the metabolism of each separately.

Glycerol

When its supply runs low, our body can use the glycerol backbone of fats to make glucose by modifying the molecule (to pyruvate), and then hooking two of these molecules together.

In the opposite direction, glucose can be split in half to make two glycerol molecules when our body needs to make fats (triglycerides) out of excess sugars absorbed from our diet.

Saturated Fatty Acids (SaFAs)

SaFAs form part of all membranes, but are mainly used as fuel. Our body breaks down SaFAs to produce the energy necessary to drive the chemical reactions that make life possible.

Fatty acids to be used for energy are brought into our cells' furnaces (mitochondria) by first being hooked up with the carrier carnitine. Enzymes within our mitochondria then snip successive 2-carbon fragments (acetates) off the acid end of SaFA molecules (the process is called beta-oxidation) and injects these fragments into our cells' main energy-producing mechanism (scientists call it the Krebs or tricarboxylic acid cycle), which 'burns' them into carbon dioxide, water, and energy. The energy drives biochemical reactions that build and maintain our body structures, or dissipates as heat that keeps us warm. Too little carbohydrate fuel in the Krebs cycle 'fire' gives the signal for beta-oxidation of fats to begin, to supply added fuel to keep the fire going. On average, 40 to 45% of our energy comes from fats, and about the same amount comes from carbohydrates.

Short-chain SaFAs such as those found in butter and coconut oil, 'burn' better than long-chain (16 or more carbon atoms) SaFAs found in beef, mutton, and pork. Long-chain SaFAs also interfere with important reactions involving EFAs, and lower our metabolic rate and our vitality.

When there are too many calories – too much refined sugar, starch, or calorie-rich, concentrated food in our diet, excess 2-carbon acetate fragments are formed. They must be taken out of the energy factory to prevent the Krebs cycle fire from burning too hot. Our body makes SaFAs out of these excess acetate fragments by hooking them end to end. It stores them as body fat.

SaFAs to MUFAs. Our body makes enzymes that insert a *cis-* double bond into long-chain SaFAs and remove two hydrogen atoms at the same time. The molecules are bent at the *cis-* double bond carbons. Now they don't stack together as well, and their melting point goes down, which makes them more liquid than SaFAs (see Chapter 7, Liquid Oils and Unsaturated Fatty Acids). For example, stearic acid (SA,18:0) an 18-carbon SaFA, which melts at 70°C (158°F) and is hard at room (20°C [68°F]) and body (37°C [98.6°F]) temperatures, is changed into oleic acid (OA, 18:1w9), which melts at 13°C (55°F), and is liquid at both temperatures. Our body changes SA to OA by inserting a *cis-* double bond between carbon atoms 9 and 10 and removing a hydrogen from each of these carbons. While SA makes platelets stickier and more likely to form flow-impeding clots in blood vessels, increasing the risk of a stroke or heart attack, OA does not have this effect. Thus our body's ability to insert that *cis-* double bond into SA can save our life.

Inserting Double Bonds. The human desaturase enzymes that insert double bonds into fatty acid chains can insert them into positions w7, w9, w12, w15, etc., but are unable to insert double bonds into positions w6 and w3 (where double bonds are found in EFAs). These enzymes therefore cannot turn SaFAs into EFAs. Because of the absence in humans, of enzymes that do this, linoleic acid (LA, 18:2w6) with a double bond at w6, and alpha-linolenic acid (LNA, 18:3w3), with double bonds at w3 and w6[1], must be provided by foods, made by plants, and why it is *essential* that they come from foods.

Although exact measurements have not been published, our body's ability to insert double bonds into long-chain SaFAs is limited. Over-consumption of sticky SaFAs (the longer the chain, the stickier the SaFAs), combined with lack of essential minerals and vitamins can lead to blood vessel degeneration, clots, heart attacks, and strokes, pulmonary embolism, circulatory problems of the extremities, and blindness in diabetes (see Chapter 5, Hard Fats and Saturated Fatty Acids).

Monounsaturated Fatty Acids (MUFAs)

Like SaFAs, MUFAs are used in our membranes, and can be chopped down to produce energy in the same way as SaFAs, and by the same enzymes.

When there is deficiency of EFAs, several double bonds may be inserted into 16- or 18-carbon MUFAs to make them up to 3 or 4 times unsaturated. At the same time, they are also lengthened to 20-carbon fatty acids. They pinch-hit for the missing EFAs, but are unable to replace them completely. A large amount of these pinch-hitting molecules – such as Mead acid (20:3w9) – in our body, compared to the concentration of EFA derivatives is one indicator of EFA deficiency (see Chapter 8, The Healing Essential Fatty Acids).

The fibers (axons) of brain and nerve cells contain enzymes that lengthen 18-carbon MUFAs up to 24 carbon atoms without inserting any more double bonds. The insulation around each axon is largely made from these long-chain MUFAs.[2] Nervonic acid (24:1w9) is one such fatty acid.

Essential Fatty Acids (EFAs)

Our body burns EFAs for energy only when an *excess* of them is present. They stimulate metabolism, increase metabolic rate and oxidation, and speed up the rate at which our body burns fats and glucose when it gets more than 12 to 15% of total calories as EFAs. In these quantities (upwards of 3 tablespoons per day), EFAs help burn-off excess fats, and help a person to lose weight and stay slim.

---

[1] Both LA and LNA also contain a w9 double bond.

[2] The nerve cell bodies and synapses of axons, however, contain enzymes that transform EFAs into very highly unsaturated EFA derivatives.

EFAs are used to make phospholipids, the main structural components of cell membranes. In biologically active body tissues (including the brain and nerve cells, synapses, retinas, adrenals, testes) and in muscles, enzymes insert several extra double bonds into EFAs and lengthen them to 20- or 22-carbon chains. Alternately, these long and highly unsaturated fatty acids can be supplied by eating the oils of cold-water fish such as trout, salmon, and sardines.

EFAs interact with proteins in the transfer of electrons and energy in biological systems. These interactions are as complex as they are fascinating. EFAs take part in so many vital biochemical reactions and biological functions that they defy enumeration. The elusive nature of energy and electrons makes transfer reactions difficult to pin down. Life is a movement of energy, dancing via electrons from one molecule tip to another, not an array of static molecular chunks. A whole book could be written on the nature and importance of these transfer reactions. Much work remains to be done (see Chapter 8, The Healing Essential Fatty Acids) before we fully understand them.

Different kinds of fatty acids take part in different kinds of reactions. Nutritional fats are *not* all alike. Some harm, and others heal. Some enhance metabolism and others hinder it. Some bring oxygen to our tissues and others choke us. Some are vital and others are fatal. The interactions between different kinds of fatty acids, the chemical changes they undergo, the functions they have in our body, and the regulation of all of these functions are precise, specific, carefully controlled, and fascinating.

Major damage occurs to our health when we depart from the fresh whole foods – and the fresh, unaltered fats and oils – that nature created for us.

35 *Vitamin & Mineral Co-factors in Fat & Cholesterol Metabolism*

The metabolism of fats and oils cannot take place without help. The helpers in fat metabolism include enzymes that are proteins made in our body, and minerals and vitamins which are essential nutrients that must come from foods.

Enzymes

Each step in every chemical reaction in metabolism (see Chapter 34, Metabolism of Fats and Oils) requires the presence of a specific enzyme, without which that chemical reaction cannot occur. Enzymes are proteins made according to our genetic master plan or DNA (deoxyribonucleic acid), via blueprints of RNA (ribonucleic acid). They are made in response to our body's need, to encourage chemical reactions to take place – reactions that could not happen without them.

Enzymes are catalysts, facilitators, 'deal makers' between molecules. Like host or hostess at a party, some enzymes introduce strangers and facilitate or dissolve molecular friendships or couplings. Other enzymes dissolve molecular associations. Enzymes facilitate social interaction between molecules. And like experts with specific kinds of skills, specific enzymes facilitate specific interactions between specific molecules in a precise way, resulting in precise chemical changes leading to precise, predictable, reliable molecular results that allow life to carry on.

Minerals

To carry out their functions, enzymes are usually allied with an essential mineral servant or aide (co-factor), which we must get from foods. For example, over 80 enzymes are known to ally themselves with zinc. Without it, these enzymes can't do their job. Many other enzymes – such as those involved with energy production – must have magnesium to function. Several enzymes require copper. Some need iron. About 20 minerals take part in functions in our body. At least a dozen of these help enzymes to function – usually bound to the enzyme (protein) molecule.

Vitamins

The second group of substances essential for enzyme function are vitamins, which must also come from foods since our body cannot make them. Vitamins are more complex than minerals, and are associated more loosely with enzymes. Thirteen vitamin co-factors, without which many enzyme-catalyzed interactions between molecules cannot take place, are essential to human health.

Co-Factors in Lipid Metabolism

Several minerals and vitamins are involved in lipid metabolism. The involvement of others remains uncertain. Important as it is, this field of study is still in its infancy.

Antioxidants. Vitamins E and carotene are necessary to keep EFAs intact in our body, to protect them from destruction by oxygen and free radicals. These antioxidants keep EFAs capable of fulfilling their important duties. Vitamin C recharges spent vitamin E so that it can be reused.

Fatty acid breakdown. To clip 2-carbon fragments (acetates) off saturated fatty acids (beta-oxidation) involves several co-factors in several different enzyme steps. Vitamins B_2, B_3, pantothenic acid, sulphur, and potassium are required in different steps of beta-oxidation of saturated fatty acids (SaFAs).

SaFAs can also be broken down in other ways. These alternate pathways of fatty acid oxidation (alpha-oxidation and others) require vitamin B_{12}, pantothenic acid, biotin, sulphur, and magnesium in order to take place.

To burn acetates into carbon dioxide, water, and energy requires vitamins B_2, B_3, and iron as co-factors. Inserting *cis*- double bonds into SaFA molecules also requires iron and vitamins B_2 and B_3.

Synthesis. To synthesize fatty acids out of 2-carbon acetate fragments, vitamins B_2, B_3, and biotin are necessary co-factors.

Prostaglandins. To change EFAs into prostaglandins, several steps, each catalyzed by a specific enzyme, are involved. Each enzyme has its own co-factor requirement. The first step requires zinc, and is blocked by excess fats, cholesterol, SaFAs, *trans-* fatty acids, processed vegetable oils, and alcohol. The second step requires vitamin B_6. The third step requires zinc, vitamin B_3, and vitamin C. If a co-factor is missing, a step in prostaglandin production is blocked. If a co-factor is in short supply, prostaglandin production is slowed down. Altered levels of prostaglandins accompany many physical and some mental ailments (see Chapter 58, Prostaglandins) with signs and symptoms similar to those of EFA deficiency (see Chapter 8, The Healing Essential Fatty Acids) and degenerative diseases (see Chapter 70, Degenerative Diseases).

Cholesterol Transport. For transport in our blood, cholesterol must be hooked (esterified) to a fatty acid, preferably an EFA. Esterification requires vitamin B_6. To change cholesterol into bile acids, vitamin C is required.

From this partial list, we see that more than half of the known essential nutrients are required for lipid metabolism. These have to be supplied by our foods in adequate, or preferably optimum quantities. If we don't get them, the metabolism of fats, oils, and cholesterol cannot take place the way it should. When that happens, we lose our health and vigor.

Deranged fat metabolism lies at the root of many degenerative diseases. This derangement may be caused by too much of the wrong kinds of fats in our diet, too much total fat, or deficiency of the right kinds of fats. It may also be due to deficiency of necessary mineral and vitamin co-factors. For health, all essential nutrients have to be in place, working together.

An example will illustrate my point. Cancer, the enigma of our time, eludes every attempt to pinpoint a single cause. It often involves fatty degeneration, something gone haywire with the way cells handle fats and energy production.

There may be changes in the fat composition of cell membranes, there may be fat droplets within cells, there may be fats surrounding tumors. In animal experiments, it has been shown that cancer can be induced by an imbalance in any one of many nutrients. Deficiency of EFAs – too many SaFAs, too many calories, deficiency of zinc, iron, oxygen, vitamin A, vitamin C, vitamins B_1, B_2, B_6, pantothenic acid, vitamin E, sulphur, selenium, and protein (especially the amino acid methionine) – can lead to cancer. The list is not complete. A diet rich in these essential nutrient factors protects animals from both radiation- and chemically-induced cancers, and can reverse human cancers.

Co-factor Deficiencies

Large scale but incomplete nutritional surveys have uncovered essential nutrient deficiencies common among humans: vitamin C, E, B_6, and A, and the minerals iron, zinc, calcium, and magnesium. EFA deficiency and deficiencies of the other B vitamins are widespread. Over 60% of the population is deficient in one or more essential nutrients. A complete survey of all essential nutrients would bring the percentage of deficiencies higher, to perhaps as high as 90 or even 95% (see Chapter 37, Orthomolecular Nutrition, and Chapter 13, Essential Nutrients).

At least 68% of individuals die from degenerative diseases.

It does not take a brilliant mind to conclude that vitamins and minerals, the co-factors of fat metabolism, deserve more attention. For health, our diet needs to be complete. It needs to contain all essential nutrients. They must all work together to maintain health and a vigorous, long life.

Individuality **36**

Each human being is unique. Each of us has somewhat different requirements for building, maintaining, and regaining health. To find optimum health, each of us must find out for ourselves what exactly those requirements are.

"When God made me, he threw away the mold!" said 'the Fonz', a TV character from *Happy Days*. The same is true for every one of us. From the shape of our noses, the fullness of our lips, the curve of our necks, the color of our eyes, hair, and skin, and the shape, size, and structure of our bodies, we are individual and unique, and our uniqueness extends to the shape and capacity of our hearts, the length and strength of our bones, the weight of our brains, the placement and structure of our inner organs, the distribution and attachment points of our tendons, and the pattern and distribution of hair follicles. Our physical uniqueness and individuality finds expression in our unique athletic abilities, our sensory capabilities, our mental and intellectual capacity, our temperament, our artistic talents, and our aesthetic sensitivities.

Biochemical Individuality

While we *all* have in common the fact that we need proteins, fats, and carbohydrates, and while we *all* need the same 50 essential substances to build and maintain a healthy body, each of us is also *biochemically unique*. We differ in our ability to digest, to assimilate, and to metabolize foods. We differ in the chemical structure of our enzymes, and we differ in the efficiency of our enzyme systems. We differ in our nutritional requirements. We differ in the quantities of each essential nutrient that leads to optimum health. We differ in our food preferences, and often our food preferences reflect our genetic and biochemical differences.

Because we are unique, there is no single diet that is right for everyone. We must each find our own optimum diet by experimenting with foods and with essential nutrients, to discover what kinds and concentrations make us feel and perform at our physical and mental best.

Playing with Foods

When we were told not to play with our foods, we got bad advice. When we were told to eat what was on our plate, that too was bad advice. Instead, we *should* play with our foods: experiment and pay attention to how different foods affect our energy levels, moods, and body. We are feeling machines. Our body continuously generates feeling information that signals our biological condition. When we ignore the biological signals generated inside our body regarding our needs, in order to heed social signals regarding foods from outside, we begin a process that removes our awareness from our own nature, leads to poor food habits, and gradually results in physical deterioration.

Experiment with foods: the quantity, the quality, the combinations, the timing, and the brands. This is safe, if we listen to what our *body* tells us in terms of feeling. It is unwise to cut out food entirely for a month just on a whim. That's a 'head trip'. It may be foolish to decide to eat nothing but fried carrots for a year (another 'head trip').[1] But try different kinds of foods and food combinations, and try different concentrations and methods of nutrient enrichment in an open-ended way. Respond not from an idea or a taste, but respond to how your body feels. Become aware of it. Learn what the feelings mean.

We began this process in childhood, with food preferences. I balked at eating parsnips; some kids won't eat steaks; my mother insisted her carrots must be cooked. Within the same family, food preferences sometimes diverge as much as those of Jack Spratt and his wife. For about one year (I was 7 or 8), I *craved* cod liver oil – couldn't wait to get my daily spoonful! Before that year and since, I've hated it. When I was poisoned by pesticides, I *craved* cayenne for several months. Only later I found out that cayenne is one of the richest natural sources of vitamins A and C, which both detoxify and help repair and renew tissues.

As life goes on, we may get tired of foods we used to like. That's part of the process of discovery. Even when we turned green from our first cigarette and became dizzy from our first drink, that was part of our experimenting and our body sending us signals. We've been doing it for a long time. Our body already stores an enormous amount of information it has learned about foods, but we may not have paid much attention. We need to explore our body's experience in a conscious and systematic way.

---

1 It is unwise to impose *any* belief structure or philosophy – including macrobiotic, vegetarian, or others – on our food supply. Sooner or later, all food philosophies lead us away from health, Because our body's needs change with changing demands (athletic, sedentary, pregnancy, etc.), and the effects of aging, we should therefore listen to our body's *feeling* signals to determine our nutrient needs.

Several books can help us in our careful experiments with what we feed ourselves. While they cannot determine our optimum individual diet exactly, they give guidelines regarding types and concentrations of nutrients to try. These guidelines have been worked out by doctors and researchers who themselves have carefully experimented with the effects of nutrients on health, and who successfully treat patients using nutritional therapy. The titles of these books are listed in the bibliography under **Nutrition and Related Topics**. Use these guidelines, your own ability to feel, think, and act, your capacity to experiment and observe, and a little patience and common sense, to arrive at the individual diet on which you feel and function at your personal best.

Examples of Individuality

Some people cannot digest fresh salads without rice, and get diarrhea on the same salads that I consider a gift from heaven. Others cannot tolerate whole grains. Two spoonfuls of whole-grain cereal will send someone I know into severe depression with crying spells, confusion, and blackouts. Yet such a grain-based diet has helped people with extreme cases of cardiovascular disease and obesity regain their health. Some people on a 'cleansing diet', of raw vegetables and fruit may get cancer, even though cancer is usually associated with diets high in saturated fats and processed foods, and 'cleansing diets', usually help reverse cancer and degenerative diseases. What is good for us depends more on what our body needs than what the experts think.

Some people get nauseous, depressed, or 'foggy' from eating *oils,* but tolerate quite well the *seeds* of flax, walnut, sunflower, and pumpkin, all of which contain 35% or more of their weight as oil. One man I worked with was unable to digest *any* kind of fat, until he discovered flax oil, which became his new delicacy. Another could not use flax *oil,* but did very well on flax grain-containing dog food made from human quality ingredients. Still others can digest all fats. These examples of biochemical individuality are based both on genetic differences and environmental influences.

There are many other possible examples. Inability to digest lactose (milk sugar) or phenylalanine (an amino acid) are examples of nutritional individuality based on genetics. Other genetic conditions, such as sickle cell anemia and hemophilia, are examples of individuality that result from single changes in the genetic material (mutations). The number of points of possible changes in the genetic material run into the millions or billions, and the possible combination of possible changes run into astronomical figures. These are the genetic roots of individuality.

Individual Differences in Nutrient Requirements

Dr. Roger Williams, the researcher who pioneered work on biochemical individuality, found that requirements of each essential nutrient can vary tenfold or more among animals. One guinea pig may thrive on 1 mg/kg/day of vitamin C, whereas another might need more than 16 mg/kg/day in order to thrive equally well.

Variations in individuals' optimums for essential nutrient show a range similar to that given for vitamin C. In human subjects, it has been shown that, to be able to function normally, people who have schizophrenia may require hundreds or even a thousand times more vitamin C and vitamin B$_3$ than the average person. The normalizing effect of high doses of these two vitamins on the behavior of some schizophrenics is so striking that some researchers have suggested that schizophrenia is a deficiency disease caused by an inordinately high requirement for these vitamins, which is not met by usual diets.

Individual differences in EFA requirements. Studies to determine individual differences in the requirement for EFAs in humans have not been carried out. The requirement for men may be higher than that for women. Further studies will likely show that the range of optimum amounts of these substances will show a spread similar to that shown for other essential nutrients, perhaps tenfold or more, which may in part explain why different writers have come up with different 'daily requirements' for EFAs. Each of us must find our optimum level by careful observation and experimentation. I check my w3 level by how my skin feels. Skin that obtains sufficient w3s feels soft and velvety to touch. Skin that is too dry needs more EFA-rich oil. In cold weather, skin dries and requires more w3 oil than in warm weather.

Minimum. While 1 or 2% of daily calories as linoleic acid (LA, 18:2w6) prevents symptoms of LA deficiency in most people, optimums are higher, and some people's requirements may be still higher. Conditions of stress or disease modify the EFA requirement, and sugars, saturated fatty acids, and other substances in the food supply increase the EFA requirement.

Optimum. As with most essential nutrients, it appears likely that an optimum for EFAs is higher than the minimum requirement. An optimum amount has been suggested as 3 to 6% of daily calories as LA, 2% as LNA, and a combined total of EFAs of at least one-third of the total fat consumed. Your exact optimum level is something you must determine for yourself through practical experience.

37 *Orthomolecular Nutrition*

Orthomolecular nutrition offers the only real hope of reversing and preventing degenerative conditions. An overview of this healing field, the foundation for a field of *true* health care (and not just disease management), should be helpful.

Nutritional guidelines given by government agencies, taught in schools, passed on in medical practice, and adhered to by people are clearly inadequate for health. The fact that at least 68% of us die from food-related degenerative conditions confirms the findings of surveys that indicate over 60% of us lack some essential nutrients. The foods we eat at home, in cafeterias, restaurants, and hospitals are key factors leading to the epidemic of degenerative diseases that has overtaken us in this century. The fact that other people who eat other kinds of foods are not prone to degenerative disease strongly suggests that our food habits are to blame. The observation that healthy people from healthy dietary backgrounds become prone to degenerative diseases soon after they adopt our dietary ways,[1] strongly underlines that suggestion. People who have been cured of their degenerative afflictions by nutritional means add the exclamation point to the strongly underlined above suggestion.

'Orthomolecular'

Orthomolecular means 'with the right molecules'. Orthomolecular nutrition and orthomolecular medicine are synonymous terms, since foods and essential nutrients are the main 'medicines' of orthomolecular practices (injections of hormones are also part of these practices). Two-time Nobel prize winner (Chemistry and Peace) Dr. Linus Pauling defined orthomolecular medicine for the U.S. Senate in 1968 as the "preservation of good health and the treatment of disease by varying the concentration in the human body of substances that are normally present in the body and are required for health."[2] Orthomolecular nutrition refers to dietary measures (food, water, air, essential nutrients) that support the functions of healthy cells.

Its definition distinguishes orthomolecular nutrition from toximolecular medicine, which is the introduction into the body of alien (toxic, destructive, poisonous, polluting) substances – the present standard in medical practice – based on what, in cancer treatment, has come to be known as the 'cut, burn, and poison' approach of surgery, radiation, and drugs. Toximolecular medicine attempts to kill unhealthy cells and invading organisms with 'magic bullets'.

For building health, the toximolecular approach is fundamentally wrong. Toxic 'magic bullets', even if they do destroy the 'bad guys', also damage healthy cells. They undermine health, rather than build it. Governments make the same mistake when they spend our money chasing criminals instead of spending it to teach social cooperation and good citizenship.

In the last 90 years of using toximolecular medical approaches, deaths from degenerative diseases have risen from 15% of the population to 68% or more, an

---

[1] After adopting our dietary ways, healthy people do not *immediately* become prone to degenerative diseases, because degeneration needs time to develop. There is a time lag of 2 to 40 years before a person's health is compromised by poor food habits.

[2] Natural substances include vitamins, minerals, essential amino acids, essential fatty acids accessory, nutrients, water, oxygen, hormones, and enzymes.

increase of over 350%. Obviously, toximolecular medical intervention is not making us healthy.

Orthomolecular nutrition has yet to gain wide acceptance by the medical establishment but, in the hands of a few courageous doctors, is chalking up impressive records of healing successes. At present, the orthomolecular approach is being practiced largely by amateurs, for the simple reason that 'professionals' have refused to give it a fair hearing in spite of volumes of research evidence for its efficacy.

But the inevitable change is coming. In the last few months, I have seen mainstream media report on the usefulness of folic acid (a B complex vitamin) to prevent prenatal nervous system defects (spina bifida); the use of vitamins and minerals to prevent cancer, cardiovascular disease, aging, and other degenerative conditions; and the use of vitamin E in doses many times greater than the government-set Recommended Daily Allowance (RDA) to prevent cardiovascular disease. Research literature of the benefits of many other nutrients is readily available in mainstream research journals.

Nationwide Nutritional Deficiencies

Nationwide surveys that measured the food intake of thousands of people in North America indicate that more than 60% of the population is deficient in one or more essential nutrients. The surveys tested only 13 of about 45 known essential nutrients, and used as their standard for adequate nutrition the RDAs, which are estimated amounts of each essential nutrient that prevent deficiency symptoms in healthy adults.

RDAs do not account for increased requirements during pregnancy, lactation, growth, puberty, activity, athletic performance, stress, infection, injury, convalescence, or aging. All of us fit into one of the listed categories for a large part of our lives. As such, RDAs are estimates, not of optimum requirements for good health, but of standards just above minimum. Also, RDAs are statistical averages, not indications of individual requirements which, as we discussed in Chapter 36, can vary for each nutrient by a factor of 10 or more. At worst, RDAs are official standards of accepted levels of substandard nutrition, inadequate to maintain optimum health for almost everyone. The present trend is toward increasing malnutrition.

The most common deficiencies found in these surveys were of iron, calcium, zinc, magnesium, vitamins C, A, E, B_6, B_2, and folic acid. Other surveys have turned up frequent deficiencies of iodine, manganese, copper, chromium (90% deficient), and selenium. W3 deficiencies may be over 90% (see Chapter 13, Essential Nutrients).

Studies carried out in hospitals have shown that over 50% of patients became nutritionally deficient and more ill from eating hospital foods, and not as a direct result of their illness. Even the diets of hospital dieticians were found to contain inadequate amounts of vitamin B_6, even when measured by the already-low RDA standard for that vitamin.

Orthomolecular Practice

When a person visits a doctor practicing orthomolecular medicine, the doctor may measure that person's nutritional status by testing blood, hair, or tissue levels of essential nutrients. These tests, relatively simple to carry out,[3] frequently indicate deficiencies. When deficiencies are corrected by improved diet and oral or injected supplements of the missing essential nutrients, usually a change for the better occurs. Large doses of certain nutrients may be used, because some people have much higher requirements of these nutrients than others.

Deficiency. Orthomolecular practice cures obvious deficiency diseases such as scurvy (lack of vitamin C), pellagra (lack of vitamin B_3), beriberi (lack of vitamin B_1), and soft bones (lack of vitamin D). Deficiency of each essential nutrient has its particular set of degenerative symptoms as our body gradually loses its ability to function and finally falls apart because of inadequate amounts of that nutrient. Symptoms of deficiency of each of the two EFAs have been listed (see Chapter 8, The Healing Essential Fatty Acids). Prolonged severe deficiency of any single essential nutritional substance has to be fatal.

Sub-clinical deficiency states, which are less severe than those that result in the classical symptoms of scurvy, beriberi, etc,. also occur. For instance, a less severe (sub-clinical) deficiency of vitamin C results in tissue weakness (e.g., bleeding and receding gums), because vitamin C is necessary to build the major component of connective tissue (the protein collagen).

Connective tissue holds the body together. Sub-clinical deficiency of zinc slows down wound healing, because zinc is required in healing functions. Subclinical deficiency of vitamin A results in proneness to infection and poor skin condition, because this vitamin has important immune functions and is necessary for healthy skin. Sub-clinical deficiency of nutrients lowers our body's ability to withstand stress.

Each essential nutrient has its own set of sub-clinical symptoms. These symptoms result in suboptimal functioning of the whole organism, lowered vitality, and feelings of malaise rather than definable disease. Over many years, often precipitated by increased stress, clinically definable diseases finally do occur. These diseases are considered by medical professionals that are untrained and unknowledgeable about the link between nutrition and optimal health to be of 'unknown cause'.

Duped medical students. To be fair to doctors, they did not *choose* to ignore nutrition when they were medical students. Their lack of nutritional education is largely the result of having had a *drug-oriented curriculum imposed on them*. Pharmaceutical companies, which have gained handsomely from this

---

[3] These tests monitor tissue, serum, and urine levels of vitamins, minerals, and metabolites of essential nutrients and other orthomolecular substances. Hair samples can be sent to laboratories for an accurate analysis of *some* of the minerals.

approach, have exercised a strong influence over the course content of medical studies and the politics of medical associations. Business considerations have duped the last 2 or 3 generations of doctors (see Chapter 58, Snake Oil and Patent Medicines).

Happily, the profession is slowly changing, largely due to demands for more natural treatments in an age where more information is available to all. An informed public has been forced to lead rather than follow the professionals. Keep up the pressure. Push your doctor to learn orthomolecular nutrition. Become an ornery patient if you are unsatisfied, or take charge of your health yourself by becoming better educated about it. Insist on natural treatments for degenerative conditions *before* accepting drugs, surgery, radiation and other invasive procedures, except in life-threatening crises.

Optimum Levels. Orthomolecular nutrition attempts to bring the levels of all essential nutrients in our body up to the minimum required level for health, and beyond that, to their optimum level for well-being, vitality, and accomplishment.

Excess. Orthomolecular nutrition also concerns itself with lowering the concentration of substances natural to the body that may be present in excessive quantities. Examples of such substances are glucose and saturated fats. We reduce the concentrations of these substances by decreasing our dietary intake of sweet and fatty foods, and by increasing exercise.

Genetics. Orthomolecular nutrition also addresses itself to genetic diseases such as phenylketonuria (PKU), whose effects can be prevented by designing a special diet low in the amino acid phenylalanine (Phe). The presence of Phe in the diet of PKU infants causes mental retardation and other problems. Genetic diseases of fat and cholesterol metabolism, which result in very high serum levels of these substances and carry high risk of cardiovascular disease and death when accompanied by inadequate vitamin and mineral nutrition, can be helped by nutrient-enriched diets that lower food content of fats and cholesterol.

Hormones and enzymes. Orthomolecular medicine uses natural hormones such as insulin, thyroxin, and other glandular products to treat patients with defectively functioning glands. Orthomolecular nutrition also uses enzymes, hydrochloric acid, bile, fiber, and acidophilus bacteria to improve digestion and bowel function. Enzyme injections can also be part of orthomolecular practice.

Large doses. Another aspect of orthomolecular nutrition is 'megavitamin' therapy, in which large doses of vitamins are taken by people who, for reasons of disease or biochemical individuality (see Chapter 36, Individuality), require larger than average amounts of certain vitamins for normal functioning. They also help those consuming diets deficient in vitamins. Mainstream medicine, which tends to view 'megavitamin' therapy with contempt (some say it just makes expensive urine), nevertheless routinely inject mega doses of vitamin B_{12} (1000 times the RDA), and have recently added mega doses of vitamin B_3 (several hundred times the RDA) to their treatment of cardiovascular disease (CVD). Research and clinical results indicate that 5 to 50 times more vitamin E than the RDA protects arteries against damage that can lead to CVD.

Plenty of evidence links different disease states, both physical and mental, with deficiencies of essential nutrients, with excesses of some nutrients, and with imbalances of the levels of various nutrients in the human body. Orthomolecular nutrition and therapy are effective because they treat nutritional problems at their nutritional source, with nutritional substances, altering the concentrations in our body of these natural substances.

Toximolecular Practice

Triumphs. Medical science has made tremendous progress in the control of infectious diseases. Smallpox, diphtheria, typhoid, yellow fever, rabies, and polio have been eradicated or controlled through vaccinations. Childhood diseases have been defeated. By controlling bacteria that cause infections, antibiotics have taken the threat out of them.[4] Medical technology has taken huge strides. Surgical techniques, life support systems, diagnostic tools, and lab tests are sophisticated. Doctors have become very skillful in their application.

Toxic drugs. However, these medical triumphs have also brought problems. One problem with medicine is our overwhelming reliance on synthetic, toxic, but patentable drugs. Toximolecular medicines *cure* no diseases. Natural organisms do not suffer from deficiencies or imbalances of unnatural toximolecular substances such as aspirins, tranquilizers, or painkillers.

Drugs may remove, mask, or 'bury' symptoms of diseases caused by other factors, and because symptoms are thus put to sleep, the use of drugs destroys our incentive to find root causes and real cures. Drugs cause many diseases ('side effects') themselves. Alien molecules disrupt the delicate, precise architectural design of our body and the life-sustaining functions based in this architecture. For example, diuretics deplete potassium, resulting in heartbeat abnormalities. Birth control pills result in water retention and behavioral changes, and deplete our body of vitamins B_6, B_{12}, and folic acid. Tranquilizers interfere with cell membrane functions, resulting in lowered vitality, sleep without rest, and increased risk of cancer. Antibiotics and cortisone both interfere with our immune system, increasing our risk of cancer. Antibiotics can also cause rashes, nausea, vomiting, anemia, joint pain, and yeast infections, as well as failure of intrauterine devices (IUDs) for birth control. Drugs used for conditions such as rheumatoid arthritis can have serious and wide-ranging side effects.

---

[4] On the other hand, antibiotics are useless against colds, flu, hepatitis, and other viral infections, and inhibit our immune system. They also select for survival, those bacteria that have developed resistance to antibiotics. The net result is that antibiotics make *us* weaker and *bacteria* stronger.

The lists of detrimental, toxic 'side' effects of all pharmaceutical drugs are very long, requiring books such as the *Physicians Desk Reference* and others to keep doctors informed. Even 'harmless' aspirin causes about 40 deaths each year from internal bleeding.

Business. But synthetic drugs, regardless of their toxicity to human health, can be patented to protect huge profits for the companies that make them. These companies often start with a natural (and therefore unpatentable) remedy or herb that affects human functions, and isolate its most potent active (effective) ingredient. Then they use chemical methods to change the ingredient's configuration slightly to make it synthetic and therefore patentable – strictly a business consideration – but also more toxic because the changed configuration won't fit our body's molecular structures like the natural molecule did (and therefore has side effects). Then the companies sell the patented, non-natural substance as a drug under patent-protected profits of as much as 600% or even more for 17 to 20 years, in preference of the natural substance. We have created business structures that mediate against natural living and our own health. In the long run, these business structures cannot work for us and must be changed.

The patented drugs are used to 'manage' (suppress) symptoms of disease. If we remember that symptoms are our body's messages to alert us that something is amiss, requires our attention, and needs to be changed, then suppressing symptoms with drugs while our health continues to deteriorate makes no sense. Worse than killing the proverbial messenger who delivers bad news, we are cutting off his tongue before he finishes his message, one that we need to hear in order to arrange for our survival and safety.

Responsibility. Another – and key – problem is that our reliance on medical technology has made us less inclined to take care of ourselves to keep strong from within, to make our bodies capable of fighting infections and other threats to health. Our reliance more on doctors and technology than on ourselves and nature has resulted in what is called the 'passive patient syndrome', a giving up of personal responsibility for health.

These are unfortunate changes. My heart attack *kills* me, but *pays* my doctor. The pain and suffering of illnesses are personal. The expenses of treatments that provide neither reversal nor cure have become financially unmanageable.

Primary health care. It is important for individuals to take charge of their own health. Since our entire body is made from food, water, air, (and light), *primary health care* cannot rest in synthetic drugs and high technology, but must be built on appropriate choices of what we eat, drink, and breathe. Primary health care through the proper use of food, water, and air to build a properly functioning body will always remain the personal responsibility of the one doing the eating, drinking, and breathing. We carry out that responsibility (for better or worse) with our knives, forks, spoons, cups, and plates.

Essential nutrients and other orthomolecular substances play key roles in primary health care. Remaining problems should be subjected to secondary intervention by drugs and medicines only *after* primary, self-responsible health care has been thoroughly put in practice.

Returning What's Missing

Major causes of degenerative diseases include nutrient deficiency, food pollution, and imbalance. Essential nutrients have been removed from the natural whole foods eaten by our ancestors (see Chapter 16, From Seed to Oil) by processing, by nutrient losses occurring during storage and transport, and by unbalanced farming methods that leave soils depleted. They have been poisoned by the addition of artificial, non-natural, toxic ingredients to our food supply. Our food choices have been influenced by a constant barrage of advertising (see Chapter 24, Advertising and Jargon).

In fact, degenerative diseases are almost always caused by malnutrition and/or internal pollution (see Chapter 90, The Biological Basis of Natural Therapies). They can be reversed and cured only by nutrient enrichment and/or detoxification. Less than 0.5% of degenerative conditions are caused by 'bad genes', but at least 68% of the population dies from degenerative conditions. Effective treatment for these diseases means a return to whole food habits followed by our ancestors, to food choices which adequately cover our known nutrient requirements, to a way of eating more in harmony with the ways of nature. Orthomolecular nutrition attempts to move us in that direction, returning to our bodies, often in concentrated form, essential nutrients that went missing from our diets.

Stress and the Battery of Life **38**

Our capacity for dealing with stress has limits. If we exceed those limits, our body breaks down and we become ill. Let us look at how our stress coping system works, how fats are involved in this system, and how we can increase our body's capacity for dealing with the physical and mental stresses of life without getting burned out.

Stress takes two forms that share biological mechanisms: *positive stress* that we *choose* to engage in, which includes challenges, romance, and sex; and *negative stress*, which we perceive as being *imposed* on us, over which we feel powerless. Positive stress strengthens us; negative stress demeans us and tears us down.

Stress and the General Adaptation Syndrome

Hans Selye received worldwide recognition for his inquiries into the nature of negative stress. He (and later, other scientists as well) showed that many different kinds of stress – cold, heat, noise, overexertion, mental and emotional stress, forced physical restraint, injury, sensory overload, toxic chemicals, x-ray and other radiation, deprivation of food or love, overeating, even pregnancy – produce a common set of biological response symptoms. From his observations, he concluded that one underlying adaptive mechanism deals with all types of stress. Selye named this common set of symptoms which occur in response to stress the General Adaptation Syndrome (GAS), and divided GAS into three distinct stages.

1. *Alarm reaction.* The organism (Selye worked with chicks, rats, hamsters, and rabbits, but similar observations have also been made with humans) displays restlessness, nervousness, 'jitters', and other non-specific and non-directed behavioral signs of agitation.

2. During the stage of *resistance,* which follows the alarm reaction, the organism actively uses its inner resources (we'll discuss the biochemical components of these resources below) to deal with the stress. Directed activity and specific biochemical functions within an organism characterize the stage of resistance, and if the inner resources are sufficient to overcome the stress, the animal adapts and recovers.

3. If stress is greater than an organism's adaptive resources, the resources are depleted, and *exhaustion* occurs. What Selye called 'diseases of adaptation' (more appropriately, diseases due to the failure to adapt) result from exhaustion, and minor additional stresses can then kill us. The most noticeable organ changes during exhaustion include enlarged stress-fighting (adrenal) glands and atrophied (shrunken) immune system (lymph and thymus). Diseases of adaptation include high blood pressure, water retention, arthritis, heart enlargement, strokes, ulcers, kidney disease, eclampsia and toxemia of pregnancy, allergies, diabetes, neurological problems, and cancer. These disease symptoms resemble symptoms of essential fatty acid (EFA) deficiency (see Chapter 8, The Healing Essential Fatty Acids). They also resemble modern-day degenerative diseases (see Chapter 70, Degenerative Diseases).

The 'Life Battery'

It appeared to Selye that there was within each organism a sort of 'life battery' that stores life current in a way similar to the way an electric battery stores electric current – a battery with a limited capacity, that runs down when used without recharging. Selye wondered what the biochemical basis of this life battery might be, and whether there was a way to recharge the battery when it ran down.

Selye did his major work in the 1940s. He was a doctor, not a biochemist, and biochemical techniques that are common now were not known then, so Selye had no way of answering his own question. It remained for others who followed to elucidate the biochemical and molecular mechanisms underlying the experimental observations that Selye made on tissue, organ, and organism levels.

The analogy of the life battery turns out to be a good one. A battery has two poles, positive and negative, between which currents of energy will flow under suitable conditions, that is, when the circuit is completed. This happens to be true for our life battery as well. It too, has two poles. Between these two poles, our life energy flows when our circuit is completed. Biochemically, the poles of our life battery are good oils and good proteins – oils rich in EFAs, and sulphur-rich proteins: oils containing many slightly negatively charged *cis-* double bonds and proteins containing many slightly positively charged sulphydryl groups. On our life battery, good oils are the negative pole and good proteins the positive pole. Between these two poles, our life currents, produced by the metabolism of carbohydrates and other molecules, flow when the circuit of essential nutrients is complete.

In biological terms, one could call good oils the female pole, because eggs and female bodies contain more of these oils, and good proteins the male pole, because sperm and male bodies contain more sulphur and more of these proteins. But both males and females need both poles for health. Present-day diets are usually protein-rich but lacking in good oils. The result of an unbalanced life battery is lowered capacity to withstand stress, easier breakdown of health, and degeneration.

The more we are stimulated and stressed, the more life current must flow between the poles of our battery, the more good oils and good proteins are used up, and the sooner our life battery runs down. Oils and proteins must be continually replaced through foods to recharge our battery, starting at birth and ending only at death.

More stress requires more oils and proteins (as well as minerals and vitamins); less stress requires less. Whenever the demand by our body for good oils and good proteins plus mineral and vitamin co-factors exceeds that supplied by our foods, our body begins to run down, and we slowly develop deficiency as our reserves of these substances are used up. With deficiency comes weakness, then sickness. The severity of the sickness depends on the severity of the deficiency. We require rest then, a chance to reorganize our resources, and good nutrition to replenish low supplies.

The cure for a run-down life battery (nutrient deficiency and sickness) involves increased intake of good oils, good proteins, and co-factors through the use of foods that are rich in these nutrients. Continuing good health requires maintaining optimum intake of all essential nutrients, to provide for the demands on our bodies of a changing environment with fluctuating levels of stress.

Protein and oils are the two most abundant substances in our cells and those of all other animals, plants, and single-celled organisms. We find them together in cell membranes, in lipoproteins that carry fats and cholesterol in our blood, and in membranes of subcellular organelles (see Chapter 8, The Healing Essential Fatty Acids). They form the main structures and functional components of our entire body.

Completing the Circuit

Vitamins and minerals, as well as other substances that our body can produce from nutrients, complete the circuit (see Chapter 35, Vitamin and Mineral Co-factors). They are the supporting cast, with oils and proteins the stars in the drama of life. Vitamins C, E, and A, and the minerals zinc, selenium, and iron are especially important, but all essential nutrients are necessary. The absence of any one of them is itself an intolerable internal nutritional stress.

The fast pace at which we live runs down our life battery. Life in the fast lane is faster, but also shorter. The better our nutrition, the longer we can stand up to this pace; the worse our nutrition, the sooner we fall apart. Degenerative diseases, fatty degeneration, diseases of civilization, Selye's 'diseases of adaptation', and what Budwig (see Chapter 63, Budwig, Flax Oil, and Protein) calls the 'fat syndrome' all refer to the same conditions, characterized by a run-down life battery. All worsen under increased stress and poor food choices, the latter being the *greatest* single stress to which we subject our bodies. Degenerative diseases share many symptoms, aggravating factors, and alleviating factors (see Chapter 70, Degenerative Diseases).

Relationship of Oil with Protein

We can get too much oil or too much protein if either is taken by itself over the long term (see Chapter 62, Oil and Protein Work Together), and we can get too little. Oil and protein belong together, work together, and protect each other.

Budwig's program for treating terminal cancer by nutritional means pre-scribes good oil and good protein together. For most of us, however, protein intake is already adequate or even too high. The addition of good oils to our diet is the critical factor.

Most biological cancer treatments limit protein intake at first, rather than increasing it, because high protein intake has toxic effects on liver and kidneys. Many people have allergic reactions to dairy products, which further compromise their immune system. A protein that does not produce allergies (such as tofu) must then be found.

Body signals. Our body knows its needs. Hunger signals us to start to eat; satiety signals us to stop. If these signals were ineffective, our eating would get completely out of proportion and we'd blow up from overeating or waste away from not eating at all.

When the natural composition of foods is altered by processing, removal of nutrients, chemical changes, artificial flavors, and additives, our hunger receptors can become confused, and our eating can get out of proportion. This can result in obesity.

Wild animals eating natural foods don't get fat. Humans who eat natural foods rich in nutrients are also unlikely to become obese. Domesticated animals that share their masters' unnatural nutrition habits and nutritional stresses also share their degenerative conditions.

The average diet of people living in industrialized countries contains ample good protein, because we live in a protein-, muscle-, and male-conscious society. The meat, egg, and dairy industries have successfully convinced us of our need for protein. Besides, proteins are present in all living tissues, and all natural foods contain protein. Protein foods are easy to store, because they can be dried or frozen, and keep well for a long time.[1]

Destruction of Protein's Oil Partner

Good oils, however, the equally necessary partner of good protein, are systematically destroyed by our methods of processing, storage and food use. Oils do not keep well, because light, oxygen, heat, and time destroy their delicate *cis-* double bonds (see Chapter 8, The Healing Essential Fatty Acids). Even refrigeration does not protect oils from destruction by light and oxygen, although freezing them solid will stop deterioration quite effectively.

Exclusion of light, air, and heat throughout pressing, filling, storing, and transporting procedures up to the point of consumption keeps good oils intact. For oil sources or for help with the design and development of machinery and processes, see Services Provided, at the back of the book.

Destroyed oils are foreign and toxic to our body. They cannot couple with good proteins, cannot recharge our life battery, and interfere with the action of oils that can recharge our battery. When the female, softening, receptive partner to protein is absent, our life battery ends up with only one pole. No life current flows, because the circuit is interrupted, and the current has nowhere to go.

The deficiency of EFA-containing oils is one of the greatest stresses in our technological way of life. We don't need huge amounts of them, but they are extremely important. 'Good' oils effectively alleviate degenerative conditions because they return the missing EFAs in their natural state to EFA-deficient diets.

---

[1] Protein deficiency *can* occur due to food allergies and digestive (usually pancreas) malfunction, in which the proteins consumed are not completely broken down and absorbed. Some elderly, poor, and mentally ill citizens also suffer from inadequate protein nutrition.

39 Antioxidants & the Fire That is Life

A balanced diet supplies foods that can provide the energy we need to live, and also provides substances which prevent that energy from doing damage to our cells.

Humans tend to get out of balance by looking at only one aspect of our life to the exclusion of others. We do it by siding with one half of an issue, and ignoring, forgetting, or even fighting the other. The story of fats and oils in human health has certainly seen its share of one-sidedness. But the entire story of nutrition and human health has also suffered from a one-sided approach.

Antioxidants – One Side of the Nutrition Story

Over the last 20 years or so, an increasing amount of attention has been given to substances popularly known as 'antioxidants' (AOs). Free radicals are like sparks coming off a fire, and AOs prevent free radical reactions (see Chapter 21, Light, Free Radicals, and Oils) from becoming uncontrolled free radical *chain* reactions (showers of sparks) that damage our cells and tissues, and lead to premature aging. Rightly, the importance of AOs including vitamins C, E, and A (carotene), and the elements selenium, sulphur, zinc, and manganese have been emphasized. Vitamin B_3, B_6, and K also belong on the list, along with coenzyme Q_{10} and dozens of bioflavonoids. All act as AOs. All are important to health. Many are removed from standard diets when grains, oils, sugarcane, beets, and other whole foods are processed. For health, the lost AOs must be replaced.

With all the attention that free radicals are getting, we are told to increase our intake of AOs to improve spark control. Some writers have even recommended decreasing our intake of substances, such as essential fatty acids, that produce the fire that produces free radicals. This second piece of advice is wrong.

It is true that we can prevent sparks by decreasing the fire. In fact, the only way that sparks can be completely prevented is by extinguishing the fire which, in our analogy, means death. I don't think we want to recommend that!

The Fire of Life – the Other Side of the Nutrition Story

The inner fire of human life results from burning (oxidizing) foods – the fuels for our life's fire. The differences between a fire and our 'fire of life' are that ours is slower, takes place in water, is driven by sunlight energy, and is enzymatically controlled to go in a particular direction that allows life to take human form. But the chemistry is exactly the same: carbohydrates (wood versus starch) or oils (petrochemical versus edible oils) are changed into water and carbon dioxide, releasing energy that was stored in the bonds of their molecules.

190

The brightness of the fire is the rate at which our body produces energy – our metabolic rate. For continued good health, it is vital that the fire of life burns brightly. When our body has used up the fuel supplied by previously consumed foods, our metabolic rate decreases. Our fire of life dies down due to lack of fuel from which to make energy. We start to feel hungry (may even feel tired, dizzy, or weak), and eat foods to replenish our body's energy-producing fuel supply. These fuels – 'pro-oxidants' – are the substances that burn (oxidize), increase metabolic rate, and increase energy levels.

The major pro-oxidants – our cells' fuel – that nature uses to build the fire of life within us are glucose, fatty acids, and oxygen. Fruit sugar (fructose) and table sugar (sucrose) are other pro-oxidants. Too much of any of the simple sugars at any one time increases the fire too much. We get antsy, energetic, and hyper, and the body releases control mechanisms to dampen the excessive fire, partly by turning excess sugars into saturated fats, which slow the fire down.

Essential fatty acids (EFAs) – especially the w3 EFA and its derivatives – are like a poker that stokes the fire, increasing oxidation and metabolic rate in a sustained way over a longer time, unlike the yo-yo effect produced by sugars. Fats include a whole range of substances that modify metabolic rate, some slowing it down and others speeding it up. Iodine (thyroid) is a regulator of oxidation rate (again, like a poker stoking a fire), which speeds up oxidation, metabolic rate, and energy production.

In order for pro-oxidants to perform their functions, a long list of vitamins and minerals is necessary, including the B-complex, vitamins, iron, potassium, chromium, magnesium, calcium, and others.

A common feature of many degenerative diseases is decreased oxidation, decreased metabolic rate, and low energy levels. Our cells (like tired people) lack the energy to do all of their housecleaning. Biochemical dust piles up, the cellular house gets dirty, and molecular wastes and toxins accumulate. Our liver, which is our main organ for detoxification, also slows down in its functions when energy levels decrease, and garbage piles up in our body even more. Under these circumstances, we want to increase the energy levels of our cells, tissues, and organs so they are fit to do their housework.

Controlling Sparks by Using Antioxidants

Our inner fire of life *must* burn fuels like glucose and fatty acids to create a bright, healthy fire to give us energy. This process creates free radicals as short-lived intermediates, a normal occurrence in energy production. But this energy-producing process is 2 to 5% inefficient, which means that some of the free radicals, like sparks from a fire, escape. They can start other fires in unintended places and are not conducive to normal biological functions (health). AOs provide spark control.

Obviously, the stronger the fire, the more sparks it produces. Here is where our intake of AOs becomes important. Increasing our intake of spark-controlling

AOs is good advice, as long as we have also built a strong fire. AOs *do* prevent free radicals from getting out of hand. They *do* slow down aging processes and neutralize toxins.

Much of nature's supply of AOs is removed from foods by processing practices geared to convenience, taste, shelf-life, and profit rather than health. Having lost AOs from foods, we must return them to our diet by replacing processed foods with whole foods, drinking freshly pressed juices, using foods super-rich in essential nutrients, or taking concentrates of these essential nutrients. A growing understanding of the importance of AOs is one of the factors that led to the growth of the food supplement industry.

Finding the Balance

The processing that resulted in losses of AOs also resulted in losses of pro-oxidants and their co-factors: complex carbohydrates, B-complex vitamins, EFAs, potassium, magnesium, calcium, iron, iodine, and others. We must return these pro-oxidants to our food supply – as whole foods or as supplements. They are as vital to our health as AOs.[1]

We must find and keep a balance between pro-oxidant fuels that keep our fire of life burning brightly, and AO nutrients that provide spark control to keep the fire from burning out of control. Both are equally important. Both are required for health.

40 Why Calorie Counting Fails & What to Do to Lose Weight

Calorie counting is a futile endeavor. There are safer and more effective ways to regulate body weight. Let us examine this proposition. Many factors besides calories affect our weight. If we fail to consider other nutrient and life-style factors, calorie counting will fail. A simpler approach – one that makes calorie tables and charts unnecessary – is more effective.

Basic Facts

The energy released for body functions when foods are oxidized or 'burned' in our body is measured in calories (more correctly Kilocalories [or Kcal], which is the

---

[1] By cutting down the trees and plants that produce oxygen – the major non-food pro-oxidant we need – we slowly choke ourselves. Better management of our planet's flora (weeds and poisonous green plants also make precious oxygen) is also key to human health.

energy necessary to raise the temperature of 1000 grams [2.2 pounds] of water by one degree Celsius [1.8°F]). Calories come from proteins, carbohydrates, fats, and alcohol. Calories in excess of our body's needs are stored as fat, and therefore all calories are potential sources of fat.

An adult person burns about 2500 Kcal daily, or just over 100 calories per hour on average. The rates may slow down to 60 during sleep and may increase to 150 during normal daytime activity. Walking and biking burn 300 calories per hour. It takes 30 hours of walking to use up 1 kg of fat (or 14 hours to lose one pound), but only 13.5 hours of intense aerobic dancing to burn a kg (6 hours per pound), because intense aerobic dancing burns 665 calories per hour. If only I could discipline myself to walk for an hour *instead* of having dessert!

The total calories (Kcal), consumed each day by men varies from 1500 to 4000 for most males; the total for females varies from 900 to 2500. The extremes are wider, and go from 0 on a water fast (with loss of weight) to over 8000 Kcal for a logger, who burns them all through work without gaining an ounce, and as high as 12,000 Kcal per day for professional weight lifters and body builders. [1] (footnote: For comparison, an elephant lumbers its way through 50,000 Kcal each day, derived from several hundred pounds of grass.)

Fat stores more than twice as much energy, at 9 Kcal per gram, as does an equal weight of carbohydrate or protein, each of which stores 4 Kcal of energy per gram. Alcohol provides 7 Kcal per gram. Our body's major energy reserve is fat, the most efficient way to carry energy, in terms of both volume and weight. Vitamins and minerals, although essential to our health, contain no calories at all.

More Facts

Each kilogram of body fat produces 9000 Kcal of energy. An average adult carries 10 kg of deposited body fats, which means a reserve of 90,000 Kcal. At 2000 to 2500 Kcal per day, this allows about 40 days without food but, since metabolic rate slows down when a person fasts, the stored fat may provide energy for as long as 85 days on a fast (but vitamin, mineral, and protein depletion may have grave consequences, such as death, and therefore extended fasting should never be undertaken lightly).

Food Sources of Calories

The food groups that supply the calories in a typical Western diet are as follows (percentage amounts listed are percentages of total calories consumed):

meat	20%	eggs	2%
refined cereals and flour	18%	alcohol	2%
refined fats	18%	dairy products	12%
sugar	17%		
high fiber foods (whole grains, vegetables, and fruit)		11%	

Another study, which breaks the Western diet down according to food constituents, concludes that this diet is typically made up as follows:

Fats provide 42% of the total calories consumed daily.[2] Of these, 18% are visible refined fats such as butter, margarine, shortenings, and oils. The other 24% are hidden in various foods.

Carbohydrates provide 46% of the total calories consumed daily. Of these, 17% are refined sugar, 20% are refined cereal products such as breakfast cereals and refined flour bakery products, 3% are alcohol, and only 6% come from complex unrefined carbohydrates.

Proteins provide 12% of daily calories.

According to the figures given above, at least 58% of the calories in the typical refined Western diet come from 'empty calorie' foods (white fats, 'white' (refined) oils, white sugar, white flour products, and alcohol), most of whose minerals, vitamins, and fiber have been removed by processing and refining.

Calories as a Source of Fat

Refined, 'empty calorie' foods are likely to cause us to gain fat. They cause us to overeat. One of the mechanisms that turns off hunger is a feeling of fullness. By the time we've filled up on these concentrated-calorie, fiber-poor foods, we've eaten more calories than we need. The excess turns to fat. When we obtain adequate amounts of all essential nutrients, biological hunger ceases. If our foods are nutrient-deficient, we may overeat until we get them, which is one reason why nutrient enrichment is important for staying slim.

Because they lack fiber and bulk, high-calorie refined foods also slow down intestinal activity. They take up to five times longer to pass through the intestinal tract than do natural, unrefined, high-fiber foods (75 hours compared to 15) and the body absorbs calories during the entire time of their constipated passage.

Foods cannot be metabolized properly without minerals and vitamins. The energy that 'empty calorie' foods contain becomes unavailable to our body and is stored as fat until (or in the hope that) we get the necessary minerals and vitamins at some later time. In the meantime, we feel hungry, and eat more. This too, turns into fat, unless minerals and vitamins are also provided.

Minerals, vitamins, and essential fatty acids (EFAs) are systematically removed from foods during refining. Their absence lowers our metabolic rate; we feel less like being active and become lethargic. Then, even if we eat less, we don't burn up the calories we eat, and get fat even on a low-calorie diet.

---

[2] The percentage of calories supplied by fats is probably higher, because of increasing consumption of fat-rich fried, deep-fried, processed, and fast foods, and sugars that turn into fats in our body.

Reasons for Failure

Calorie counting as a way of keeping weight down does not work. It is easy enough to count the calories, but counting calories is not the same as burning them, just as thinking about exercise is not exercising. There are so many factors that modify the rate at which our body burns calories that simply regulating the number of calories we consume is ineffective in the battle against the bulge.

Caloric burns. The caloric values of foods printed in books assumes that foods containing them are completely burned or oxidized. In practice, our body burns some foods better than others, and there are individual differences in food-burning ability. The caloric value of fats is overrated, because fats, especially when present in large amounts in the diet, may not be completely burned to carbon dioxide and water. Instead, they oxidize partially and produce ketones, which are like charcoal that is left when wood is not completely burned to ashes (or like carbon deposited on the pistons of an engine whose fuel-air mixture is unbalanced). Until our kidneys get rid of them, ketones suppress appetite. This is why fats are used in some reducing diets. Long-term presence of ketones from such diets can damage our kidneys and liver. Be cautious in using high-fat reducing diets.

EFAs and other highly unsaturated fatty acids contain 9 calories per gram, but our body uses them for structural, hormonal, and electrical functions rather than for energy. At high levels of intake, EFAs increase metabolic rate and increase fat burn-off, resulting in loss of weight. Here are 'fats' that can help you become slim.

Metabolic rate differs from one person to another, from one time to another in the same individual, and varies with the total nutrient mix. Genes, hormones, nutrition, exercise, and state of health affect metabolic rate. Some people are born with a high metabolic rate and never gain weight no matter how much they eat. Thyroid activity affects metabolic rate over a wide range, from hyper- (overactive) or increased metabolic rate, down to hypo- (underactive) or lowered rate. The slower the rate, the less calories are burned, and the easier it is to put on weight. EFAs, B-complex vitamins, and minerals including potassium, iron, magnesium, calcium, and manganese, increase the efficiency of oxidation, and raise metabolic rate, energy, and activity level.

Carnitine, which carries fatty acids into the cell's furnaces (mitochondria), can help burn fats for weight loss. Carnitine is especially helpful for vegetarians whose normal foods are low in methionine and lysine, from which our body can make carnitine.

State of health. Our state of health alters our metabolic rate. During fevers and infections, much more energy is burned than when a person is healthy. In late stages of cancer, tumors eat most of the body's stores of energy, resulting in loss of weight. This kind of weight loss we want to avoid.

Growth and convalescence. During childhood, calorie-containing protein and fat molecules are built into body structures. After injury, proteins and fatty acids are used to rebuild cellular structures and new tissues, rather than being used for energy, and the metabolic rate is increased. These examples illustrate a false assumption made by calorie counters, that calorie-containing foods are useful only for energy production.

Stress increases the body's fat-burning rate. Some people lose 10 pounds in just a few days of serious worry. Other stresses also stimulate the body's fat-burning mechanisms.

Activity burns more calories than sedentary living. An hour of exercise keeps our metabolic rate elevated for 12 to 16 hours. The length of time per day spent awake makes a difference, as we burn more calories when we are awake than when we are sleeping. The level of mental activity affects the use of calories. Our brain, although it is only 2% of the body's weight, uses 20% or more of total calories burned by our body.

Environmental conditions affect the rate at which calories are used. Our body responds to changes in temperature, season, and climate, increasing or decreasing metabolic rate to keep body temperature constant. Clothing conserves more or less calories, depending on what it is made from, how thick it is, and how much of our body we cover with it. Our body loses more heat swimming in cold water than when surrounded by air of the same temperature, because air conducts body heat away less rapidly. Shivering also increase fat-burning.

Hunger and satiation factors also influence whether the foods we eat keep us fit or fat. Different foods are digested, absorbed into our body, and made available for use at different rates, and therefore have different hunger-stilling values. Fats may take as long as 5 to 8 hours to be digested, proteins take about 3 to 5 hours, and complex carbohydrates take about 2 to 3 hours. Refined sugars take only 30 minutes. Even though fats contain twice as many calories as carbohydrates, they keep hunger satisfied three times as long, and may therefore result in less weight gain than lighter diets.

Starvation and exercise. Calorie restriction (crash diets; starvation) for weight loss is self-defeating because, when we starve ourselves, our metabolic rate decreases. Then we need even less food to get fat than before. On the other hand, regular exercise increases metabolic rate, and is therefore one of the most reliable ways to lose fat.

Refined sugars and sugars from honey, syrups, and sweet fruit are absorbed rapidly, flood our blood and, to prevent toxic reactions, our body quickly turns them into fat. Then we get hungry again, overeat, deposit more fat, and get hungry once more. Hunger usually wins hands down over our strongest resolutions to restrict our calorie intake. A built-in basic drive, it demands that we eat until we get what our body needs for its functions. If this drive was weak, we would get absorbed in other pursuits, forget to eat, and starve to death.

Overeating undernutrition. Refined foods deficient in essential nutrients can lead us to overeat, and fatten us in the process. Also, refined foods take less work and energy to digest than whole foods, leaving more calories for fat production.

Addiction to taste. Finally, calorie-counting doesn't work because few of us have the patience to systematically weigh out our food portions without cheating. We eat for enjoyment – far more with our eyes and our palate[3] than we do with our rational mind. We prefer the pleasure of eating to the pain of restricting ourselves. We people of Western nations live in a century of feasting uninterrupted by scarcity. Eating is one of our greatest passions.

Habit. On top of all this, most people eat out of habit at regular, clocked intervals, before actually experiencing hunger. One writer claims that the difference between slim and overweight is this: slim people eat only when hungry, eat whatever they like, and stop when the hunger subsides. Overweight people constantly think about food and dieting, eat whenever they see food, and stop eating when all the food is gone. According to this counselor, to lose weight one needs only to learn to think like those who are slim. He recommends counseling for a change in thinking.

High-Technology Weight Control

Liposuction literally means 'sucking fat' out of the body. It is a cosmetic surgery process performed by doctors in which body fat tissue is vacuumed from the body. While it effectively removes fat from the body (injuring tissues in the process and leaving scars), it does nothing to change the conditions by which the extra fat was gained. It is therefore symptom control rather than effective treatment toward natural health. The latter requires increased exercise, changes in eating habits (possibly including certain nutrient concentrates), and changes in the way we think about food.

Stomach stapling, another medical intervention, is a procedure that decreases stomach volume. It then becomes painful to overeat. The procedure does not address the activity, nutrition, and life-style issues at the root of overweight.

Removal of part of the intestine as a method of weight loss, lost favor some time ago. This surgery decreases the absorption of nutrients, allowing people to overeat without gaining weight. The technique produced many complications, and was abandoned. Some people died from malnutrition when a part of their intestine that was critical for the absorption of a certain nutrient was removed, making them unable (for the rest of their lives) to absorb that nutrient. As with the other two high-tech methods, this medical intervention did nothing

---

[3] We also eat for reasons that have nothing to do with hunger, health, or survival. Some weight loss clinics focus on identifying *social-psychological* reasons behind overweight — what goal is the extra weight serving? — and to find another way to reach that goal, so that the person becomes free to let go of the now purposeless extra pounds.

for exercise, nutritious eating, or biological thinking.

Two other methods that have been tried are **jaw wiring** and the **insertion of a balloon into the stomach** to prevent eating and lessen stomach capacity.

Health improvement requires increased care for ourselves, according to the laws of biological functioning of the cells and tissues that make up our body. It is less likely tobe attained by quick-fixes.

Calorie Counting and Health

Aside from overweight – an important risk factor in most degenerative conditions – there is another aspect of calories and health.

The energy value of foods has importance in diets. There have to be enough calories for our body's energy requirements. But 20 minerals, 13 vitamins, and fiber (none of which contain any calories) are also essential for health. Their presence or absence can also change the rate at which energy is produced (or calories burned). Calorie-counting does not take into consideration our need for these vital nutrients (see Chapter 13, Essential Nutrients).

In twentieth century fad and junk foods, it is easy to get the perfect number of calories every day and at the same time to suffer from malnutrition that causes degeneration of cells and tissues. Our body falls apart, molecule by molecule, unraveling the fabric of the body. Degenerative disease bridges our journey from the refined food feast to the graveyard. Our incidence of malnutrition, when all essential nutrients are considered, may be more than 90% of the entire population.

In the midst of plenty, 30% of us are fat and starving. We get plenty of calories but insufficient essential nutrients. People in poorer nations that can't afford refined foods and still eat 'primitive' whole food fare of preindustrial man are better nourished than we.

When the nutrient content of our foods is altered and out of balance, it follows that our hunger mechanism and our body will also be out of balance. In that case, our calorie-counting will not help us.

A Simple Solution

When our food feasts are natural, nutrient-rich, and fiber-rich and we eat only what we need to still our hunger (eat to live rather than live to eat), then hunger takes care of our caloric needs, essential nutrient requirements, EFA and fuel needs, tastebuds, ideal body weight, and physical health, regardless of the changes and conditions through which we pass in our lifetime (see Chapter 74, Overweight and Constipation).

When we use our body for regular physical activity – which is what it was specifically designed for – we can maintain both a trim body shape and fitness into old age.

Blood Cholesterol = Plasma Lipoproteins = HDL, LDL, & Lp(a) 41

Revolutionary new findings about cholesterol and cardiovascular health can conquer the number one killer of affluent people – cardiovascular disease – which affects two-thirds of the population. We review these new findings, as well as cholesterol dogma, and methods of measuring serum (blood) cholesterol.

Cholesterol in Transport

The 7 grams (half ounce) of cholesterol present in our bloodstream[1] is found, together with triglycerides, phospholipids (see Chapter 9, Triglyceride Fats, and Chapter 10, Phospholipids and Membranes), carotene, vitamin E, and proteins, in carrier vehicles called *plasma lipoproteins*.

Two groups (fractions) of lipoproteins play different roles. One fraction, made up of four sub-fractions, the most prominent of which is called low-density lipoproteins (LDL, sometimes called 'bad' cholesterol)[2] carries cholesterol and fats (triglycerides) from foods and our liver to our cells. The other fraction, called high-density lipoproteins (HDL, sometimes called 'good' cholesterol) carries cholesterol from cells back to our liver, where that organ changes cholesterol to bile, excretes both into our intestine, and eventually discards them with our stool.[3] Total blood cholesterol is all cholesterol in transit, being carried by the different lipoprotein vehicles, to and from our cells.

Measuring Blood Cholesterol Levels

For the last 30 years, doctors have measured our blood cholesterol levels as predictors of cardiovascular risk. These measurements are turning out to be better for business than for prediction. Let's look at them here, before we consider newer and more promising methods.

The most common method is to simply measure total serum cholesterol level. This measurement lumps the 'good' HDL and 'bad' LDL fractions together. Total blood cholesterol is considered a general indicator of risk of cardiovascular

---

[1] The total body content of cholesterol is 150 grams (5 ounces).

[2] The other 3 sub-fractions are called very low density lipoprotein (VLDL), intermediate density lipoprotein (IDL), and chylomicrons. Their interrelationships are complex. They exchange material among themselves, and also with the HDL fraction. In addition, a more recently discovered lipoprotein called lipoprotein(a) or Lp(a), which resembles an LDL vehicle but also carries a repair protein, is getting attention as a key factor in the development of atherosclerosis and peripheral arterial disease.

[3] This is the major route by which our body gets rid of excess cholesterol.

disease (CVD), but can be inaccurate. For example, low total cholesterol consisting of low protective HDL coupled with high 'bad' LDL inaccurately indicates a low risk of CVD. On the other hand, high total cholesterol consisting of high protective HDL coupled with high 'bad' LDL would inaccurately indicate a high risk of CVD.

A better indicator of CVD risk might be to measure both HDL and LDL levels. A few years ago, most doctors took this measurement only if specifically asked to do so, but today it is commonly done. The ratio of total cholesterol /HDL is also common now. According to the old dogma, a ratio of 3.5 or lower indicates low risk of CVD.

Changing measurements. Cholesterol used to be measured as milligrams of cholesterol per deciliter (a tenth of a liter, or 100ml) of blood volume, or mg/dl. Doctors considered a reading of 200 mg/dl or lower to indicate low risk of CVD. They considered 240 mg/dl dangerous enough to warrant medical intervention. The average heart attack patient measures 244 mg/dl.

Recently, the medical profession introduced a new measurement for blood cholesterol, in millimoles of cholesterol per liter of blood, or mmol/L. The new measurement is more complex and more difficult for non-technical people to understand than the old measure. Just as we are beginning to master the old system, all the numbers change!

A level of 200 mg/dl becomes 5.15 mmol/L in the new system; 240 mg/dl becomes 6.20 mmol/L; 244 mg/dl is now 6.30 mmol/L. To roughly convert the old measure (mg/dl) to the new measure (mmol/L), divide the old number by 39.

The new measure can be confused with the total cholesterol/HDL ratio, because the numbers are similar in size. You can tell them apart because the ratio is just a number, while the new measure is in mmol/L.

According to Old Dogma

Both HDL and LDL fractions have vital functions to fulfill, but in opposite ways. According to the 'cholesterol theory' of cardiovascular disease – the accepted dogma of the medical establishment – a high 'good' HDL level (50 to 75 mg/dl) in our blood indicates that the system for removing excess cholesterol is functioning well, and preventing the accumulation of cholesterol in our arteries. We are therefore protected from cholesterol deposits in our arteries and from cardiovascular disease. A high 'bad' LDL level (above 120 mg/dl), on the other hand, indicates that our system is being overloaded by cholesterol from food, from synthesis, and/or from too-slow removal. This excess cholesterol is being deposited in our arteries, and is increasing our risk of high blood pressure, heart attack, and stroke.

According to Newer Research

Nutritionists suggest that the measurement of blood cholesterol is a fad. Cholesterol consumption has remained about constant over the last 90 years, while CVD has skyrocketed. Factors which are as closely related to CVD as blood cholesterol include consumption of sugars, fats, additives, and *trans-* fatty acids. Drugs that lower cholesterol without reducing heart attacks or deaths also indicate that cholesterol is not the real issue here.

The data of the continuing Framingham study, which correlates cholesterol levels with cardiovascular deaths by following the population of the town of Framingham, Massachusetts for several decades, is open to interpretations that involve essential nutrients.

Nutritionists link CVD to vitamin, mineral, and EFA deficiency, and to lack of antioxidants (AOs). Years ago, it was already known that high doses of a natural substance, the vitamin *niacin* (B$_3$), protect our heart. According to Dr. A. Hoffer (the pioneer of work with high doses of niacin in the treatment of schizophrenia), niacin protects us, not by its cholesterol-lowering effect, but by its AO action against the toxic effects of oxidized adrenaline (adrenochrome). It may also modify prostaglandin levels. More recently, vitamin C and other AOs have attracted much attention for their heart-protective roles.

Any condition that impairs the 50-member biochemical orchestra from playing the biochemical symphony of life also compromises the functions of our heart and arteries. Deficiency of essential nutrients (such as magnesium and potassium) may prevent necessary cardiovascular functions from being fulfilled, and can thereby lead to a collapse of function severe enough to cause death. Drugs and other poisons can also interfere in biochemical functions of our heart to the extent of functional failure and death.

Nutritionists see the cholesterol 'problem' as due to disruptions in the normal biology and biochemistry of life. Different kinds of disruption can lead to high cholesterol levels, cholesterol deposits, high blood pressure, and other symptoms of CVD.

When we eat foods containing all essential nutrients in optimum quantities, avoid contaminating our body with toxic substances, and live active life-styles in harmony with nature, most of us can forget about cholesterol. Blood cholesterol levels take care of themselves if we eat fresh, nutrient-rich, toxin-free, fiber-rich natural foods. Animals in nature and human generations, until the last two or three, took no measurements, yet had few cholesterol or cardiovascular problems.

Since cholesterol is not essential, we can *both* optimize our intake of minerals, vitamins, fiber and EFAs *and* lower our food intake of cholesterol That way, neither the theoreticians, nor our own body, can argue.

Caution: Low cholesterol and cancer. Low cholesterol levels are associated with increased cancer. Cholesterol-lowering programs and drugs can also increase cancer incidence. Researchers suggest this may result from decreased delivery of vitamin E and carotene to our cells as the level of cholesterol – carrying vehicles in our blood decreases, and suggest that before embarking on a cholesterol-lowering program, people should supplement with these two cancer-protective nutrients for at least two weeks. That way the cells are enriched with carotene and vitamin E. Both are non-toxic.

Teaching Old Dogma New Tricks

In spite of new findings, the dinosaur of old dogma continues to lumber on in medical practice. Economics rather than health or truth drive the old beast. The practice of medicine, contrary to idealistic notions, popular belief, and the desperate hope of the ignorant and seriously ill, is not about care (which comes from our heart), or cure (which must be preceded by accurately identifying the cause of an illness or condition and knowing what health is,), but about making money.[4] Much future profit is invested in the old dogma. Change comes slowly and is strongly resisted.

The new findings question the entire approach to cholesterol and CVD, and will one day provide practical approaches to CVD that can actually reverse and cure the number one killer of our time. Here are the main findings.

Oxidized cholesterol. Recent findings show that only *oxidized* LDL cholesterol damages arteries and leads to atherosclerosis. When our body's normal, food-borne AOs (vitamins C and E, carotene, selenium, and sulphur) which normally prevent and repair oxidative damage in our bloodstream and cells, become depleted, cholesterol and fats (triglycerides) become oxidized and cause damage to arteries. Oxidation also uses up AOs further lowering already low levels. We prevent and reverse oxidized cholesterol by increasing our intake of AOs.

Lp(a) and its adhesive protein apo(a). It has been found that a lipoprotein known as Lp(a), which looks like LDL but carries an adhesive repair protein known as apo(a), is a strong risk factor for CVD. Measurements on which cholesterol dogma is based have erroneously lumped LDL and Lp(a) together. Disassociated from Lp(a), LDL appears to be only a weak risk factor. This means that LDL has been wrongly blamed for damage done by Lp(a). Lp(a) often increases when vitamin C levels in our blood decrease, and usually decreases when vitamin C levels increase.

Apo(a), a protein carried by Lp(a), is an adhesive protein used for tissue repair. It, together with other repair proteins (fibrinogen/fibrin), thickens our arteries. It is interesting that vitamin C, which builds strong arteries, lowers apo(a) and fibrinogen/fibrin levels in our blood. W3 fatty acids also lower blood fibrinogen/fibrin levels, and preliminary findings indicate that they also lower blood apo(a).

Drs. Matthias Rath and Linus Pauling (see Chapter 37, Orthomolecular

---

[4] In my first year medical class, 58 of 60 medical students were there primarily because medicine is a well-paid profession. The 59th, a Mennonite, wanted to do missionary work in Africa. The 60th – myself – wanted to know what health is, and left because medicine taught only about illness.

Nutrition) suggest that a process that produces the CVD which kills us must also have enormous survival value to not have been discarded by evolutionary processes. They speculate that apo(a) protects our arteries from damage due to vitamin C deficiency (scurvy) by thickening them. From an evolutionary perspective, it is better to die of CVD after producing children than of scurvy before we have had a chance to reproduce. Rath goes even further, and suggests that apo(a) is the factor that made us the dominant species on our planet due to its roles in human fertility, tissue and organ differentiation, and the development of the human brain.

Increased intake of vitamin C (several grams per day) and other AOs can keep Lp(a) and apo(a) levels down, reverse scurvy, build strong, thin arteries with strong connective tissue, and reverse and cure cardiovascular disease. Mineral ascorbates are the best form in which to take vitamin C.

Vitamin C, free radicals, and artery damage. Vitamin C, the strongest AO normally present in our body, is water-soluble and easily replaced by eating vegetables, fresh fruit, or supplements. It snags free radicals, preventing them from doing damage. Vitamin C also recharges vitamin E (which in turn recharges carotene), which snags free radicals in oil-soluble membranes. Vitamin C also recharges sulphur-containing glutathione, which snags free radicals that made it through the membrane into a cell. According to Pauling, vitamin C is (therefore) the most important AO in our body, and increased intake of vitamin C plays the key role in preventing and reversing atherosclerosis, heart attacks, and strokes.

Back to nature. All of these findings point in the same natural (orthomolecular) direction. Improved intake of essential nutrients is the primary treatment of choice in cardiovascular diseases. Drugs should be a last resort, used only after the primary treatment has been fully put into practice.

CVD is so widespread, and its prevention and reversal by means of a complete and thorough nutritional program are so simple and so important, that it merits a separate book.

Red Wine and Heart Health

In Europe, ground water is so polluted that no one drinks it. They drink bottled water instead. In France, however, a different custom has developed. Children above age three drink red wine. Sounds like a stupid idea, because alcohol is toxic. It produces aldehydes and free radicals, which damage arteries and liver, and should therefore lead to both cardiovascular disease and cancer. But French kids do not show an increased incidence of these, and the rate of deaths due to CVD in France is about half that of North Americans. Why?

Researchers recently discovered that the pigment in red grapes and red wines are bioflavonoids (polycyclic proanthocyanidins to biochemists) with excellent antioxidant, as well as artery-, and liver-protecting properties. The red pigment is now being marketed as a supplement in North America.

A similar pigment, this one green, is found in Japanese green tea, which people eating sushi drink in liberal quantities. This natural pigment is now being marketed as a 'nutraceutical', a new name for natural substances with therapeutic effects.

Over 600 bioflavonoids are known. Most plants and whole foods contain them. But processing often removes or destroys these helpers of heart, artery, and liver health.

The Fats of Life

Fats in Food Products

We begin this section by examining the health benefits (and failings) of different kinds of diets. Many popular diets are less than healthy, and some can kill you. After we rate the diets, we go on to examine the fats contained in specific foods from many plant and animal sources. This section gives you practical information that will help you buy foods that contribute to wellness.

Later in the section, we visit the butter-margarine controversy, and take a look at the greatly maligned 'tropical fats'. We end the section with a chapter on hidden junk fats and fat substitutes.

Quality of Products

Heal

Udo's Choice Oil Blend
hemp (but may fail drug screens)
flax
soybeans
fish
walnuts
seaweed
sunflower seeds
sesame seeds
almonds
wild birds
filberts
venison
chicken
fresh, mechanically pressed oils in amber glass
evening primrose oil
eggs
butter
lamb
beef
roasted nuts and seeds
dairy products
pork
refined oils
refined starch
sugar
fried oils
margarines, shortenings
alcohol

Kill

Diet Controversies 42

Let us take a short walk through different diets that traditionally sustained human populations on different parts of the globe. We will show the involvement of fats and oils in these diets, and begin a process of looking more closely at how the fats present in our foods impact our health.

Some nutrition writers suggest that by nature man is a hunter who, since the dawn of our species, has lived on a diet high in animal proteins and fats. These writers, mostly North American or European and affluent, cite evidence of primitive hunting spears, arrows, animal bones, and other artifacts of the hunt found around remnants of fire pits in archaeological sites on all continents. They use historical records of the past to confirm their personal preference for diets high in meats.

Equally vociferous, and marshalling a similarly impressive set of evidence, are writers who claim that man was always a gatherer of seeds, grains, roots, nuts, berries, and herbs. Seeds and implements for crushing and preparing seeds have also been found in archaeological digs. Three-quarters of the world's present population lives on a diet based around vegetables and grains (including rice, millet, corn and beans, buckwheat, wheat, rye, oats, barley, spelt, triticale, sorghum, quinoa, and amaranth). These people consume few animal products. Eggs, meat, blood, or milk products are special treats for festive or religious occasions.

It is not clear why these two sets of writers insist that man should have been rigidly one or the other. Survival is a practical matter, and it makes sense that during millions of years of history, climactic changes, and migrations, our ancestors ate whatever they found in their environment and climate. In a state of affluence, we can afford to speculate. In a state of hunger, we eat what we can find and catch.[1]

---

[1] Our teeth are less able to tear flesh than those of meat-eating animals (carnivores), and less able to grind than those of vegetarian animals (herbivores). Our intestine is longer than that of carnivores and shorter than that of herbivores. Our body is less powerful than that of carnivores, making us less capable to catch and kill, and slower than that of most herbivores. Biologically speaking, we appear to be mixed eaters (omnivores).

A third set of writers considers man's original foods to have consisted mainly of raw fresh greens, with some flowers, fruits, and roots, and an occasional inadvertent supplement of under-leaf insect eggs or worm. Gorillas, chimpanzees, and orangutans live on such foods. This kind of diet required no tools or fire, and would have left little archaeological evidence of its existence.

Climatic Differences and Diet

In tropical climates, vegetables, fruits, and seeds are the foods easiest to obtain. Tropical people would have favored them. Vegetables and fruits are rich in minerals, vitamins, enzymes and fiber, but low in fats. Their seeds contain ample fats.

Plains grow grasses and grains, and plains people became gatherers and later, farmers. Plains also provided lean, low-fat animals such as buffalo, antelope, gnu, and other wild cattle. So, on early plains, we find hunters who followed the animals, herders who tamed these grazing animals and lived on meats, blood, and milk, and farmers who grew food plants.

People of the North depended mainly on high-fat, high-w3 animal and fish foods. Winters were long and cold, and vegetation was sparse.

People along coasts, lakes and rivers included fish in their food supply. In each area, man adapted himself to the foods available, and learned the skills required to live.

Seasonal differences in diets. Seasonally too, there were differences. Summer grew fresh, perishable vegetables and fruits rich in minerals, vitamins, and water lost as sweat in summer heat. For winter, seeds, nuts, grains, roots, and dried foods were stored. Storable foods contain concentrated energy, the fuels that keep us warm in cold weather – starches, proteins, and fats.

Animal-based diets. Traditional Inuit and Northern Native diets come closer to being animal-based. The people ate virtually the entire animal. Organ meats such as liver, eyes, gonads, adrenals, and brain were preferred to muscle meats. Some organs were eaten raw. Nutritional analysis – which became possible only in recent history – confirms that organ meats are superior to muscle meats, being richer in EFAs, minerals, and vitamins, and of equal protein quality. Stomach contents (including lichens, mosses, seaweed, and plankton) of animals were also eaten. In summer, the people collected herbs from the almost barren land. These bits of vegetable matter provided fiber and vitamin C, which are difficult to obtain in sufficient quantities from animal sources.

Plant-based diets. Completely vegetarian (vegan) traditional diets are unknown. Insects and their eggs provided animal products, as did the occasional trophy of rat, gopher, or possum. Dairy products were commonly used in some parts of the globe.

Many people relied on greens and grains for their main meals, but occasionally got their hands on meat, eggs, fish, milk, or blood. Grain eaters got vitamin B_{12} – an animal product required in only minute quantities and virtually absent from plant products – from insect-infested grain kernels, dried insects crushed in grains, or from insect eggs. Modern methods of grain storage use fumigants to prevent insect infestation, and thereby rob vegans of a source of vitamin B_{12}.

Changes in Dietary Preferences

Changes in our food habits took place over history, especially in the last one hundred years. Processing became widespread. Many traditional and time-tried balanced and healthful food habits were lost.

Organ meats have taken a back seat to muscle meats that are low in several minerals, several vitamins, and both EFAs.

After domesticating wild animals, changes through breeding and feeding took place. Commercialization of a limited range of stocks resulted in limitations in diversity, quantity, and quality of fats in animal foods. Processing brought about changes in the fat, mineral, and vitamin content of foods, as well as introducing into our food supply many substances foreign to human body chemistry.

Shortsighted farming methods deplete soils of minerals, decreasing the mineral content of foods grown in these soils. Unripe harvest prevents full nutritional content from being developed. Transport and storage result in nutrient losses. Processing takes the heaviest nutritional toll.

Food consumption is also influenced by religious, philosophical, moral, ethical, and faddish considerations. In times of plenty, we can afford to indulge in speculations, and to base our food choices on these speculations. Statements such as: "Taking the life of conscious creatures is wrong!" and "I don't think that anything that died in agony can be good food for humans!", are valid ethical considerations, but during famines, they usually occupy a position of low priority. These considerations are not based on the rigors of nutritional science which, at its best, deals objectively with the essential components of human nutrition, their minimums and optimums for health, and digestible sources of these essential nutrients in nature. Nutritional science takes the side neither of vegetarians nor meat eaters, but attempts to improve the health of both through better food choices based on nutritional information.

In the following chapters, we examine the fat content of different diets and foods. We can observe how the fat content of our diet has changed over history. This may give us insight into why present diets that *appear* to be the same as past diets, now result in diseases of fatty degeneration.

43 *Rating Oils in Diets*

Some diets build and maintain healthy bodies. Others do not. In this chapter, we rate the most common diets for oil content and their ability to maintain or rebuild health.

High-Complex Carbohydrate, Low-Fat Diets

The Pritikin diet (developed at the Pritikin Longevity Center in California) is the most popular of many high-complex carbohydrate (80%), low-fat (10% or less) diets. The newly popular Dean Ornish's diet is another. A third is nutritionist Paavo Airola's diet, which is similar to Pritikin's diet in its makeup, but contains less protein and a better balance of oils.

Pritikin and Ornish's diets work for people who overate themselves fat and sick on a typical affluent Western and North American diet rich in protein, white flour, white sugar, and super-rich (over 40%) in hard and altered fats. Pritikin-type diets are mostly whole-grain and vegetable diets plus a little fruit, with meats used mainly as condiments. They reverse many of the degenerative changes in cardiovascular disease, obesity, diabetes, rheumatoid arthritis, hypertension, and senility.

Once a person becomes healthy, Pritikin-type diets may be dangerously low in fats. Fat-soluble vitamins A, D, E and K require fat (or oil) for absorption, which is impaired when total fat intake is 5% or less. Pritikin's diet comes too close to that lower limit (food at the Pritikin Longevity Center contains only 7% fats), especially for older people whose digestion and absorption are suboptimal. Diets containing less than 5% fats are correlated with cancer in places like the Philippines, most likely due to impaired absorption of vitamins A and E, which protect against cancer-causing free radicals.

W3s have been shown to inhibit tumor incidence and growth. Pritikin and Ornish's diets are low in w3s, to which they pay no attention at all. The fats in their diet programs contain essential fatty acids (EFAs), but there may not be enough of them because of the low total fat content.

For people who spend time outdoors in sunny, warm climates like California, sunshine may compensate to some extent for a low supply of EFAs, but in winter, in northern latitudes, and in smoggy and indoor environments, more EFAs are required. A diet that contains 15 to 20% of calories as fat (one-third to one-half of that as EFAs) and a balanced w6:w3 ratio is more likely to ensure health over the long term.[1] For hot southern tropical climates and summers, the

---

[1] All other essential nutrients, including the antioxidant minerals and vitamins, must also be optimized for optimum health.

Pritikin diet's grain content may be too high. A lighter fare of fresh fruit and vegetables needs to be emphasized. People who spend their time in air-conditioned rooms under artificial lights may need more EFAs than Pritikin's diet supplies, even in the tropics.

An engineer, Pritikin developed his diet to meet his own needs. He was obese and had clogged arteries in his 40s, and he reversed both conditions. His arteries were clean when he was autopsied in his 60s. But Pritikin died of suicide after battling leukemia.

Pritikin's diet is a step in the right direction for this generation's over-fat, over-processed way of eating. However, in the long run, it may kill those who are not overfed.

High-Protein, High-Fat Diets

High-fat, low-carbohydrate diets include Atkins, Stillman, and Drinking Man's diets. These diets assume that man has always been a hunter, which is open to debate, and that he has always eaten a diet high in protein and fat, which is not true (see Chapter 46, Meats).

High-protein, high-fat diets may be a short-term way around grain intolerance for people that have developed allergic reactions to grains (especially wheat). But systematically improved, enriched, and balanced nutrition is necessary to reverse such allergies (when they *can* be reversed). Avoidance of the offending food(s) might be necessary in some cases.

High-protein, high-fat diets are weight reduction diets that promise the loss of pounds and inches while we eat all we want. They work because fats are digested slower and suppress appetite longer than carbohydrates (especially refined carbohydrates). Fats also produce ketones, which reduce hunger even more. Refined carbohydrates, a large part of many overweight people's diets, are omitted completely from the menu or allowed only in small quantities. This is the best way for *some* people to eat. People differ in their food requirements for health.

High-protein, high-fat diets are basic Western 'meat and potatoes' diets without the potatoes. High-fat diets can lead to ketone-induced kidney damage. Too much protein produces an excess of ammonia – a toxic protein breakdown product that can damage the liver, kidneys, and brain before the body turns it into less harmful urea. Excess urea is part of the cause of gouty arthritis. High-protein diets also increase chances of developing allergies, because proteins are potent allergens. Food allergies may result in digestive and absorptive problems, nutrient deficiencies, and immune impairment common to allergies.

EFA intake is not considered at all in these diets. The fats they contain are usually rich in saturated fatty acids (SaFAs) which are associated with cardiovascular disease and diabetes, and moderately with cancer.

Traditional Northern Diets

Inuit and Northern natives adhering to traditional diets consume mostly animal foods rich in fats and proteins, but are free of most of our common degenerative diseases.[2] They do suffer strokes due to lack of vitamins C and E, and kidney damage and osteoporosis due to high protein. The fats in their diets come from fish and marine mammals containing large concentrations of highly unsaturated w3 fatty acids.

When these people lose their traditions and adopt Western diets, they lose their immunity to the degenerative diseases common to Western cultures.

The Affluent Western Society's Diet

Most people consuming the foods eaten by affluent Western people suffer degenerative diseases sooner or later, no matter which race they belong to or where on earth they live. Few people are genetically immune to damage from Western diets containing over 40% hard and altered fats, 40% refined carbohydrates, and only 6% complex carbohydrates.

People who move to the West from places and diets free of degenerative disease, and people who adopt the Western diet wherever they live, begin to degenerate within one generation after they adopt the Western life-style. The Western diet contains too much SaFAs and altered fatty acids, too much protein, too much w6 oil, too little w3 oil, too few minerals and vitamins, too few antioxidants, and too little fiber.

Before the industrial revolution, white flour had to be made by slow, time-consuming sifting methods. Only the rich could afford white flour, and only the rich suffered degenerative diseases. By designing mass production machinery for the process, white flour production has become very efficient, and we can all now afford the flour that produces the ailments due to nutrient deficiency. A folk saying tells us that if we want to be healthy: "Though you be rich like a king, eat like a pauper."

Reconciling Differences

We reconcile the fact the one high-fat diet protects against, while the other high-fat diet fosters degeneration, by differentiating between healing (EFA-rich) and killing (saturated and chemically altered) fats, and between nutrient-rich natural and nutrient-poor processed foods (see Chapter 13, Essential Nutrients).

Diets free of refined sugars, which turn into SaFAs and rob our body of vitamins and minerals necessary for fat digestion and metabolism (see Chapter 6, The Sugar-Fat Connection), support health. Diets free of refined and altered oil products support our health. Diets low in SaFAs and altered fats, which interfere

---

[2] Japanese fishermen and West Coast North American Indians on traditional fare, similar to that of these Northerners, are also free of most degenerative diseases.

with EFA functions, support health. Diets free of processed foods that lack many vitamins and minerals support health. Diets free of de-natured fat products support health. Diets rich in enzymes support health. Diets containing nature's rich endowment of essential mineral and vitamin co-factors support health. Diets containing both EFAs or their derivatives in adequate amounts and right balance support health.

Diets high in SaFAs and altered fats, which interfere with EFA functions, interfere with health. Diets containing refined carbohydrates add to the load of SaFAs and are also deficient in vitamins and minerals. Diets low in refined carbohydrates are an improvement over diets that contain them in larger quantities.

People who cannot tolerate certain complex carbohydrates (grains) may do better on a fat and protein diet, but the fats in such diets should be chosen to contain one-third to one-half of their fatty acids as EFAs or EFA derivatives. Both EFAs are present in hemp, flax, and fish oils, and are also present in soybeans. Beef, mutton, pork, cheese, and butter are poor sources of EFAs, and margarines and shortenings are unreliable sources of EFAs as well as being toxic.

A diet deficient in essential nutrients can be prevented from leading to degenerative diseases if properly nutrient-enriched with whole foods, fresh juices, super-foods, or concentrates of essential vitamins, minerals, and EFAs.

How Fat are Your Foods? **44**

Everything that lives contains fats and oils, because everything that lives is made up of cells, and all cells are surrounded by membranes containing phospholipids which, as we learned in Chapter 10, Phospholipids and Membranes), contain fatty acids. Since our foods are ultimately derived from living plant and animal materials, all natural foods contain some fats.

All cells contain smaller sub-units or 'little organs' (organelles) specialized for particular functions. Organelles, too, are surrounded by membranes containing phospholipids containing fatty acids. This chapter's overview of the fats and oils contained in foods will be extended in the chapters that follow.

Membrane Fats

Membranes account for 1 to 3% of a cell's total weight. They contain between 20 and 80% phospholipids. Our red blood cells contain about 45% phospholipids and 55% proteins in their membranes, whereas our nerve cell membranes (myelin sheath) contain 80% phospholipids and only 20% proteins. Membranes of organelles – nuclear membrane, inner membrane of mitochondria, and lysosomal membranes – contain 25% phospholipids and 75% protein. Liver cell membranes and membranes of endoplasmic reticulum contain about 50% each of phospho-lipids and protein.

Plants: leaves, stems, flowers, and roots. Oils found in low-fat parts of plants (all but their seeds) are found largely in the plants' cell membranes. These cells contain 1% or less fats. According to the U.S. Department of Agriculture's *Handbook #8 on the Composition of Foods,* plants contain the following percentages of fats by weight:

cucumbers, potatoes, beets, celery, kohlrabi, squash	0.1%
cabbage, carrots, lettuce, garlic	0.2%
dandelion greens, watercress	0.7%
kale, collard, lamb's quarters	0.8%
seaweeds	0.3 - 3.2%

Oils in the green parts of plants are EFA-rich. More than half (60 to 70%) of the fatty acids of dark green leaves are the essential, triply unsaturated w3, alpha-linolenic acid (LNA, 18:3w3), which is especially concentrated in the membranes of green, chlorophyll-containing, photosynthesizing organelles (chloroplasts). Here, LNA takes part in processes by which plants capture sunlight energy and store that energy in the bonds of the molecules they make – sugars, starches, proteins, and fats. The energy stored in the bonds of these molecules is the energy we need to live. We eat leaves, stems, roots, or flowers of these plants, and in our body the sunlight energy stored in their molecules is slowly released through the process of respiration (oxidation). This energy powers the molecular motors of our life. Indirectly, all life on earth depends on the ability of chlorophyll to trap, harness, and store sunlight.[1] The meat we eat is either made from plants (herbivores are made from plants) or from flesh made from plants (carnivores are made from meat made from plants).

The membranes of other parts of plants contain up to half of their fatty acids in the form of w6 essential fatty acid (EFA), twice unsaturated linoleic acid (LA, 18:2w6). Both EFAs in all living plants are in the all *cis-* state. EFAs degenerate rapidly when cells die, so it is best for health to eat much of our plant material fresh; freshly cooked and immediately eaten vegetables are also okay. Leftovers lose nutritional value with time through oxidation processes. Cooking can destroy more than half the vitamin C present in fresh, raw vegetables, as well as a percentage of the B complex vitamins.

Plant *seeds* are rich in fats or oils in the form of triglycerides.

Fruits are similar to vegetables in oil content. A few of these are listed in the following table with their percentage of fat content by weight:

---

[1] Our life also depends on the ability of plants to 'fix' carbon from carbon dioxide, and to release the oxygen we need to live.

214

peaches, grapefruit	0.1%
apples, apricots, gooseberries, oranges	0.2%
lemons, figs, crab apples, cherries	0.3%
pears and mangoes	0.4%
blueberries	0.5%
blackberries	0.9%

The oils in fruits are similar in fatty acid content to non-green parts of plants. They contain less LNA than green parts of plants, but both EFAs are present.

Our body converts fruit sugars into saturated fatty acids if we eat more fruit sugar than we can burn-off in immediate activity. Fruits are therefore more likely to fatten us than green vegetables, because their sugar content is higher.

Fruit *seeds* are usually fairly rich in fats or oils in the form of triglycerides.

Fats from Fat-Storing Cells

In addition to less than 1% phospholipids found in *all* cell membranes, larger quantities of triglyceride fats or oils are found in special fat-storing cells found in the seeds, nuts, and kernels of all plants – grasses, grains, legumes, shrubs, and trees – as well as in animal and human tissues. Figure 41 shows some major sources of different kinds of fatty acids.

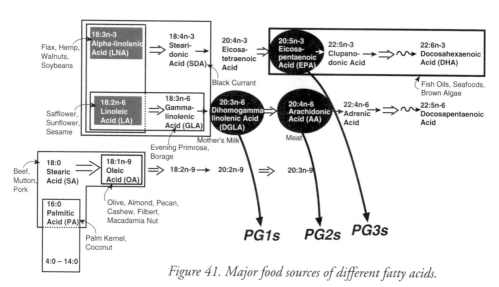

Figure 41. Major food sources of different fatty acids.

Depending on what percentage of the total cells are fat cells, a seed or tissue can contain from less than 2% to over 70% fats and oils.

Grains usually contain between 1 and 3% oils. A list of the quantities of oil found in grains follows:

amaranth	0.5%	wheat	2.0%
wild rice	0.7%	buckwheat	2.4%
barley	1.0%	millet	2.9%
rye	1.7%	sorghum	3.3%
rice	1.9%		

The oils contained in grains are about half LA, and contain only a little LNA. They spoil rapidly when grains are broken, pressed, or ground into flour. Store-bought rolled oats are often rancid during summer months. You can *smell* the rancidity.

To prevent flour rancidity during long storage time on shelves and in warehouses, oils are removed from seeds in modern milling practices (along with minerals, vitamins, fiber, and some protein), leaving starch greatly lacking in essential nutrients. Insects cannot live on this flour – refined flour starves *them* too – hence refinement helps protect against insect infestation. But we do not need this kind of protection from insects, because we now know other ways to effectively control pests, allowing us to retain in grains the nutrients *we* need.

Whole grains can be cooked without destroying their EFAs, but once cooked, they begin to deteriorate.

Legumes vary widely in oil content. A list follows:

lentils	1.1%	chick peas	4.8%
peas	1.3%	soybeans	18.0%
mung and lima beans	2.0%	peanuts	47.5%

Soybeans and soybean oils contain both EFAs. Peanuts, which are not nuts but legumes (more pea than nut) grow underground and are prone to infection by a fungus that produces highly carcinogenic aflatoxins. Peanuts contain no LNA, and only modest quantities of LA. Contrary to popular belief, they contain no arachidonic acid (20:4w6), but instead contain 2 to 4% arachidic acid (20:0), which is a long-chain saturated fatty acid melting at 75°C (167°F). The popularity of peanuts is commercial. Nutritionally they are overrated. Peanut oil is stable and keeps fairly well.

Cooking legumes does not destroy their oils, but their nutrient value is gradually lost if, after cooking, they are left standing.

Nuts and oil seeds vary widely in oil content. A list is given below:

chestnuts	1.5%
corn	4.0%
coconut, flax	35.0%
sunflower seeds, pumpkin seeds, cashews,	
safflower, sesame seeds	40 - 50%

almonds, pistachios, pine nuts	55%
brazil nuts, walnuts, filberts	up to 60%
macadamia nuts	71.6%

The oil content of nuts and oil seeds varies from year to year and with the area of cultivation. Northern plantings produce more oil, more EFAs, and more LNA (if any) in their seeds, to ensure adequate energy for sprouting seeds in colder climates.

Olive oil is pressed not from the seeds but from the flesh of olives, which contains 12 to 20% low-EFA oil. The olive pit also contains oil, but this is not used.

The kinds of fatty acids present in nut and seed oils vary widely. Some have no LNA, and some have very little LA in their oils. Others contain one or both in varying proportions (see Chapter 50, Oils in Seeds). Nature covers whole nuts and seeds with shells and/or skins that exclude light and air from the oils they contain. They keep for a long time without spoiling. *Broken* nuts and seeds have lost this protection.

Oils from plant sources contain virtually no cholesterol. A few oils contain traces, but the amount is so small that it can be ignored as a source of cholesterol in human nutrition.

Oils also vary in their degree of rancidity (damage by oxygen), measured by their peroxide value (PV). The PV of olive oil is usually around 20 milliequivalents per kilogram (meq/kg).[2] The PV of corn oil is often over 40 or even 60. Other oils generally range from a PV of 0.1 (if the oil has been made with exceptional care) to 10. The PV level at which an oil becomes unpalatable varies from as low as 2 for flax to over 40 for some refined oils. PV therefore measures damage by oxygen, not necessarily taste.

Eggs. Whole eggs contain about 11% fats. The yolk contains about 30% fats and oils by weight. The egg white is fat-free. An egg also contains about 250 mg of cholesterol. One third of the fats in *natural* free range eggs is EFAs.

The fats found in eggs vary with the foods the chicken eats. If it forages for its own food, the yolk contains both LNA and LA, but if it is fed man-made, EFA-poor chicken feed, then the yolk of their eggs will also be EFA-poor (see Chapter 49, Eggs).

Dairy products. Dairy products vary widely in fat content, as the following list indicates:

---

[2] meq/kg is a measure of the number or rancid molecules per kg of product; between 2 and 3% of oil molecules are damaged by oxygen to get a PV of 100. At this level of oxidation, an oil is totally unpalatable. In the commercial oil trade, the PV is often given without the units of measurement [meq/kg].

cow milk	3.5%	dry cottage cheese	0.3%
goat milk	4.0%	low-fat cheeses	10% or less
human milk	4.0%	normal and process cheeses	20-30%
reindeer milk	19.6%	fancy cheeses	30%+
butter	81.0%	cream cheese	35%

Fatty acids in dairy products are mostly long-chain saturated and monounsaturated, and short-chain saturated. From butter, about 500 different fatty acids have been isolated, many of them present in only trace amounts.

Fats in dairy products, but not human milk (which is not exactly a dairy product!) contain *trans-* fatty acids (up to 6% in summer and 3% in winter) produced from the LNA and LA present in grass by bacteria that live in the stomachs of cattle. The main *trans-* fatty acid in dairy fat is *trans-* vaccenic acid (t18:1w7), with a double bond between w carbons 7 and 8. This isomer is easier to digest than *trans-* fatty acids found in margarines.

Dairy products are poor sources of EFAs (see Chapter 51, Butter Versus Margarine).

Seafoods. Shellfish are lowest in oils. Fish oil content ranges between 1 and 18%, as the following list illustrates:

scallops, frog legs	0.3%	cod, snapper	1% or less
abalone	0.5%	whale	7.5%
shrimp, octopi	0.8%	sardines	8.6%
mussels	1.4%	mackerel	15.0%
lobster, crab, oysters	2.0%	eel	18.0%
roe (eggs) of cod, pike, shad, haddock, herring			2.3%
salmon, sturgeon, steelhead, lake trout, shad, herring			10.0%

In general, the warmer the water, the lower the oil content of the same kind of fish. Atlantic herring cooled by the Arctic current have 11.3% oils, while Pacific herring warmed by the Japanese current have only 2.6% oils. The fat content of fish can also vary greatly with age, season, and spawning activity.

The oils of some fish and seafoods are rich in highly unsaturated w3 oils, which are useful in arthritis, heart disease, and cancer. W3 fish oils lower elevated blood triglycerides, may lower cholesterol, and protect against fatty degeneration of inner organs. These oils are extremely sensitive to destruction by light, oxygen, and heat, and must be protected to retain their therapeutic value.

Not all marine animals and fish contain highly unsaturated fatty acids. Warm-water (tropical) fish, sharks, and other slow-moving fish contain more monounsaturated fatty acids. Some fatty acids found in fish may be toxic (see Chapter 19, Other Toxic Products).

Among highly unsaturated w3 fatty acids found in sardines, trout, salmon, and mackerel are two of special note: five times unsaturated eicosapentaenoic acid (EPA, 20:5w3), and six times unsaturated docosahexaenoic acid (DHA, 22:6w3). Very low melting points (between -40 to -50°C; -40 to -58°F) equip fish containing them for living in icy cold water. These oils – nature's biological antifreeze – keep fish and marine animals from freezing solid at low temperatures, and provide the high energy necessary for fish to get away from warm-blooded predators pursuing them in freezing cold water. The oils also pull into their body the oxygen necessary for life functions. Water does not contain much oxygen; the extremely oxygen-loving oils are vital for reactions involving oxygen[3] in cold water animals.

Animals and humans who eat these fish and marine animals incorporate the w3 fatty acids into their own body fat. In humans, oils containing EPA, DHA, and other highly unsaturated fatty acids that are extremely oxygen-loving can prevent and reverse degenerative diseases resulting from over-consumption of saturated and monounsaturated fatty acids (such as 16:0, 18:0, 16:1w7, 18:1w7, and 18:1w9) that interfere with cell oxidation or respiration (see Chapter 55, Oils from Fish and Seafoods). In addition, EPA is the precursor of series 3 prostaglandins (see Chapter 58, Prostaglandins) with beneficial effects on our kidneys, arteries, immune system, platelets, and triglyceride levels.

Meats from land animals. As the following list shows, wild animals carry less fat than their domesticated counterparts.

rabbit (wild)	5%	caribou (wild)	5%
rabbit (domesticated)	8%	reindeer (domesticated)	20-40%
venison (wild)	3-5%	sheep (wild)	5%
moose (wild)	1-3%	sheep (domesticated)	20-40%
beef (domesticated)	18-41%	pig (wild)	1.3%
		pig (domesticated)	35-60%[4]

Wild animals also have a higher percentage of EFAs in their fat. Beef and lamb fats contain almost no LA or LNA; their fats consist mainly of saturated and monounsaturated fatty acids. Pork fat contains up to 10% LA and a little LNA, but is undesirable for other reasons (see Chapter 46, Meats).

Fowl. Goose and duck are around 30% fat, chicken around 20 to 25% fat. Turkey is slightly leaner than chicken. Wild birds are leaner than domestic birds.

---

[3] Oxygen is 8 times more soluble in fats than in water, and far more attracted to highly unsaturated than to less saturated fatty acids.

[4] Pork gets so fat that on the train ride to slaughter houses in Europe, as many as 10% of the animals die of heart attacks. They literally choke on their own fat. A Japanese prophecy states that Western civilization will die of asphyxiation. By our choices of the kinds and amounts of fats we consume, we are fulfilling that prophecy.

Most of the fat of birds is just under their skin; the meat itself is only 7% fat. This is why doctors recommend skinned chicken or turkey over beef, lamb, and pork for people who need to decrease their fat consumption. Fowl fat contains up to 25% LA – which helps metabolize saturated fats – more than beef, mutton, or pork fats.

Organ meats are lower in fat and higher in EFAs than muscle meats. Liver contains about 4% fat, brain about 9% fat, heart about 6 to 10% fat, and kidney about 6% fat. Organ meats are also richer in essential vitamins and minerals than muscle meats, and are therefore preferable to muscle meats from a nutritional point of view.

Meat concoctions. Sausage meats vary in fat content, from 20 to 38% (by weight) for salami, 27% for bologna, 37% for blood sausage, and 50% for some pork sausages. Weiners are about 43% fat. Fats in these products are mostly saturated. Some of them also contain refined starch as fillers or 'extenders' and sugars for taste which, when converted to saturated fat, adds to the load of saturated fatty acids that our body must manage. For health, these high-fat meat concoctions are never recommended. The percent of calories from fat in these concoctions is very high – often more than twice the weight percentage of fats.

Processed foods. A potato contains 0.1% oil. If the potato is cut into sticks and deep fried, the French fries contain 13.2% oil, most of which has been picked up from the overheated oil in which they were fried. A potato cut into thin slices and turned into a crunchy potato chip contains 39.8% partially hydrogenated fat, containing up to more than one-third *trans-* fatty acids. In addition, part of the potato has been burned. Clearly, the natural composition of a potato is drastically changed by these processes. A 'natural' potato chip is anything but natural, if 'natural' means 'the way nature made it'.

Hundreds of processed products on the market contain hidden fats, sugars, starches, and salt. Colorings, flavorings, preservatives, and other additives not found in nature are also used liberally. They can interfere with the delicate workings of our natural biological systems, because they do not fit the highly specific structural or functional requirements of these systems. These hidden and unnatural substances comprise an unwelcome addition to our diet and a detriment to our health.

Cholesterol in Foods 45

Saturated, sticky, land animal fats and cholesterol in foods, and especially the combination of both, increase *some* people's serum low-density lipoprotein (LDL) cholesterol levels. This happens when the quantity consumed and absorbed from foods or made by our liver exceeds our cells' capacity to absorb and use, and our liver's ability to metabolize[1] and discard, the cholesterol carried in our blood.

Old research claims that high LDL levels enhance the buildup of atherosclerotic plaque, narrow our arteries, and finally kill us by a stroke, embolism, or heart attack (cardiovascular accident) resulting from narrowed arteries and sticky platelets, which do *not* happen by accident! Antioxidant, mineral, and vitamin deficiencies probably have more to do with cardiovascular 'accidents' than with LDL levels in our blood (see Chapter 41, Blood Cholesterol). In addition, only 30% of the population is subject to increasing blood cholesterol from increased cholesterol consumption. The other 70% are protected by an efficient regulating mechanism that has their body producing less cholesterol when they eat more, and producing more when they get less of it from their foods.

In deference to outdated dogma, let's find out which foods contain cholesterol, and how much. *All* cholesterol comes from animal sources. If you want to be sure of minimum (zero) cholesterol intake, strict vegetarian (vegan) food habits are your ticket – no meat, no eggs, no dairy products: these three contain cholesterol.

Bad Combination

For the 30% who respond to dietary cholesterol, animal products that are rich in both saturated fats and cholesterol raise LDL cholesterol levels. Although cholesterol consumption has remained about constant for the last 100 years, and therefore cannot be the *primary* cause of increases in cardiovascular disease (300%) and cancer (500%) in that time period, it may worsen problems caused by sticky, hard, saturated fats, and in later stages of CVD, is found in deposits that narrow the arteries. Beef and mutton muscle meats are highest in saturated fats. Pork contains enormous amounts of fats. Inner organs of animals are higher in cholesterol than muscle meats, but also contain more EFAs, which hook up with (esterify) cholesterol and aid, to some extent – the exact extent has never been measured accurately enough to be agreed upon – in the metabolism and transport of cholesterol.

Include sugar on the list of substances that increase the risk of 'cardiovascular accidents', because they turn into saturated fats. Also include honey, syrups, and even too much sweet fruit. Also include refined, hydrogenated tropical fats.

---

[1] The liver's capacity to metabolize cholesterol is also influenced by the presence or lack of the minerals and vitamins required to do so.

On the other hand, several minerals and vitamins decrease our risk of 'cardiovascular accident'. Of special note are B complex and C vitamins; chromium, magnesium and several other minerals; and mineral and vitamin antioxidants.

Cholesterol Content of Foods

The amount (in mg) of cholesterol in a 100-gram portion (3.3 ounces) of various foods is as follows:

brain	2000+	cheese	100
egg yolk	1500	lard	95
whole egg	550	veal	90
kidney	375	beef, pork, fish	70
liver, caviar	300	mutton	65
thymus, butter	250	chicken	60
oyster, lobster	200	ice cream	45
heart	150	cottage cheese	15
shrimp, crab	125	milk	11
cream	120		

Supplements and Fiber

It bears repeating that the effect of dietary cholesterol on our health depends on whether we are one of the 30% uncompensating absorbers, whether our sources of cholesterol also contain saturated fats (dairy, beef, lamb, pork) or EFAs (seafoods, internal organs), whether the nutritional status of other essential nutrients is optimal or deficient, and whether the diet contains phytosterols that block cholesterol absorption. Unless these food issues have been adequately addressed, and the kinds of fiber[2] that bind bile acids and cholesterol in our intestine and remove them from our body are included in our list, we should indulge in high-sugar, high-fat, high-cholesterol items far less than is the custom in Western industrialized nations.

Seafoods

Of cholesterol-containing foods, cold-water animals and fish are least troublesome for our heart, arteries, and immune system. While the combination of sticky, hard saturated fatty acid-rich fats and cholesterol are involved in every type of fatty degeneration, high levels of highly unsaturated, anti-sticky (dispersing), liquid w3

---

[2] Examples of fiber which binds cholesterol are: pectin, found in apples, potatoes, beets, and carrots; gums and mucilages found in flax, okra, psyllium husks, beans, and oats; and lignin, found in whole grains, cabbage, peas, tomatoes, strawberries, and pears. Seaweeds containing algin are excellent foods for binding cholesterol, as well as being good sources of minerals and vitamins. Cellulose does not bind cholesterol.

fatty acids from fish like salmon, trout, mackerel, and sardines protect against fatty degeneration, fat aggregation, and cholesterol deposits (see Chapter 55, Oils from Fish and Seafoods).

Meats **46**

The commercialization of meat production illustrates most clearly how taking control of our food supply (domesticating, breeding, and artificial feeding) has affected its nutritional content and our physical health.

Diseases of fatty degeneration afflict mainly people who eat diets high in beef and pork, and spares people who live on natural complex carbohydrate diets made up of mostly vegetables and grains. Fatty degeneration also passes by people who eat meat from wild animals or fish. Beef and pork are not the only sources of fatty degeneration, however. *All* foods processed and altered from their natural state carry part of the story of fatty degeneration.

Writers who evidently like their steaks and pork chops suggest that meat and fats cannot possibly be the problem since man has been a hunter from the beginning. Even accepting man's hunting ancestry as true (which is open to debate), and notwithstanding the fact that man today does not exactly 'hunt' his steaks in the old sense of the word (at great expense of energy and exercise with bow and arrow, spear, or stone implements), there is another important factor that is usually overlooked by meat-loving writers: a comparison of the kinds and amounts of fats present in the meats of domesticated animals and their wild (natural) counterparts.

Fat Content of Meats

When we compare their fat content, we discover that domesticated animals contain far more fat than the wild animals our ancestors hunted. If we compare the fatty acids contained in domestic animals with their wild counterparts, we find important differences here as well.

Beef contains between 18 and 41% fat (by weight; double that for an estimate of percentage of calories from fat); mutton contains between 20 and 40% fat; pork runs between 35 and 60% fat. In comparison, venison and moose usually carry about 2 to 3% (maximum 5%) fat. Wild sheep are muscular and sleek with 5% body fat; they could not survive for long in nature if they carted a lot of fat around. Wild pigs carry only 1 to 3% fat. In spite of cold winters, even wild animals in the far north carry little extra fat. Wild caribou have only 3% fat, but domesticated reindeer go up to almost 20% fat. In short, domestication and breeding has increased the fat content of the 'hunter's diet'. Beef was specifically inbred to produce meat with a marbled appearance, which results from (unnatural) hard fats deposited within muscle tissue, which was said to improve both taste and moistness. Rabbit meat went from 5% or less fat in wild, to 8% in domesticated animals. The same trend of increased fat holds for all food animals that we have tamed.

Table D1 shows results of a study comparing fat contents of pigs and cattle.

Table D1. Total fat content of domestic and wild pigs and cattle.

	Domestic		Wild
	Pig	Heavy Hog	Warthog
Fat (%)	38	46	1.3
Lean (%)	50	44	82
*Protein/Fat	1/3	1/4	10/1

	Western			East African		
	Domestic Beef		Wild	Dom.	Wild	
	Fat	Lean	Venison	Zebu	Eland	Buffalo
Fat (%)	35	25	2	1.8	2	3
Lean (%)	50	55	76	71	79	75
*Protein/Fat	1/3	1/2	7/1	7/1	6/1	5/1

* Protein/fat is not the same as lean/fat because
   a) both fat and lean contain both protein and fat
   b) muscle tissue contains 80-85% water, whereas fat tissue contains only 30-50% water

Note that nomad cattle of East Africa, domesticated but not inbred, are as lean as their wild counterparts. When writers claim that the high meat diet of Africans does not predispose them to degenerative diseases, this is true. But when they claim that therefore beef won't hurt us either, this is false. The fat content in these two diets is markedly different.

Fatty Acid Composition of Meats

Beef and mutton contain large quantities of sticky, saturated and monounsaturated fatty acids, which explains why fats such as tallow are hard. Pork also contains mainly saturated and monounsaturated fatty acids, but also some linoleic acid (LA, 18:2w6), making pork fat (lard) softer than beef and lamb fats.

Table D2 shows the results of a study in which researchers measured the content of different fatty acids in both wild and domestic cattle and pigs.

Domestic cattle contain 80% non-essential fatty acids: 40% saturated fatty acids, made up of 28% palmitic acid (PA, 16:0) and 12% stearic acid (SA, 18:0); and 40% monounsaturated oleic acid (OA, 18:1w9). Beef fat contains only 4.3% essential fatty acids (EFAs) and EFA derivatives: 2.1% linoleic acid LA (18:2w6);

Table D2. Fatty acid content of wild and domestic cattle and pigs fats.

	Fatty Acids (percent of total fat)					Derivatives of	
	Non-Essential			Essential		Essential	
	Saturated		Monounsat.				
	16:0	18:0	18:1w9	18:2w6	18:3w3	20:4w6	22:6w3
Cattle							
Wild	16	20	21	16	5	8.2	3.2
Domestic	28	12	40	2.1	0.8	0.7	0.8
Pigs							
Wild	18	9.6	9	32	5	8.7	3.6
Domestic	24	13	34	10	0.5	0.4	0.5

0.8% LNA (18:3w3), and 1.5% EFA derivatives. Saturated and monounsaturated fatty acids compete for enzymes that metabolize EFAs (see Chapter 8, The Healing Essential Fatty Acids). We might guess that a ratio of 80 non-essential fatty acids to 2.9 EFAs is not ideal for health.

Critical Ratio

Tests have shown that in an oil containing 69 parts OA (18:1w9) to 3.5 parts LA (18:2w6), OA completely inhibits the EFA activity of the LA present in the oil. In percentages, this would be an oil containing 5% LA and 95% OA. This is the 'critical ratio'. It means that although our enzymes prefer to work on LA, large quantities of non-essential fatty acids compete successfully for enzyme attention and crowd out the LA from getting this enzyme attention.

Beef. The ratio of OA to LA for beef fat is 40:2.1 (69:3.6), about the same as the critical ratio. The LA in beef fat therefore cannot function. That's not the end of the bad news. Our body converts saturated fatty acids into unsaturated ones: 16:0 becomes 16:1w7 and 18:0 becomes 18:1w9. These also compete with LA for enzymes which normally elongate and desaturate LA to make prostaglandins and other vital long-chain derivatives. Thus the ratio of OA to LA for beef fat is potentially 40(18:1w9) + 12(18:0) + 28(16:0) to 2.1 or 80:2.1, much lower than the critical ratio of 69:3.5. This means that eating beef fat can be worse than getting no LA at all. Its long-term consumption inhibits the function of the main EFA in our body. Beef fat might therefore be called an EFA robber.

In *wild cattle*, the ratio of non-essential fatty acids to LA is 57:16 (69:19), which is 5 times more LA than the critical value of 69:3.5. Clearly, there is enough LA in the fat of wild cattle to be active in humans, and not so many non-essential fatty acids that they cancel out the LA's ability to function.

Pigs. The ratio for domestic pigs is 71:10 (69:9.7), whereas the same ratio for free-living warthogs is 37:32 (69:59.7). Although LA activity still occurs on a diet high in pork[1] the ratio in wild pig is far better and therefore has far higher LA activity. Refined sugars, refined starches in desserts and confections, and saturated and altered fats in junk foods also add to the load of non-essential fatty acids, and even further decrease the amount of LA still able to function. This needs to be considered when serving, say, pork chops with apple sauce, followed by dessert.

Effects on EFAs and health. EFAs produce prostaglandins that help regulate blood pressure through their effects on arterial muscle tone (see Chapter 58, Prostaglandins). They keep blood vessels elastic and affect platelet stickiness. EFAs are also necessary to metabolize cholesterol (see Chapter 8, The Healing Essential Fatty Acids). EFA-derived prostaglandins also regulate kidney function, inflammation response, and immune function.

Functional deficiency of LA hampers cholesterol metabolism, hardens arteries, raises blood pressure, impairs kidney and immune function, and alters tissue inflammation response. From our consideration of the fat content of the three most commonly eaten meats, such problems are fostered by 'normal' foods eaten by affluent Westerners.

The traditional Inuit diet, rich in both meat and fat, does not produce the above problems of fatty degeneration. The fatty acids found in their foods (see Chapter 55, Oils from Fish and Seafoods) have a better ratio of non-essential to essential fatty acids as well as being rich in w3s. Inuit do get osteoporosis, attributable to their extremely high protein intake, and burst blood vessel strokes, due to lack of vitamins C and E.

A Hopeful Note

With the present volume of press being generated on the role of high-fat diets in heart and artery disease, stroke, high blood pressure, and kidney failure, the meat industry is starting to listen. The American Heart Association, American Academy of Science, and other official and government bodies recommend decreasing our consumption of red meats.[2] Leaner red-meat animals are being produced by feeding them lean grass instead of fattening grains before they are slaughtered. One could also import and grow East African Cattle to solve the problem. Beef crossed with buffalo (called 'beefalo'), which contains less fat, is available in some restaurants.

But we have a long way to go before our meat contains the natural 3% of their weight as fat and the natural fatty acid ratios. If we, as consumers, keep demanding lean red meats (3 to 5% fats), we can push the meat industry to produce red meats that will not kill us.

---

[1] Other compelling reasons for avoiding pork include toxic substances, viruses, and parasites in its meat.

[2] In truth, there's nothing wrong with the red meat, but a lot wrong with the white fat bred into these animals. Before their slaughter, they are fattened on grain (grass keeps them, as salads keep us, leaner) for heavier profits, because animals are sold by weight.

Mother's Milk and Dairy Products 47

Mother's milk is the primordial, perfectly prepared, nutritionally balanced baby food for the first six months of life. Its origin reaches back through the dark shadows of the past, to a time when reptiles evolved into mammals that hatched their eggs within the safety of their own bodies instead of just laying them, running off, and leaving the hatchlings to fend for themselves.

Young mammals were better protected than young reptiles and had a better chance of survival with the extra maternal care, one reason why mice survived and dinosaurs perished. Mother's milk goes back to the time when cold-blooded reptiles became warm-blooded furry mammals, an adaptation that made them able to move fast even in cold climates, at a time when the earth's climate was cooling off. Like flies and spiders, reptiles slow down when the temperature drops.

Human Milk

As time progressed, the little reptiles-cum-mammals changed, through many new forms, to give rise to . . . us. That's if you believe in evolution. If not, then mother's milk has been around since the time of Eve. In either case, mother's milk as human food has been around as long as we have, and only the last few generations in recent civilized history have worshipped the breast as an anatomical ornament while feeding their children ersatz out of a bottle. Doctors miseducated by the 'better living through chemistry' gang had a lot to do with that unhealthy change.

According to figures published by the World Health Organization, mother's milk contains about 4.4% fat, of which an average of 8% is LA (18:2w6). Other figures show mother's milk to contain 3.5 to 4.0% fat. It has very little gamma-linolenic acid (GLA, 18:3w6) but contains dihomogamma-linolenic acid (DGLA, 20:3w6), an intermediate in the production of series 1 (PG1) prostaglandins (see Chapter 58, Prostaglandins). DGLA may be converted to arachidonic acid (AA, 20:4w6)[1], the parent of series 2 prostaglandins (PG2). DGLA is absent from most other human foods, and is not present in dairy products. Mother's milk ensures the newborn of a plentiful supply of prostaglandins with beneficial effects on blood pressure, clotting ability, kidney function, and immune system function. Among other things, it gives the baby a healthy cardiovascular start into its new world.

---

[1] Rats convert LA into AA readily. Under normal circumstances, humans do so only slowly (stress appears to increase the human conversion rate). Since the original experiments were done with rats, confusion resulted in scientific circles when rat results were automatically assumed to also apply to humans.

Studies have measured the content of different fatty acids present in mother's milk. They vary widely, depending on the fats present in the mother's diet. Table D3 shows pooled results of these studies.

Table D3. Fatty acid composition of human breast milk.

				Fatty Acids (percent of total fat)						
10:0	12:0	14:0	16:0	16:1	18:0	18:1	18:2	18:3	w6 long	w3 long
*2.5	8	11	25	2	6.2	30	9.2	0.9	0.9	1.3
**omnivore			27.6		10.8	35.3	(6.9)	(0.8)		
**vegan			(16.6)		(5.2)	31.3	31.7	1.5		
**Japanese			22.2		(5.5)	(27.9)	13.0	2.5		
**American			21.9			7.6	37.7	14.5	1.9	

Numbers in parentheses are lower than average.
Numbers underlined are higher than average.
* Average from studies carried out by FAO/WHO
** Values reported by Tinoco

It is especially interesting that breast milk of strict vegetarian mothers is very high in LA (18:2w6), and low in sticky saturated 16:0 and 18:0 fatty acids. Strict vegetarians have less than one-quarter the average rate of death from cardiovascular disease. It appears that their protection from this disease starts early in life.

Japanese (and Inuit) have a higher milk content of w3 fatty acids than North Americans. This results from their high intake of oils from fish, marine animals, and seaweed, and protects these people too, against cardiovascular disease, starting from an early age.

Cow's Milk

Cow's milk averages about 3.5% fat, a little less than human milk, and its history as human food is quite old. It is praised in East Indian scriptures over 5000 years old, and cheese-making equipment has been unearthed in old stone age dwellings in Switzerland, also from about 5000 years ago. The actual use of dairy products probably dates back much further into prehistory. A typical milk fat sample has the fatty acid composition shown in Table D4.

Table D4. Fatty acid composition of cow's milk.

				Fatty Acids (percent of total fat)						
4:0	6:0	8:0	10:0	12:0	14:0	16:0	18:0	18:1	18:2	18:3
3	2	2.5	1	5	10	30.6	12.5	26.9*	3.1	1

*Includes 3 to 6% *trans*- vaccenic acid (t18:1w7)

Fatty acid content of cow's milk can be modified by diet to increase 18:2w6 and 18:3w3 content. This is more difficult to achieve in cows than in humans, because bacteria in one of the cow's four stomachs destroy both EFAs by hydrogenating (saturating) them. For this reason, cow's milk is almost always low in essential fatty acids (EFAs).

To prevent this bacterial destruction of EFAs, a cow's food must be specially coated and processed by an expensive, time-consuming, economically unfeasible procedure. The milk that results from this endeavor is higher in EFAs, but tastes like formaldehyde, a cancer-causing preservative fed to cattle to knock out the bacteria in the cow's stomach that destroy the EFAs present in its food. Is industry trying *too* hard to make a better dairy product?

About 500 different fatty acids have been isolated from cow's milk so far. Most are present in only minute quantities. Cow's milk fat contains short-chain fatty acids (4:0 to 10:0) which are easy to digest, but is higher than human milk in sticky, saturated 16:0 and 18:0 fatty acids, and much lower in EFAs.

Other Milks

Goat's milk contains about 4% fats, and these fats are richer than cow's milk in short-chain fatty acids, making goat's milk easier to digest than cow's milk. Goat's milk, like cow's milk, is low in EFAs because goats also have EFA-destroying bacteria in their stomachs.

All ungulates which, besides cows and goats, include sheep, camel, water buffalo, llama, zebu, reindeer, caribou, moose, elk, and deer, produce low-EFA milk.

Ass' and mare's milk are EFA-rich. In Gengis Khan's Mongolia, mare's milk was fermented to make 'koumiss'. This high-w3, high-energy fuel powered the conquests of the Mongolian hordes, and made them feared adversaries. The fermenting bacteria, kept secret for generations, were wrested from a Mongolian warrior king by a Russian paramour, who brought them to Russia, where they were then used to ferment cow's milk to make the original 'kefir'.

An analysis of mare's milk shows why it had such a good reputation for enhancing health. It contains a whopping 38.4% of its fatty acids in the form of the w3 superunsaturated EFA, alpha-linolenic acid (LNA, 18:3w3),[2] and almost no sticky 18:0. The figures are given in Table D5.

Table D5. Fatty acid composition of mare's milk.

Fatty Acids (percent of total fat)				
16:0	18:0	18:1	18:2	18:3
19.9	1	18.6	7.4	38.4

[2] Unlike cows, horses have only one stomach, with no saturating bacteria in it. Their diet, of course, is the same grass. What a difference a bacteria can make!

Kefir sold in 'modern' trade is the EFA-poor cow's milk product. EFA-rich fermented mare's milk is far better for health. The high content of LNA in horses is also reflected in the makeup of their serum, where it is found associated with proteins. Horse serum was used experimentally in the 1950s to dissolve hard tumors. This research led to the use of flax oil to dissolve tumors in humans (see Chapter 59, Flax).

Milk fat of animals from cold far northern areas is very rich in w3 long-chain fatty acids. These are required to supply the energy chemistry to keep warm. Polar bear milk contains 31% fat, dolphin milk contains 19% fat, and harp seal milk contains 50% fat. Dolphin milk contains almost 15% of its fats as long-chain w3 superunsaturated 20:5w3 and 22:6w3, and 1.2% as w6 polyunsaturated 20:4w6 and 22:5w6. Harp seal milk contains about 10% of its fatty acids as long-chain w3s and w6s. Dolphin and harp seal milk contain very little sticky saturated stearic acid (18:0).

Polar bear, dolphin, and seal milk are unlikely to become human food in the near future, but the information shows that the fatty acid profiles of both food supply and milk of each species are similar. Both are adapted to the needs of climate (see Chapter 67, Oils and Sunshine), and differ from one species to another. The information we gather from studying the milk of these animals further corroborates which fats cause fatty degeneration and which fats prevent and heal it, and why traditional Inuit were free of these diseases while we are not.

Dairy Products Other Than Milk

By extracting water, removing all or part of the fat from milk, and/or fermenting it, we make products whose fat content varies from less than 1% fat, such as skim milk and dry cottage cheese; to close to 50% fat, such as gourmet and cream cheeses (see Chapter 44, How Fat are Your Foods?).

The fatty acid profile of fats in dairy products is similar to that of milk. All dairy products are low in EFAs. They contain nothing to alleviate fat problems of human beings and, taken in excess, enhance these fat problems. They raise triglyceride and cholesterol levels. They increase platelet stickiness. Although they contain good protein and calcium, and may taste delicious, they leave a lot to be desired from the point of view of fats, oils, cholesterol, and human health. They are also low in the minerals magnesium, iron, and zinc.

The cholesterol in dairy products, combined with sticky fatty acids, creates a burden that must be carried by fat-dispersing w3s and w6s, which must come from another source. Although human milk contains cholesterol, it also contains the dispersing w3 and w6 EFAs that help keep cholesterol from oxidizing and damaging the walls of our arteries. Human milk is therefore better adapted for human health than the milk that the cow, and her relatives produce.

In contrast to beef, whose muscle meat is streaked with fats throughout (bred especially for this effect), birds carry the bulk of their fat just under the skin. It is easy to separate fowl fats from their meat, and this is a reason for their nutritional superiority to fattened beef and pork.

Fat Content

Table D6 gives the fat content of different parts of birds most commonly eaten.

Table D6. Fat content of common fowl.

	Fat Content (percent of total weight)				
	Total Fat	**Skin**	**White Meat**	**Dark Meat**	**Innards**	**Linoleic Acid (18:2w6)**
---	---	---	---	---	---	---
Turkey - young	14.7	39.2	0.4	2.6	6.6	15-20%
- old	14.7	39.2	1.2	4.3	6.6	15-20%
Chicken	17.9	28.9	1.9-3.7	4.7-7.5		20-25%
Goose	31.5		7.1			
Duck - domestic	28.6		8.2			
- wild	15.8		5.2			

Turkey meat without skin is the leanest and driest poultry. More fats make meats more 'moist'. White meat contains less oil than dark meat, and is therefore drier. We verify this fact for ourselves every Thanksgiving.

The skin of poultry is loaded with fat. People on low-fat diets should eat only the meat and leave the skin. The figures in Table D6 show the difference in fat content of meat and skin.

Young birds are leaner than older ones. Like humans, domesticated turkeys apparently get middle-aged spread. Inner organs contain more fat than muscle meats, but less than skin.

Fowl contains 25% w6 EFA (LA, 18:2w6), more than beef (about 2%) or pork (up to 10%), but far less than good oil seeds. Fowl contains far less w3s than oily fish and far less LNA than oil seeds like flax and hemp.

Goose and duck have more oil in both meat and skin than do chicken and turkey. Goose grease was used traditionally for frying in place of lard.

Domestic birds have higher fat content than wild birds, as with other animals. This is also true for birds like pheasant, quail, and pigeon. Fat wild animals perish quickly. Changes in commercial poultry raising practices resulted in increased fat content of birds. Cooped chickens are fatter than free-range birds.

Nursery Wisdom

A nursery rhyme tells us that:

Jack Spratt would eat no fat.
His wife would eat no lean.
So twixt them both,
They cleared the cloth
And licked the platter clean.

Nutritionally speaking, Jack Spratt and his wife had a useful arrangement. He avoided fat, and she wasted no food. He kept his arteries clean, thereby avoiding a coronary or stroke. She ate the fats. Her estrogen hormones (or periodic blood loss) protected her from cardiovascular disease until menopause. This old traditional nursery rhyme is based on a sound practical understanding of fats.

In practice however, men consume slightly *more* fats than women. Women avoid eating fats more for mistaken cosmetic reasons[1] (mustn't be fat!) than for health. This is unfortunate, because men are more prone than women to get fat clogging their arteries and die of cardiovascular disease more frequently. Better stick to nursery wisdom!

49 Eggs

Eggs are (or were, before their commercialized production) a balanced, rich source of nutrients. Primarily, eggs are designed for making new birds rather than for our culinary pleasure. To make a new bird, the egg must contain all the minerals, vitamins, proteins and fats necessary to create a fully formed, hatchable, living chick.

Wild Birds' Eggs

Our ancestors relished an occasional feast of eggs whenever they succeeded in stealing eggs from birds before the latter brooded and hatched them and the young birds flew away. For primitive man, eggs were a *rare* delicacy. Since they did not keep birds, they had to first find, then pilfer, the hidden nests of birds. Birds laid seasonally, and only a few eggs every year, so eggs were available only in spring and summer. Eggs were nutritionally rich.

---

[1] The underlying notions are that fats make you fat, and that slimness is attractive. The first notion is not true; the second is a matter of taste. Rembrandt, Michelangelo, and the Renaissance painters, as well as many less artistically gifted, present-day men prefer their women 'pleasantly plump'!

Domestication

As we domesticated birds, we made changes in their food supply. We fed them grains and other household discards. Second, we sheltered them, so their egg laying capacity increased, and our consumption of eggs became possible on a more regular basis. Even then, winters were eggless, a time of rest for the chicken, to gather its resources for the next breeding, laying, and hatching season.

Eggs contain about 11% fats. The yolk contains about 30% fats by weight; the white is fat-free. An egg contains about 250 mg of cholesterol.

Commercial Egg Production

When we turned egg production into an 'intensive' business, we made more changes. One of these was the introduction of chicken feeds 'scientifically' formulated to maximize egg production – to 'get *everything* out of the chicken'. These feeds replaced grains, living insects, and live plant materials that birds obtained in the wild.

We learned how to keep chickens alive and producing in the least labor-intensive situation. This resulted in the laying 'battery', where hens spend their entire life indoors, eating and laying till they die. Antibiotics were added to feeds to keep cooped-up chickens 'healthy', which means safe from epidemics of infections that can spread like wildfire through crowded quarters, and which can kill many chickens very quickly.

The composition of chicken feed was changed to increase shelf life. Nature protects nutrients in grains and seeds from spoiling by using meticulous, ingenious, precise, molecule-by-molecule packaging. To obtain fresh greens, free chickens foraged in the barnyard. Lacking nature's packaging genius, we couldn't protect some of the more sensitive ingredients from spoiling when we formulated feeds that need to be stable during long transport and storage times in warehouses and retail stores. To accommodate this commercial consideration, we took out some of the easily spoilable nutrients.

The easily spoilable EFAs linoleic acid (LA, 18:2w6) and alpha-linolenic acid (LNA, 18:3w3), which are present in the natural chicken diet of grains, seeds, and greens, were replaced by more stable, non-essential oleic acid (OA, 18:1w9). The result of this change was eggs higher in OA, but lower in LA and LNA; and eggs with the same amount of cholesterol, but less EFAs to transport and metabolize it properly in our body.

With the 'refinement' of commercial chicken feeds, plant sterols, which reduce the cholesterol content of eggs by up to 35% and are found naturally in all vegetables, were removed from the chickens' diet. Commercial eggs therefore contain more cholesterol than home grown barnyard eggs. Refined, dried foods are also subject to deterioration by oxidation of essential nutrients and by time.

Eggs, considered for centuries a most nutritious food, have been attacked during the last 35 years as a possible source of cardiovascular 'accidents' – one name for heart attacks and strokes.[1]

Over the course of years, our 'improvements' in commercial methods enabled us to produce – cheaply and by the millions – eggs whose yolks are almost colorless, almost tasteless, and unhatchable. Not exactly the proverbial 'good egg' anymore. Like humans, chickens in concentration camps don't perform their best, because they are not in a healthy situation. Like us, healthy chickens require sunshine, whole fresh foods, fresh air, and room to move. Then they lay healthy eggs.

Free Range Eggs

Health-conscious consumers have created a market for a return to more 'primitive' small-scale methods of egg production. Free-range eggs come from free-ranging chickens. These chickens are fed commercial mash because without it, egg production would be too low, and the price too high. But free-range chickens also run around and forage for themselves. The difference in taste and yolk color is remarkable. Although precise biochemical analyses to compare the nutritional merits of the two types of eggs have not been performed (no one has volunteered to support the needed research), the difference in taste and color points to differences in nutritional content. To compare the nutritional qualities of 'battery' and free-range eggs would be a worthwhile project for a budding young researcher.

Where I live, it is illegal to advertise free-range chicken eggs. If such advertising were allowed, the Egg Marketing Board might have to explain the difference and they don't want to have to do this. Perhaps because they might end up with egg on their faces?

Eggshell color is not an indicator of nutritional value. Like brown eyes, brown eggs are determined by a gene. The *nutritional value* of the egg depends on what the chicken ate.

It is possible to 'doctor' the color of egg yolks with beta carotene, but this is not usually done because beta carotene is expensive (bottled oils are sometimes doctored with carotene or other dyes). Cheap artificial dyes could be used, so it is wise for consumers to know the source of their eggs. Free-range eggs are usually found in natural food stores and on farms.

Since free-range eggs cannot be advertised and there is no government control, someone could sell battery eggs as free-range. If you can afford a piece of

---

[1] Despite its high cholesterol content, statistics of egg use and cardiovascular disease (CVD) seem to exonerate the egg from blame for the rise in deaths from CVD. In the years from 1950-1965, egg consumption dropped from 390 to 315 per person per year, while deaths from CVD rose from 215 to 292 per 100,000 population, suggesting that *not* eating eggs causes CVD. One has to be careful, however, with these statistics, since many factors besides egg consumption, including time lag between consumption and disease development, need to be taken into account.

land, keep your own chickens. Then you know what they are eating. You can feed them grains, vegetable peels, and other kitchen refuse, and let them find the rest of their food by scratching. That way, you can avoid using commercial feeds.

A bad egg is not the chicken's fault. The chicken can only make eggs as good as the feed it gets. When it is free to pick its own food, it makes great tasting, nutritious eggs.

Free-ranging chickens lay few eggs in winter, because winter is their time of rest. In keeping with the flow of nature, free-range eggs are hard to find between November and February. To make eggs go around when the chickens quit for the year, eggs were traditionally pickled or 'jelled' in glass jars. Even without the benefit of a university education, chickens have always known that winter is not a good time to hatch eggs.

Oils in Seeds 50

The seeds of most plants contain oils[1] that serve as high-energy starter for seedlings. Like a chicken's egg, a plant's seed must contain enough energy for sprouting a whole plant, and for growing first root, first stem, and first leaves, which then take over the functions of drawing water and minerals from the soil, drawing sunshine from the sun, and conducting the water and minerals up and the sunshine down to grow to maturity. Oils in seeds are the mother's breast for seedlings until the new plant becomes independent. They are nutrient-rich – an excellent source of health-providing nutrients.

The tougher the conditions, the more oil the seed needs to store. The colder the climate, the more superunsaturated w3 essential fatty acids (EFAs) it contains in its oils to increase its metabolic rate. The amount of oil and the fatty acid composition varies widely between different species from different climates.

Oil Content
The amount of oil found in different kinds of seeds and nuts varies from 4% for corn to over 70% for pecans. There are wide variations in oil content of seeds from the same kind of plant in different years and from different locations, so tables give only typical values.

Fatty Acid Composition
Table D7 lists fat content and fatty acid composition of common (and not so

---

[1] Seeds also contain protein, fiber, minerals, vitamins, enzymes, and water, but our focus here is on their oils.

common) oil seeds.

The EFA-richest oils are hemp, kukui, chia, and flax oils. These oils contain both EFAs.

Best oils.

The best oils are unrefined, and taste like the seed from which they were mechanically (expeller) pressed without solvents. These oils must be made with care and stored in opaque containers, protected from light, oxygen, and heat. Nutrient-wise, they are superior, but they must be consumed fresh before they spoil. Fresh oils from superior seeds should be available freshly pressed, protectively packaged, and quickly delivered in such a way that consumers get them unspoiled.

Hemp seed oil comes from the seeds of the marijuana plant. From their childhood in Russia, my parents remember huge, lush fields of dark green hemp plants. The fiber was used to make hemp rope; the seeds were used to make delicious 'hemp butter' that puts peanut butter to shame for nutritional value; the leaves were ploughed back under as organic fertilizer. No one smoked the plant! Hemp oil contains 19% of the three times (super) unsaturated alpha-linolenic acid (LNA), 18:3w3; 57% of the twice (poly) unsaturated linoleic acid (LA), 18:2w6; and 1.7% LA-derived, three time (poly) unsaturated gamma-linolenic acid (GLA), 18:3w6. Its unusually well-balanced profile means that one could use it for a lifetime without ever suffering EFA deficiency. Its content of GLA makes it unique among edible seed oils.

Flax provides the best therapeutic oil for people with w3 deficiency-related fatty degeneration, because it contains the largest amount of LNA, the most strongly dispersing EFA. LNA helps disperse deposits of saturated fatty acids and cholesterol, which like to aggregate and make platelets sticky. To be good for health, flax oil must be fresh and not exposed to light, oxygen, and heat, because these three agents destroy LNA rapidly. In the long run, flax oil can be *too* rich in LNA, leading to LA deficiency.

Pumpkin seed oil is dark green and delicious, but difficult to obtain. Depending on the variety of pumpkin, it may contain from 0 to 15% LNA and from 45 to 60% LA. Unfortunately, most commonly available kinds contain no LNA.

Unrefined **walnut** oil has a delightful flavor, but is difficult to find fresh. Most walnut oil being marketed is refined.

Unrefined **soybean** oil is a high-quality oil, but the yield from mechanical pressing is low (only 18% of the bean is oil). Fresh, unrefined soybean oil is delicious. It is an excellent source of EFAs, lecithin, phytosterols, and other natural factors that inhibit some kinds of cancers.

Most of the soy oil in commercial trade is refined and partly hydrogenated, destroying the LNA it contains to prevent off flavors due to deteriorating LNA. Strains of soybean with lower LNA content are being developed to improve soy-

Table D7. Fat content and fatty acid composition of seed oils.

Name	Fat Content (%)	Fatty Acid Composition (% of total oil)					Other Information
		18:3n-3	18:2n-6	18:1n-9	18:0	16:0	
almond	54.2		17	78	5		
avocado	12		10	70	20		
beech	50		32	54	8		
brazil	66.9		24	48	24		
cashew	41.7		6	70	18		
chia	30	30	40				
coconut	35.3		3	6	3%	± 10%	18% 14:0 myristic / 14% short chain fatty acids / 50% lauric acid 12:0
corn	4		59	24	17		
cottonseed	40		50	21	25		toxic ingred.
evening primrose	17		81*	11	2	6	
filbert	62.4		16	54	5		
flax	35	58	14	19	4	5	
grape	20		71	17	12		
hemp	35	20	60**	12	2	6	may fail drug screens
hickory	68.7		17	68	9		
kukui (candlenut)	30	29	40				
macadamia	71.6		10	71	12		
neem	40	1	20	41	20		extremely bitter
olive	20		8	76	16		
palm kernel	35.3		2	13		85	
peanut	47.5		29	47	18		toxic fungus
pecan	71.2		20	63	7		
pistachio	53.7		19	65	9		
pumpkin	46.7	0-15	42-57	34	0	9	
rape (canola)	30	7	30	54***	7		
rice bran	10	1	35	48	17		
safflower	59.5		75	13	12		
sesame	49.1		45	42	13		
soybean	17.7	7	50	26	6	9	
sunflower	47.3		65	23	12		
walnut	60	5	51	28	5	11	
wheat germ	10.9	5	50	25	18		

* Includes 9% GLA
** Includes up to 2% GLA
*** Includes up to 5% erucic acid

bean oil shelf stability. When such strains become commercial, we will have diminished the quality of an excellent oil. Soybeans are more nutritious than refined oil.

Instead of breeding LNA out of soybeans, it makes more sense to preserve the nutrient value of oils, and develop better technology for protected pressing and sheltered packaging, storage, and transport to ensure that good oils reach consumers fresh. The technology and methods to deliver such oils are now available. It just needs to be more widely applied. I help manufacturers with the details of building and conversion.

Fresh, unrefined **wheat germ** oil has a nice taste. Most wheat germ oil being marketed is old and rancid, and tastes awful. Wheat germ oil contains some LNA, and is a rich source of a 28-carbon fatty alcohol (octacosanol),[2] which protects heart function and may help nerve regeneration. Wheat germ oil is also one of the richest natural sources of vitamin E.

Good oils

The next five oils lack LNA, the w3 EFA. Therefore they should be used in conjunction with LNA-containing oils. Our body's need for LA, the w6 EFA (18:2w6), is higher than its need for LNA, and these oils supply good quantities of the major EFA.

Unrefined **safflower** and **sunflower** seed oils are available in natural food stores alongside refined oils. Generally they are sold in transparent bottles that expose them to light on display shelves. These oils would be better in opaque containers, safe from light, air, and heat.

Sesame seed oil has a pleasant natural flavor, and is easy to press without heat. For health, it should be unrefined and untoasted. Sesame oil contains natural preservatives (sesamol, sesamin) that stabilize this relatively LA-rich oil, so it keeps longer than expected.

Rice bran oil is another stable w6 oil. Unrefined rice bran oil is a rich source of natural waxes and sterols that lower cholesterol levels. Unfortunately, its black color makes it look rather unpleasant.

None of the above oils should be used for frying, because EFAs and other natural constituents of these oils are destroyed by high temperature (see Chapter 22, Frying and Deep-Frying). These oils are for salads, salad dressings, mayonnaise, and yogurt, and can be added to freshly prepared dishes such as hot vegetables and hot grains. To improve health, preferred habits such as frying with oils must be changed. These habits, traditionally handed down from parent to child, or learned from modern food trends, do not support the health we seek.

Evening primrose oil (EPO) is used therapeutically. It is sold in small cap-

---

[2] Octacosanol, like EPA, is considered a drug in Canada, but wheat kernels, wheat germ, and wheat germ oil, all of which contain it are considered foods.

sules in natural food stores. It is more expensive than bottled oils, because we're paying for research and research staff. The oil is usually solvent-extracted, but expeller-pressed EPO is now available. EPO is always refined.

EPO and other therapeutic oils such as **borage** and **black currant** contain LA and GLA, a triply unsaturated w6 EFA derivative. Under certain conditions of illness and dietary deficiency, our body may be unable to make GLA from LA, and EPO can compensate for this inability. GLA provides benefit for arthritis and premenstrual syndrome. As much as 10 to 25% of affluent populations could benefit from its use. GLA is an intermediate in the production of prostaglandins (see Chapter 58, Prostaglandins) with important hormone-like regulating functions affecting heart and arteries, menstrual cycle, glands, kidneys, joints, mental function, and metabolic rate (see Chapter 57, Evening Primrose, Borage, and Black Currant Oils). In addition to GLA, black currant oil also contains LNA and the first w3 derivative of LNA, which is called stearidonic acid (SDA, 18:4w3).

Mediocre W6 Oils

Corn oil is usually solvent-extracted (corn contains only 4% oil) and refined, but occasionally one can obtain mechanically pressed, unrefined corn oil pressed from corn germ. But corn oil is usually partially rancid, with a peroxide value (PV) of 40 to 60. Most other oils have a PV of less than 10.

Grape seed oil is similar to corn oil, and has no special advantages over other oils. It is rich in w6s and contains no w3s. We'd have to eat a lot of grapes to collect enough seeds to press a teaspoon of oil, but if we buy seeded instead of seedless grapes and crunch up the nutritious seeds instead of throwing them away, our digestive system will extract their unrefined w6 oil without destroying its quality or losing the vitamins and minerals they also contain. Grape seeds are used for pressing oil because as waste products in wine and juice operations, they are cheap starting material.

Oils for Skin

Almond, apricot, and **prune** oils are similar in their fatty acid profile. All are high in oleic acid, making them monounsaturate oils. Almond oil is rich in vitamin E, and stable. Its stability and fine aroma makes almond oil valuable as a skin and massage oil. EFA-rich oils are better for our skin, but become rancid when applied to skin from outside. The best way to oil our skin with EFA-rich oils is from inside, by eating them.

Neem oil is good for skin because it contains natural ingredients with anti-fungal, anti-bacterial, antiseptic (germicidal), fever-reducing (anti-pyretic), anti-inflammatory properties. It is also an excellent repellent of mosquitoes, sandflies, and other noxious insects, and kills lice and fleas. Neem oil has been used to heal eczema, acne, psoriasis, dry skin, and dandruff. The oil kills athlete's foot fungus, ringworm fungus, thrush, vaginal yeast, and candida. Neem oil is used in some skin creams, shampoos, soaps and toothpastes.

Monounsaturated Oils

Rape and **mustard** seed are monounsaturated oils that contain small amounts of both EFAs. Unrefined, these oils have a spicy flavor due to glucosinolates (sulfates) that make the oil range in taste from bearable to unpleasant. Therefore they are usually sold refined. Rape and mustard seeds contain up to 40% erucic acid which was mistakenly thought by the Canadian government to cause heart damage in humans (see Chapter 20, Erucic Acid). They have been removed from our market. In India and China, they continue to be used (unrefined) without apparent damage to health.

Canola oil, the low erucic acid rape seed (LEAR) oil that replaced high erucic acid rape (HEAR) and mustard oils in North America, contains less than 5% erucic acid. Like soybean oil, canola oil is sometimes partially hydrogenated, destroying its LNA to prevent off flavors due to LNA deterioration.

Peanut oil is a stable, high monounsaturate oil. If peanuts are fungus-free, the oil is fine. Peanut oil is available as a true batch-pressed unrefined oil with a wonderful peanut aroma. But peanuts (and therefore their oil) may contain carcinogenic substances made by a fungus that grows in damp peanuts (see Chapter 19, Other Toxic Products). This fungus can also infest other damp grains and seeds, but peanuts are most susceptible because they grow underground.

Avocado oil is a monounsaturated oil that is usually sold refined. It is similar to olive, peanut and almond oils in its EFA and monounsaturated fatty acid content.

Olive Oil

Olive oil is rich in monounsaturates but low in EFAs. Reasons for its popularity over thousands of years of history include stability (important in a Mediterranean climate before refrigeration), and ease of pressing from soft olive flesh without requiring high pressure equipment (important before high pressure oil-pressing equipment was invented).

A major reason for olive oil's reputation for health is that *virgin* olive oils are the only unrefined oils sold on the general mass market. Olive oil still contains phytosterols, chlorophyll, magnesium, vitamin E, carotene, other substances present in seeds and natural unrefined oils, and important 'minor' ingredients unique to olives (see Chapter 54, Virgin Olive Oils). This fact alone makes olive oil the *only* mass market oil presently worth recommending. All other mass market oils, being refined, bleached, and deodorized, are nutrient-poor. Their natural antioxidants, natural flavor and odor molecules, pigments, oil-soluble vitamins, and plant sterols were largely removed during processing.

Olive oil contains about 80% monounsaturated fatty acids, 8 to 10% LA (w6), and about 1% LNA (w3). It is therefore not a rich source of EFAs, which must be provided by other oils. Besides its use in foods, olive oil is used, along with fresh lemon juice, to flush toxins from the liver. Its usefulness in this application has declined in recent years. Unrefined oils richer in both EFAs more effectively relieve overworked livers.

Seed Oils that can be Heated

Butter, and tropical fats – **coconut, palm, palm kernel, cocoa,** and **shea nut** – are safest for frying, because they contain only small quantities of EFAs. The saturated fatty acids contained in oils are inert and therefore heat-stable. Heat does not destroy them in the same way as it destroys EFAs, which heat turns into poisonous breakdown products that interfere with EFA functions (see Chapter 22, Frying and Deep-Frying). Butter and tropical fats are best used *un*hydrogenated. Only small amounts should be eaten, as they are sticky, hard, saturated fatty acid-containing fats.

Tropical oils got a bad reputation for increasing cholesterol and triglyceride levels that supposedly cause cardiovascular disease. An unconfirmed rumor suggests that the soybean industry financed the successful campaign against tropical fats to kill imports and increase soybean oil sales. Tropical oils used in their country of origin have been shown in several studies to *decrease* cholesterol levels. The difference in results may be due to several causes: deterioration in tropical oils during storage (oxidation); processing (hydrogenation); differing experimental design; or a combination of the above. Raw tropical oils are rich sources of vitamin E and tocotrienols, which help protect arteries from damage leading to CVD.

Bad News

Other oils in table D7 have one or more of several possible problems. **Cottonseed** oil contains toxic natural ingredients as well as pesticide residues. Other oils are rich in monounsaturated and saturated fatty acids, but poor in EFAs. Still others are commercially unavailable.

Whole Seeds

Seeds are nutritionally balanced. They provide the best way to get fresh oils. In addition to EFAs, seeds also contain vitamins, minerals, proteins, fiber, and many important minor seed-specific ingredients. Good quality seeds are our most reliable sources of the freshest possible oils. Only if we need more than 2 tablespoons of oil, which is common in the treatment of degenerative conditions, do we need to rely on bottled oils.

In view of the nutritional value of seeds, we ought to consider chewing the seeds of fruits and melons. People from many older cultures, including traditions like Hunza and parts of Russia famous for health and long life, eat seeds as a normal practice. In India, papaya seeds are eaten for both their nutritional value and their tonic effect on nerves. They have a slight peppery nip, reminiscent of radishes and watercress.

We should seriously reconsider our habits of both processing and throwing nutrient-rich seeds away.

51 *Butter versus Margarine*

Is butter better than margarine? This question sustains a marketing battle waged in the media by dairy boards and oil processors. Everyone loves a good controversy. This one has become a good advertising tool for both sides, keeping both products on our mind. Let's look at the health effects of butter and margarine in light of what we know about fatty acids and their metabolism in our body.

Butter

About 500 different fatty acids have been isolated from butter. Butter contains butyric acid (4:0) and other short-chain fatty acids (6:0, 8:0, 10:0), which are easy to digest. Score 1 point for butter.

Butter is low in essential fatty acids (EFAs), containing only about 2% linoleic acid (LA, 18:2w6) and virtually no alpha-linolenic acid (LNA, 18:3w3). Human milk fat, in contrast, contains between 7 and 14% LA and up to 2% LNA. The milk fat of vegetarian mothers contains up to 32% LA and 3% LNA. Since the composition of human milk provides a natural standard for humans, and butter fails to meet that standard, take 1 point from butter.

Butter contains about 9% stearic acid (SA, 18:0), 19% oleic acid (OA, 18:1w9), and 38% palmitic acid (PA, 16:0), a total of 66% of its total fat content. These three compete for the enzymes that metabolize LA and LNA and, in excess, can interfere with the functions of EFAs, especially if the latter make up less than about 5% of total fat content. Take 1 point from butter.

A pound of butter contains about 1 gram of cholesterol, a substance required by all of our cells. Some people's cholesterol level increases from eating cholesterol-containing foods. Others' cholesterol levels are unaffected by dietary cholesterol. According to old dogma, elevated (oxidized) cholesterol levels are associated with atherosclerotic deposits – made of proteins, fats, cholesterol, calcium, and other materials – in our arteries, and deaths from heart attack, stroke, and kidney and heart failure.

Newer research blames North American diets' lack of antioxidants, minerals, vitamins, and fiber for failures in cholesterol metabolism. While we hold butter blameless for these dietary inadequacies, butter lacks factors required for its own metabolism (oil seeds do contain these factors). Take 1 point from butter.

Butter concentrates pesticides about 5 to 10 times more than oils of vegetable origin. Take 1 point from butter.

Dairy farmers use antibiotics,[1] in both cattle feed and injections. These find their way into butter. Antibiotics encourage the growth of yeasts and fungi (including candida) in humans, and can cause allergies, tiredness, sugar craving (to feed candida), hypoglycemia, skin afflictions, and other conditions. The use of antibiotics also kills susceptible bacteria, allowing antibiotic-resistant bacteria to thrive. Their resistance factors can be transferred to disease-causing bacteria. These findings, just starting to get attention, have ominous implications. Take 1 point from butter.

Butter contains up to 6% *trans-* fatty acids. *Trans-* fatty acids are produced by bacteria in the stomach of cows, and are mainly *trans-* vaccenic (t18:1w7) acid, which is more easily metabolized than most *trans-* fatty acids found in hydrogenated oils, fats, shortenings, and margarines; therefore they constitute a *minor* risk to health. Take 1/2 point from butter.

Butter can be used for frying and other high-heat applications because its mainly saturated and monounsaturated fatty acids are relatively stable to light, heat, and oxygen. Its low content of EFAs is an advantage here. Score 1 point for butter. Total score for butter: plus 2, minus 5.5 = minus 3.5.

If butter comes from an organic farm, it contains no antibiotics or pesticides. Then it scores -1.5. If our diet contains the necessary nutrients, cholesterol is not a problem. Then butter breaks even.

That's what butter is. A neutral fat, not good, not bad. Useful for frying and easy to digest. But not necessary and, in excess, dangerous.

Margarine

Margarine contains few short-chain, easily digestible fatty acids. Take 1 point from margarine.

The oils from which margarines are made contain ample EFAs. But partial hydrogenation destroys many of these EFA molecules, or changes them into altered substances. The finished product is low in EFAs and contains toxic molecules. Take 2 points from margarine.

Margarine's non-essential 18-carbon fatty acids compete with the EFAs it still contains, further lowering the functional amount of EFAs in the product. Take 1 point from margarine.

Margarine contains no cholesterol. Score 1 point for margarine. But like butter, margarine lacks the minerals and vitamins for its metabolism. These were left in the seed cake as well as processed out of the oil, and are not present in margarine. Take 1 point from margarine.

Margarine contains less pesticides than butter. Take 0 points from mar-

---

[1] Before the advent of antibiotics, farmers kept cattle healthy by feeding them cooked flax mash and other natural, nutrient-rich foods.

garine. Margarine contains no antibiotics. No point for or against.

Margarine contains *trans-* fatty acids in substantial amounts. Some samples of margarine tested contained 60% *trans-* fatty acids.[2] *Trans-* fatty acids have properties different from natural *cis-* fatty acids, interfere with EFA functions, are concentrated in heart tissue, burn slower than *cis-* fatty acids and, for this reason, may help cause cardiovascular disease. Take 1 point from margarine.

Hydrogenation produces dozens of other non-natural chemicals. Many are toxic or have not been adequately studied to determine their effects on human health.

Almost 10 pounds of altered fat substances are consumed each year by each person, more than twice the amount of all other food additives combined. More than half of these altered fat substances come from margarine. Take 2 points from margarine.

Margarine is a source of unwelcome aluminum (and nickel) in our foods. Aluminum is a serious concern, associated with senility, osteoporosis, and cancer. Take 1 point from margarine.

Margarine is not suitable for frying, because the double bonds (unsaturated fatty acids) it still contains are further denatured by heat, light, and oxygen. If you fry with margarine, take 1 point from margarine. If you don't use margarine for frying, no point for or against.

Margarine is often advertised in a misleading way as high in polyunsaturated fatty acids, which the public equates with good health because EFAs are polyunsaturated. However, some of margarine's polyunsaturated fatty acids (PUFAs) are non-natural, chemically altered PUFAs that are bad for health. Take 1 point from margarine.

The water present in margarine[3] – almost 20%[4] – slowly destroys double bonds, creating altered products during storage, transit, or display. Take 1 point from margarine. Total score for margarine: plus 1, minus 11 or 12 = -10 or -11

Other Possibilities

It is possible to make margarine without pesticides.

It is also possible to make margarines without *trans-* fatty acids (such as the brand name *Becel,* in which refined sunflower oil is hardened with refined tropical fats). Margarines and shortenings containing *trans-* fatty acids are dangerous to health. The more we consume, the more dangerous they are. They're completely harmless if we leave them on the shelf.

Spreadable oil-water reverse emulsions that contain no *trans-* fatty acids, no

---

2 Some of these margarines contained less than 5% of the essential linoleic acid (18:2w6).

3 Butter also contains about 20% water, but since saturated fatty acids are not altered by water, butter loses no points on this count.

4 Water is an inexpensive ingredient.

cholesterol, no tropical fats, no hydrogenated products, and plenty of EFAs may appear on the market. They are made by mayonnaise technologies, usually using fully refined deodorized oils with salt, flavor, and preservatives added. These emulsions may be preferable to margarines in terms of health. They cannot be frozen or heated without coming apart, which somewhat limits their applications. How good they are for health depends on their freshness and the freshness and quality of the oils and other ingredients used.

In countries like Spain, people spread neither butter nor margarine on bread. Instead, they cut a tomato in half, squash the open tomato into their bread to close the holes, and then pour fresh virgin olive oil directly onto the bread. In Italy, people simply dip their bread in virgin olive oil. That solves the butter and margarine question for them, and gives them better health.

The Trophy Goes To . . .
Butter wins easily on taste, digestibility, usefulness for frying, and naturalness. Lower cost is the main factor favoring margarine, but the key issue – how to get optimal amounts and balances of both w6 and w3 EFAs, and avoid the killer saturated and hydrogenated fats – is not addressed by butter, margarine, becel, or new spreads.

History of Butter and Margarine
Our story of butter and margarine would be incomplete without historical perspective. Butter has been part of man's diet since cows were domesticated thousands of years ago. Degenerative diseases on a large scale are more recent in origin, having risen from rarity to epidemic proportions in the last 100 years, while butter consumption decreased. It is unlikely that butter, the cholesterol it contains, or the cows that provide us with both are to blame for the meteoric rise of degenerative disease.

The history of margarine is shorter. It began in France under Napoleon III, who was looking for a cheap source of fat for the 'cheap' classes of people in his country: the army, the navy, and the poor. He held a contest in 1867, inviting inventors to submit recipes and samples. Professor Hippolyte Mege-Mouris won the contest by mixing beef fat (suet) with skim milk to create the first margarine. The concoction tasted awful. As late as 15 years later, in 1882, poor working housewives were being dissuaded from using this 'artificial butter' because "its taste is disagreeable, and it is harmful for health."

Since then, the story of margarine has been twofold: experiments to concoct tastier mixtures; and the hype of image-making campaigns to free margarine from its image as the 'poor people's butter' and to dress it up as 'heart-healthy'.

The most common starting materials for margarines today are cheap seed oils: refined cottonseed, soybean, canola, and corn oils. Sometimes fish and whale oils are also used in mixtures of several oils. Hydrogenation makes it possible to chemically 'harden' any liquid oil to the desired plastic consistency (see Chapter 17, From Oil to Margarine).

The image-making campaign has been largely successful. Margarine is far cheaper than butter to make and, although it costs less to buy, leaves large profits for manufacturers, with money left over to continue image making (see Chapter 24, Advertising and Jargon).

52 *Tropical Fats*

Tropical fats, which were called tropical 'oils' in the past, have received much negative attention since 1988. That year, an ostensibly self-styled champion spent a million dollars placing ads in major newspapers across the country to connect these 'killer fats' to high cholesterol, heart attacks, strokes, and other cardiovascular conditions. One man against the monster.

The image of the little guy against an entire industry is appealing. The ploy worked. Although the facts he used were wrong, (don't expect cardiovascular deaths to plummet because tropical oil use is down) the public was convinced. Sales of tropical oils dropped through the floor. People who used them in chocolates substituted the same saturated fats from other sources and with different names, since chocolate melting range and texture (or 'mouth feel') require them. More important than the facts was that the names of the same material from other sources (fractionated oils) did not link them with 'evil' tropical oils.

Tropical 'oils' are still used in non-dairy coffee creamers, which people now use with greater trepidation than before – the same product plus, now a small amount of mental stress due to the negative image tropical 'oils' have recently acquired. They are also used in commercially prepared baby formulas, partly because babies don't read labels, and partly because babies need some fat in their diet, and tropical oils are about the most stable fats known. They contain almost no essential fatty acids (EFAs).

More recently, in 1993, a champion *for* tropical fats has also surfaced. This champion wants to minimize essential fatty acid (EFA) intake to 0.5% of calories because of their tendency to form free radicals that can do damage. This extreme view does not line up with the clinical effectiveness of EFAs in fresh, natural oils. One-sided, alarmist views are always dangerous. Try to develop a balanced view, because life is a balancing act of many factors, including many different fatty acids with very different properties.

In Nature

Tropical 'oils' which include coconut, palm, palm kernel, cocoa, and shea nut, have traditionally been used by the people living in the regions where they grow for a very long time. They are used fresh as dietary staples. The tropics are not known for high incidence of heart attacks and strokes. If anything, tropical regions show a lower incidence of degenerative diseases than the temperate climates in which Western civilizations developed these same diseases.

In these tropical areas, the fats contained in the nuts and kernels that are their source were used in their natural state. Oil and protein were present, along with minerals, vitamins, and fiber. The oils were high in vitamin E, tocotrienols (vitamin E-like substances), carotene, and nut-specific unique ingredients.

To make tropical 'oils', nuts and kernels are crushed, and the fat (oil) is separated from the protein, minerals and fiber. The 'oil' still contains some minerals and most of the oil-soluble vitamins (E, carotene, tocotrienols). Tropical 'oils' have been part of a healthy tropical diet for thousands of years.

In the Lab

Research findings of the effects of fatty acids on serum cholesterol are now detailed and specific. EFAs (18:3w3; 18:2w6) lower cholesterol. Oleic acid (18:1w9) may not lower cholesterol, but does not raise it either. Saturated stearic acid (18:0) found in beef, lamb, pork, and dairy products does not raise cholesterol, probably because our body converts excess 18:0 to oleic acid. Tropical 'fats' do not contain substantial quantities of any of these good or harmless types of fatty acids.

On the other hand, both chemically pure palmitic acid (16:0) and chemically pure myristic acid (14:0) have been shown to increase cholesterol. Lauric acid (12:0) neither raises nor lowers cholesterol. Lauric acid has anti-microbial properties (though it is not unique since there are thousands of anti-microbial molecules in nature). Caproic, caprylic and capric acids (6:0, 8:0, and 10:0), which are fatty acids used to make medium-chain triglycerides (see Chapter 65, Medium-Chain Triglycerides), are used for energy, and lower cholesterol slightly. Tropical oils are nature's richest sources of saturated fatty acids from 16:0 down. Fractions of tropical oils rich in lauric and myristic acids are used to give margarines better melting properties.

Several studies indicating that tropical fats increase cholesterol have also been carried out in labs around North America. But studies carried out in Malaysia, the world's major source of palm oil, indicate that palm oil lowers cholesterol. It is likely that the Malaysian product is fresher and more natural.

In the Boardroom

It is difficult to separate science from advertising. Science, which in its best sense is the unbiased inquiry into the nature of things, is no longer (perhaps was never)

Truth gets less support than profit. Government, processed foods giants, oil sellers, and the business of drugs and medicine all have their hands in the pie of vested interests. Greed further clouds already shortsighted human vision.

Deception, an art more ancient than technology, has been perfected by industries. Half-truths and deception, the stuff of advertising that generates sales, make liberal use of the scientific format. 'Infomercials' look like research reports complete with references, but serve sales rather than the search for accurate information.

In the Confusion

If what we hear and read is suspect, we can still put our trust in nature. Fresh, coconuts and coconut oil are a different species from the hard white stuff called 'coconut oil' that we find in glass jars in stores. Three factors contribute to the difference between them.

The first factor is time. With time that involves exposure to light and air, contact with metal in ships' hulls, pipelines, and pumps, there is gradual deterioration of double bonds, oxidation, free radical formation, and loss of vitamin E, carotene, and tocotrienols. The effect of these changes to tropical oils on our cholesterol levels should not be overlooked.

Second, raw coconut oil may be refined and deodorized in the same way as most other commercial oils, removing vitamin E, tocotrienols, and carotene, and allowing for the formation of processing artifacts such as *trans-* fatty acids, polymers, cyclic substances, and others. The possibility that these artifacts lead to increased cholesterol has not been seriously investigated.

Third, much of the coconut oil is hydrogenated, becoming hard; hence, tropical 'fats'. We know that *trans-* fatty acids produced during hydrogenation increase cholesterol and LDL, and lower protective HDL. Hydrogenation also destroys the vitamin E, carotene, and tocotrienols not removed by refining and deodorizing processes. It also adds traces of aluminum and nickel to the fat.

There may thus be a great difference in the material tested in its country of origin and the material tested in laboratories in North America, even though both call their product coconut oil, coconut fat, or coconut butter. Research did not identify the exact composition and condition of the material used in tropical fat studies. Obviously, it should.

In the meantime, I eat fresh coconuts (when I can find them) with gusto. I love their taste. I avoid the stuff in jars. My cholesterol on a worry-free, natural diet measures between 160 and 180 mg/dl (4.10 to 4.65 mmol/L by the new measurement described in Chapter 41).

Hidden Junk Fats and Fat Substitutes 53

Hidden fats make up almost half of all the fats we eat. The fact that we can't see them makes them more dangerous than the fats we *can* see, because it is more difficult to accurately gauge our consumption of these substantial sources of fats.

Hidden fats are found in a wide range of processed foods such as sausages, hamburgers, fried and baked goods (bads?), confections, candy, ice cream, desserts, and many others.

Most of the fats used in processed foods have one of several possible problems: they may be fats discarded from slaughter operations; they may be cheap and toxic, such as cottonseed oil; they are always refined and deodorized; they may be partially hydrogenated; they are often overheated; and they may be oxidized due to exposure to air and careless handling.

Hidden fats are *never* the essential fatty acid (EFA)-rich, unrefined, fresh oils that are recommended for health.

Since we never know the sources or amounts of hidden fats, our best way of avoiding hidden fats is to avoid processed foods to a greater degree and to move more and more in the direction of fresh, whole foods like vegetables and grains.

Fat Substitutes

Fats are said to enhance the flavor and palatability of the foods that contain them. This is one of the justifications of the industry for using so much fat in foods.

Since fats and oils have been getting more criticism, and what with weight loss and fat phobia, industry has invested great effort to come up with fat substitutes. Criteria for acceptance include that they should produce the same texture in the mouth, and should be calorie-less, calorie-poor, or at least lower in calories than fats. They should also be non-toxic and 'safe' (no obvious toxicity).

Several products now being marketed fit these criteria, and some have obtained the blessing of the American Food and Drug Administration for experimentation and/or food use. No doubt there will be more such products in the future. Chemistry has become a highly sophisticated, capable tool. The giant processed food companies that sell fats also service the fat substitute market.

Fat substitutes do not yet have much history. We know that they mainly pass through our intestine undigested, and are discarded in the stool. We do *not* know their long-term effects. These long-term effects are important to consider, because people who use them for weight and fat reasons will be consuming them for a long term. How do they affect stomach acid and bowel enzyme function on the molecular level? We don't know, but some of them decrease the absorption of oil-soluble vitamins A, D, E, And K. How do they affect the absorption of each essential nutrient from our intestine? We don't yet know. How do they affect the bacteria that maintain the health of our intestines? We do not know. Do they irritate the intestinal lining when used in the long term? We have no answers yet.

Fat substitutes can help affluent, indulgent populations to continue to live out of touch with nature and not change health-destroying habits that, besides causing overweight, cause other health problems, too. Fat substitutes may help slow down the deterioration that follows culinary indulgences. Fat substitutes may also help non-affluent people who do not yet know (or care) enough about health to refrain from eating junk fat foods – probably the fats industry's largest customer base. Fat substitutes may actually help these people in the short term.

Besides the unknowns regarding fat substitutes, there is the issue of our responsibility for our habits and our health. Fat substitutes do little to encourage self-responsibility for living in line with nature.

Finally, the environmental impact of yet another industry that consumes energy, produces waste, and occupies space that once belonged to nature's green plants must be considered. Since the benefits of fat substitutes can also be obtained by the use of natural, low-fat, fiber-rich foods, we should question the wisdom of this industry.

New Research – New Fats

Fat Finding Missions, Breakthroughs, Applications

This section begins with a new look at the basis of the benefits of olive oil on health. It then goes on to therapeutic oils from fish and seafoods, and includes a chapter on snake oil that highlights why 'modern' drug approaches fail.

A chapter on therapeutic evening primrose, borage, and black currant oils is followed by a chapter on powerful fat-derived prostaglandin hormones on health and one on therapeutic w3-rich flax, then a chapter on the most perfectly balanced oil yet found in nature which, although it comes from the hemp (marijuana) plant, cannot produce an intoxicating effect.

The combination of oils with protein in nutritional therapy is described, and the work of German researcher Johanna Budwig is outlined, followed by a chapter on recipes that use therapeutic oils. Chapters on medium-chain triglycerides and alkylglycerols are followed by one on oils, sunshine, and geography, and the importance of light to health.

The last chapter in the section looks at other nutrition and life-style factors that round out the use of oils and nutrients to build good health.

Therapeutic Oils

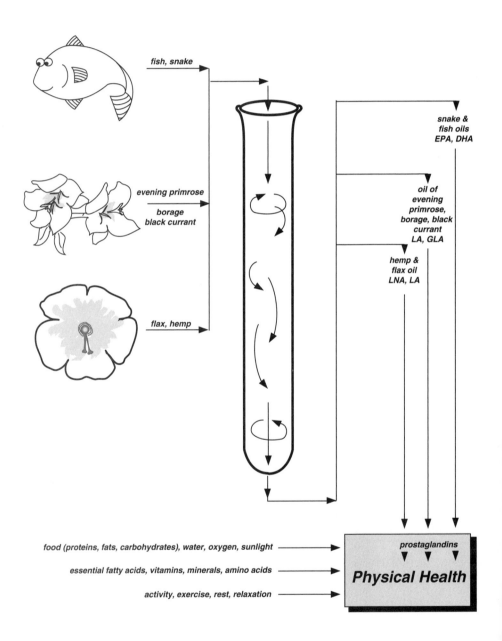

fish, snake

evening primrose

borage
black currant

flax, hemp

snake &
fish oils
EPA, DHA

oil of
evening
primrose,
borage, black
currant
LA, GLA

hemp &
flax oil
LNA, LA

food (proteins, fats, carbohydrates), water, oxygen, sunlight

essential fatty acids, vitamins, minerals, amino acids

activity, exercise, rest, relaxation

prostaglandins

Physical Health

Virgin Olive Oils 54

Unrefined versus Refined

The story of olive oil carries an important message for consumers and healers. It illustrates the *remarkable difference between refined and unrefined oils* from the vantage point of human health. That story has received almost no attention in medicine and media. It deserves a serious hearing.

Research with olive oil shows that this 'fruit oil' (pressed from the flesh of the olive fruit rather than its seed) protects against cardiovascular disease. It has also been shown in animal studies to positively influence the architecture and functions of the brain. It is also associated with low cancer incidence and general good health. What gives virgin olive oils these positive effects?

A Question of Virgin Quality

Olive oil made by simple traditional processes is known as *virgin* olive oil. It is made from whole, ripe, undamaged olives. It is made without heat. It is an unrefined oil that still contains many natural factors unique to olives. Through industrial processes like degumming, refining, bleaching, and deodorizing these natural factors are removed. Olive oil, which thereby loses its virgin quality, becomes *non-virgin*, refined, olive oil. But don't expect to find oils labeled 'non-virgin' or 'refined'.

If an olive oil is not labeled 'virgin', it is non-virgin refined olive oil. The same is true for other oils – if they are not labeled 'unrefined', they are refined, deodorized oils which have suffered nutrient losses and molecular changes that negatively affect human health.

Heat and Genetic Damage

Unsaturated fatty acids are anti-mutagenic (saturated fatty acids do not have this protective capacity). This means that they can protect the genetic material in our cells from damage (mutations) caused by toxic chemicals or destructive rays. More than 80% of the fatty acids that virgin (unrefined) olive oils contain are protective, unheated, mainly monounsaturated and some essential unsaturated fatty acids.

When these protective unsaturated fatty acids are heated above 150°C (302°F), not only do they lose their protective effects, but they become mutation-causing themselves. Virgin olive oils are the *only* mass market oils that have not been heated above 150°C.

All bland-tasting, refined, deodorized, colorless oils have been heated to temperatures far higher than 150°C (see Chapter 16, From Seed to Oil). This suggests that processing heat has much to do with the increased cancer incidence that is associated with increased use of refined, bottled, mass market oils. Virgin olive oils' heart-protecting effects can be found in other aspects that depend on their unrefined nature.

Fatty Acids

Essential. Linoleic acid (18:2w6) in olive oil ranges from 3.5 to 20% (averaging 10%), while alpha-linolenic acid (18:3w3) ranges from 0.1 to 0.6%. These figures prove olive oil to be one of the poorer sources of essential fatty acids (EFAs), which must therefore be supplied by other oils. Cholesterol-lowering w6s and triglyceride-lowering w3s cannot be the reason for olive oil's effects on health, because they are present in only small quantities.

Non-essential monounsaturated. Oleic acid (18:1w9) in olive oil ranges from 63 to 83% (averaging 75%). Palmitoleic acid (16:1w7) ranges from 0.5 to 3% (averaging 2%). These are monounsaturated non-essential, stable fatty acids (MUFAs). They keep quite well – important in Mediterranean climates before refrigeration – and account in part for olive oil's prominence throughout history.[1]

MUFAs neither raise nor lower blood cholesterol, and cannot therefore account for olive oil's health effects. An excess of MUFAs will raise blood triglycerides, which should make the oil increase cardiovascular risk, but it has been shown that olive oil actually *lowers* cardiovascular risks.

Non-essential saturated. Palmitic acid (16:0) in olive oil ranges from 7.5 to 18% (averaging 10%). PA raises cholesterol levels. A PA level of 10% in an oil is higher than average, but olive oil *protects* arteries rather than damaging them. It also contains about 2% stearic acid (18:0), which neither raises nor lowers cholesterol levels.

In addition, olive oil contains traces of several other saturated fatty acids, none of them of note. Although all of its fatty acids are common to all oils and are used by our body in cell membrane structures and as fuel, the beneficial effects of olive oil cannot be ascribed to its fatty acid profile.

Phospholipids. Olive oil contains little lecithin (a phospholipid consisting

---

[1] Other reasons for the popularity of olive oil over thousands of years of history include the ease with which it can be obtained from the soft flesh of the olive – important before the invention of high-pressure oil-presses; and its beneficial effects on health.

of fatty acids, glycerol, and phosphate), which is good for health. There is nothing special here to explain the benefits of olive oil to health.

'Minor' Components

The 'minor' components in *virgin (unrefined) olive oil* have major health benefits. They constitute only about 2% of the total, and most of them are removed when virgin olive oil is degummed, refined, bleached, and deodorized. Of the minor components present in virgin olive oil, some are common to many different kinds of unrefined oils, while others are unique to olive oil.

Common minor components. *Beta carotene* (pro-vitamin A) and *tocopherols* (vitamin E) are antioxidants that are present in most fresh, unrefined vegetable seed oils. Olive oil contains 88% of its vitamin E in the form of alpha-tocopherol. Vitamin E has protective effects on our heart and arteries. Much of it is removed when oils are refined.

Magnesium-rich *chlorophyll* is found in unrefined green oils such as olive, hemp, pumpkin, and avocado. In smaller quantities, chlorophyll is also present in most other unrefined oils. Magnesium deficiency is common in patients with cardiovascular disease. Chlorophyll (and with it, the magnesium it contains) is removed when oils are refined.

Squalene, a precursor of phytosterols, is the main hydrocarbon present in olive oil. Squalene, also found in other unrefined oils, is heart-protective in its fresh, unoxidized state, and is removed when oils are refined.

Phytosterols are present in olive and other unrefined oils. Beta-sitosterol is the main phytosterol (95%), but stigmasterol and campesterol are also present in small quantities. Phytosterols protect against cholesterol absorption from foods, but are removed from oils during degumming, refining, bleaching, and deodorizing.

Seed-specific minor components unique to olive oil. These components are also removed when virgin olive oil is processed into bland, processed, refined, deodorized olive oil.

Since olive oil is the only common, mass-marketed *unrefined* oil at present, seed-specific minor ingredients in olive oil have been more extensively studied (by the olive oil industry) than the seed-specific minor ingredients found in unrefined versions of oils that are mass marketed only in their refined, deodorized forms. But even for olive oil, the roles of these 'minor' components with complicated names have not been fully elucidated.

Triterpenic substances are modified sterols. They include several groups: *triterphenethyl alcohols, monohydroxy* and *dihydroxy triterpenes,* and *triterpenic alcohols,* all of which are present in olive oil. Among the members of these groups are cycloartenol, alpha- and beta-amyrin, 24-methylene-cycloartenol, and erythrodiol. *Hydroxy triterpenic acids* including oleanolic, maslinic, and ursolic acids, and their derivatives, are also found in olive oil. Because of their chemical structure, these substances are good candidates for being credited with the cardiovascular benefits of olive oil but, so far, little research has been conducted on them. Oil refining and deodorizing removes these substances.

Polyphenols present in olive oil are responsible in part for the color of the oil. They also have antioxidant properties that help stabilize the oil, and may also have antioxidant properties in our body. One polyphenol (oleoeuropein) found in olive oil lowers blood pressure. Hardly any research has been conducted into the health effects of olive oil's polyphenols. Polyphenols largely disappear during processing. Refined, deodorized oils contain far less of them.

Further substances can be found in the water fraction of olives. When this fraction is removed from the freshly pressed olive oil-water mixture, these substances, which include some that stabilize the oil, remain in the oil. These substances too, are candidates for olive oil's health effects.

Finally, more than 100 volatile compounds that give olive oil its characteristic aroma and flavor have been identified. The health effects of these volatile substances have not been studied.

Other Oils. The minor components found in most other unrefined oils remain largely unexamined. Each oil has its own natural set of minor components with their own unique properties. In the complex dance of molecules that is the play of nature, each molecule has a chemical personality that defines its actions and uses. Many of these can affect our health. When we remove them by processing, and then consume the processed products, we have no idea what we do to ourselves.

Virgin (Unrefined) versus Non-Virgin (Refined) Olive Oil

All *virgin* olive oils are unrefined. High-quality, undamaged olives must be used to make virgin oils. Virgin olive oils – the only *un*refined oils easily available on the mass market – can be recommended for health. 'Extra virgin' means highest quality, and strict guidelines are followed in determining whether an olive oil may be called 'extra virgin'.

If olives are damaged or bruised, they (and the oil they contain) begin to spoil, and the oil pressed from them is of such poor quality that it must be degummed, refined, bleached, and deodorized – resulting in olive oils that are equivalent to other cheap, mass market oils in quality. These oils, like other mass market oils, have been changed from anti-mutagenic to mutagenic by overheating, and their minor ingredients have been removed. Avoid these oils completely.

Health Effects of Olive Oil

Membrane health is critical to cell, tissue, and organ health. It affects every cell in our body, because all cells have membranes surrounding them. Studies carried out with virgin olive oil show that it helps membrane development, cell formation, and cell differentiation.

Virgin olive oil improves brain maturation and function in animals deficient in EFAs. These results can probably be generalized to humans, because brain development and function are generally similar in animals and man.

In patients with peripheral artery disease on fat-lowering diets, a switch from corn oil (refined) to virgin olive oil (unrefined) for six months resulted in significantly decreased 'bad' LDL cholesterol, and significantly increased 'good' HDL cholesterol. In other words, virgin olive oil performed better than corn oil for these patients.

Monounsaturated fatty acid-rich virgin olive oil has also been shown to reduce the production of cholesterol gallstones (compared to high-polyunsaturated, refined corn oil) and to favor bile secretion, which improves elimination of the toxic end products of liver detoxification and improves digestion of fats.

The minor components in olive oil also have some specific beneficial effects:
* *Beta-sitosterol* lowers high cholesterol levels.
* *Triterpenic acids* have healing and anti-inflammatory effects.
* *Caffeic* and *gallic acids* stimulate the flow of bile.
* *Gallic acid* also inhibits lactic dehydrogenase activity in the liver (a sign of liver malfunction).
* *Phenolic compounds* protect against peroxidation of fatty acids and cholesterol.
* *2-phenylethanol* (present in many unrefined oils) stimulates the production of fat-digesting enzymes in the pancreas.
* *Triterpenic acids (oleanolic* and *maslinic* – found only in olive oil) also stimulate these pancreatic enzymes.
* *Cycloartenol,* stored in the liver, lowers the amount of circulating cholesterol and increases bile excretion (in studies done with rats).
* A combination of *2-phenylethanol* and *triterpenic acids* slows down cholesterol digestion (cholesterol ester hydrolysis) and decreases cholesterol absorption from foods.

Unfair Comparison Studies

Many studies have now been carried out to compare the effectiveness of different oils on serum HDL and total cholesterol levels and other cardiovascular risks. Olive oil performs well in these studies.

What is not usually pointed out is the fact that *unrefined* olive oil is compared to *refined* versions of other oils. This is an unfair comparison. It would be more instructive to compare the health effects of:
1. virgin unrefined olive oil with refined deodorized olive oil;
2. virgin unrefined olive oil with unrefined oils from other seeds; and
3. unrefined oils from other seeds with refined oils from the same seeds.

Such studies have not been systematically carried out. They would identify which beneficial effects of oils are due to the minor components present in unrefined oils, and which effects can be ascribed to essential and other fatty acids.

Summary

Olive oil is a time-tested, stable, health-enhancing oil. It is a poor source of EFAs (especially w3s, which are more amply supplied by other oils), but an exceptional source of stable monounsaturated fatty acids and a rich source of unique minor components with health value. If our EFA requirements have been met, olive oil is excellent for improving and maintaining health because of its natural minor components.

It would be helpful for consumers to recognize that it is the minor components in olive oil that actually bring about its beneficial effects. The study of the minor components in other unrefined oils also holds promise for providing information useful for the enhancement of human health.

55 Oils from Fish and Seafoods: EPA and DHA

Fish oils bring to mind the cod liver oil I used to get in winter when I was a kid. It's hard to forget the 'fishy' smell and taste (which are caused by rancidity). I remember losing nightly battles with my parents, tearfully surrendering, and swallowing yet another slug of the greasy liquid off the old aluminum spoon, gagging on it once again – all this to get my Northern winter ration of vitamins A and D. "Why must it taste so awful to be good for health?" I asked. They had no answer. During one winter of my childhood, however, I craved and looked forward to cod liver oil.

Cod liver oil now comes in capsules. Only the occasional burp reminds us that it's still the same rancid fish oil. We've come a long way in our knowledge of cod and other fish oils regarding their benefits to health, but manufacturing practices still need to be improved.

Toxic Fish Oils?

Not all fish oils are special in their health-enhancing capacity. Oils of some fish contain fatty acids that may not be good for us. An example is cetoleic acid (22:1w11), found in herring and capelin oils, which makes up between 12 and 20% of the oil these fish contain. Cetoleic acid is also found, in smaller quantities in the oils of menhaden and anchovetta, and to some extent also in cod liver oil (did the child sense something that the parents missed?). Cetoleic acid has been suggested by some to be toxic to heart tissue because it resembles erucic acid, but this suggestion has not yet been verified, and erucic acid has now been found to be relatively harmless (see Chapter 20, Erucic Acid).

So-so Fish Oils

Many fish oils are neither toxic nor especially beneficial. Low-fat and warm-water fish fall into this 'kettle of fish'. While these fish contain nutritious protein, their oils have no special nutritional merits. Oolichan and smelt oils, prized by North American natives, were their versions of 'olive oil from the sea'. They contain few essential fatty acids (EFAs) but keep well. They were stable oils for dipping foods and making pemmican – a dry, non-perishable, meat-based food – to take on long journeys.

Wonderful Fish Oils: EPA and DHA

Some fish oils are associated with clean arteries and freedom from fatty degeneration. The health secret in these oils was discovered only recently, and revolves around two w3 fatty acids called eicosapentaenoic acid (EPA, 20:5w3) and docosahexaenoic acid (DHA, 22:6w3), respectively.

What makes these oils special? Both EPA and DHA are normal constituents of our cells. They are especially abundant in brain cells, nerve relay stations (synapses), visual receptors (retinas), adrenal glands, and sex glands – the most biochemically active tissues in our body.

EPA and DHA can be manufactured by healthy cells from the essential w3 fatty acid, alpha-linolenic acid (LNA, 18:3w3), which is found abundantly in flax, hemp, and several other seeds. However, degenerative conditions may impair our body's ability to make EPA and DHA from LNA for the same reasons that these degenerative conditions impair its ability to make the w6 long-chain fatty acids[1] (see Chapter 57, Evening Primrose, Borage, and Black Currant Oils).

In certain populations and a few individuals, EPA and DHA can also overcome the effects of mutations that have destroyed the ability of their cells to convert LNA to EPA and DHA. Populations affected might include some West Coast North American native, Inuit, Oriental, Norwegian, and Welsh-Irish – people who traditionally lived along cold-water coasts and included fish as a staple in their diets. The number of people affected is likely to be less than 2% of the population, and certainly less than 10%, but the individuals affected would require a dietary source of EPA and DHA.

EPA and DHA, come from cold water fish and other northern marine animals. Fish can make EPA and DHA from the w3 EFA, alpha-linolenic acid (LNA, 18:3w3), but get much of their EPA and DHA from brown and red algae which manufacture EPA and DHA from carbohydrates – sugar, starch, cellulose, etc.

EPA and DHA reverse the negative health effects of lack of w3 fatty acids due to deficient diets by adding a few capsules of fish oils containing these wonderful fatty acids. Even better, we can eat fresh (raw) fish whose oils contain high-

---

[1] W3 and w6 essential fatty acids require the same enzyme system to make their corresponding long-chain derivatives.

quality fresh, unspoiled EPA and DHA.

More recently, brown and red algae have begun to be grown commercially for EPA and DHA. These living little factories make 10 to 14% of long-chain w3s (on dry weight basis) and can be used as excellent, high-quality food sources of EPA and DHA-containing triglycerides. They also serve as starting material for making the free fatty acids EPA and DHA for clinical uses.

EPA and DHA, being highly unsaturated, have a strong urge to disperse. They have extremely low melting points (-54°C [-65°F]; and -44°C [-47°F], respectively), and will not harden or aggregate. So strong is their tendency to move apart from other EPA and DHA molecules that they help prevent aggregation of saturated fatty acids that like to stick together. EPA and DHA thus help keep saturated fatty acids and cholesterol dispersed.

Platelets. EPA and DHA keep our platelets from getting too sticky. The result is less likelihood of clots that can cause heart attack or stroke.

Arteries. EPA and DHA also appear to lower apo(a) and fibrinogen levels in our arteries. These two repair proteins are involved in the proliferation of atherosclerotic tissue in arteries. Lowered levels of these repair proteins result in less atherosclerosis, and more fully open arteries.[2]

Blood triglycerides. EPA and DHA can lower high triglycerides by up to 65% (by 75 to 50 mg/dl in one study). They may somewhat lower cholesterol level and low-density lipoprotein (LDL), and lower very low-density lipoprotein (VLDL) by half (from 12 down to 6 mg/dl in the same study). Exactly how is still a mystery. High cholesterol, triglycerides, LDL, and VLDL levels are associated with cardiovascular disease: high blood pressure, atherosclerosis, heart and kidney failure, stroke, and heart attack.

Blood pressure. EPA lowers elevated blood pressure through the effects of series 3 prostaglandins (PGs) made from it, which block the production of blood pressure-raising series 2 PGs made from w6 fatty acids.

Hormone effects. From EPA, our body makes PG3 prostaglandins (see Chapter 58, Prostaglandins) and leukotrienes, which help prevent strokes, heart attacks, and other problems that involve clot formation, such as pulmonary embolism and cardiovascular complications accompanying diabetes, which can result in gangrenous limbs and blindness. The presence of EPA helps prevent our cells from making too many PG2 clot-forming prostaglandins.

Cancer. In some animal studies, w3 fish oils inhibited growth and metastasis of tumors. Negative experimental results with w3 fish oils in cancer treatment are likely due to poor product quality (rancid oils) or the use of fish oils low in w3 fatty acids. Trout, salmon, mackerel, sardines, tuna, and eel are the richest sources of w3 fatty acids. The oils must be fresh for good results. They deteriorate rapidly.

---

[2] Vitamin C, cysteine, niacin, vitamin E, coenzyme Q10, and lysine are other critical factors that help prevent and reverse atherosclerosis.

Conversion of LNA to EPA

The rate at which the average human body can convert LNA to EPA has been measured in one study using normal adults to be 2.7% per day of the LNA administered – nutritional intake of co-factors necessary for conversion and PG production was not measured.

Since 80% of the population gets less than recommended amounts of al least one of the co-factors, optimum quantities of essential nutrients, especially vitamins B_3, B_6, and C, magnesium, and zinc might even boost the conversion of LNA to EPA and its conversion into PG3s above 2.7% per day.

A person's fat deposits should contain 2% LNA (2.4% is normal in bodies built from traditional diets). This amounts to 200 grams of LNA available for conversion in a normal person's 10 kg of body fat. Using the 2.7% figure, the body can make 5400 mg of EPA, as much as one would get from about 18 large (1000-mg) capsules of the w3-richest fish oil. Sellers of fish oil who claim that conversion of LNA to EPA and DHA in humans is not fast enough may be protecting sales rather than telling the truth, since they recommend only 3 capsules per day.

If a person has no w3s in their body but takes 2 tablespoons of flax oil each day, of which 50% is LNA, their body can make 378 mg of EPA, which is what two large capsules of fish oil will supply. In w3 supplementation after long-term deficit, 3 to 5 tablespoons are often used. The LNA in this oil can be turned into as much EPA as 3 to 5 large capsules of fish oil will supply. The advantage is that the EPA made in our body is fresher. LNA-containing seeds and oils are available in fresher conditions than fish oils because they are simpler to produce (less processing). They are also more stable, and are less likely to contain toxic ingredients like polychlorinated biphenyls (PCBs).

A few people might be genetically unable to make the conversion. These people would require fish or their oils in their diet.

Dietary saturates, monounsaturates, *trans-* fatty acids and cholesterol all slow down conversion, and deficiencies of vitamins B_3, B_6, C, magnesium, or zinc also inhibit conversion.

Most people don't get much LNA in its natural state in their diet. The richest sources of LNA come from flax, chia, and hemp seeds and their oils, which are new to the marketplace.

Government 'Protection'

In spite of many scientific studies showing beneficial effects of EPA and DHA on cardiovascular health, fish oils are still waiting for the official 'green light' in the U.S. In Canada, *all* essential nutrients are considered drugs rather than foods – an ill-considered notion, considering their low toxicity compared to drugs. The U.S. Food and Drug Administration concluded in 1993 that sellers of w3 (flax and fish) oils may not make claims for the usefulness of w3s to establish cardiovascular

261

health. I believe they will change their stand when they distinguish the results obtained from studies using poor quality oils, studies using low w3 oils, and poorly carried out studies, from results obtained in well-designed studies using fresh, w3-rich oils.

Foods and drugs. Foods and components of foods (essential nutrients) should be administered by a government body separate from that which deals with drugs. Pharmaceutical drugs are dangerous, toxic, unnatural substances with a narrow range between effective dose and fatal dose. They should be tightly controlled, and used as little as possible. Foods and their essential nutrient components are relatively safe even in large quantities. They have been self-administered since the days of Adam and Eve. Foods build and maintain health in the first place, starting from conception. They also reverse, cure, and prevent degenerative diseases whose origins lie in malnutrition and deficiencies. Until non-toxic foods and toxic drugs are separated under the law and administered separately (which may take years), Canadians can get EPA and DHA supplements from the U.S., and citizens of both countries can eat fish containing these oils or get their EPA and DHA from sushi, which luckily for us, is still considered food by bureaucrats. And even if we *can't* make any claims, our hearts and arteries *will* be (secretly) in better shape.

Grocers and doctors. In the same way as the administration of foods and drugs should be separated, the fields of nutrition and medicine should be separated. Farmers, grocers, and nutritionists practice primary health care through foods, and should be allowed to make *legitimate* health claims for their food products. As long as doctors rely on the practice of drug-oriented disease management without paying attention to primary health care through the appropriate use of foods, water, and air, your grocer will likely be able to do more for your health than your doctor. As doctors learn to use foods to heal, they may be able to catch up with the excellent level of service now provided by farmers, green grocers, and natural healers.

Which Fish?

The richest sources of EPA and DHA are high-fat (10 to 15%) cold-water fish like salmon, sardines, mackerel, trout, and eel. EPA and DHA make up between 15 and 30% of the oils found in these fish. The measured w3 fatty acid content of different types of salmon ranges between 18.9 and 31.4% of total fat content.[3]

Low-fat (1 to 4%) fish like pike, carp, and haddock contain EPA and DHA in much smaller quantities.

How Often?

EPA and DHA from fish take about 2 to 3 weeks to be completely metabolized in

---

[3] Their w6 content measured between 1.6 and 3.6% of total fat content.

our body after being consumed. Their triglyceride-lowering, platelet-'unsticking', and artery-protecting effects last the same length of time. To maintain these protective effects, fresh w3 fish should be eaten at least every 2 weeks. The Catholic custom of fish on Fridays may have had health benefits before it degenerated to fish 'n' chips – low-fat fish and potatoes, both deep-fried in damaged and damaging oils.

Good fish would be fresh, high-fat fish that contain EPA and DHA. They should not be fried. It is best to boil them whole, so that their oils are not destroyed by light, oxygen, or high temperature. They can be eaten raw as sushi or sashimi[4] (decked with edible gold for art's sake) made from fish which are kept fresh by deep freezing and served in Japanese sushi bars. Preserved this way, fish oils give maximum health benefits.

Unlike chicken and turkey, high-fat cold-water fish are best eaten with their skins on. The oils we want are found under their skin, especially behind the gills, around the fins, and along the belly.

Other Sources of EPA and DHA

Seals contain about 3.5% EPA and 7.5% DHA in their fat tissue. Dolphins and whales have between 1 and 3% of each in their blubber. Penguins carry about 3% EPA and 9% DHA in their body fats.

Tiny animals (zooplankton, krill, copepods) and tiny plants (phytoplankton, algae) that live in oceans and lakes are food for fish and marine animals. These are rich in w3s such as LNA, EPA and DHA. Polar bears eating marine animals that live on plankton have about 7% each of EPA and DHA in their fat.

Oils from scallop, clam, oyster, and squid contain from one-quarter to one-half EPA and DHA. Since their total oil content is less than 2% of their weight, they are minor sources of w3 fatty acids.

Functions of EPA and DHA

As already stated, EPA and DHA help keep our arteries clean, our platelets less sticky, and cold-water animals fluid in freezing cold water. EPA is the starting material for making series 3 prostaglandins, which have beneficial effects on blood pressure, cholesterol and triglyceride levels, kidney function, inflammatory response, and immune function.

EPA and DHA have other functions. In our retinas, these highly active fatty

---

[4] Fish that carry human parasites are not served raw by properly trained sushi chefs. Such fish include cod and other bottom-feeding fish that live close to the shoreline, where both hosts in whom the parasites grow – fish and humans – have regular contact. Open ocean fish that have no contact with humans can be eaten raw because they do not carry parasites active in humans. As a second precaution, sushi chefs freeze fish at -40°C (-40°F) to kill any parasites they carry.

acids are involved with the conversion of light energy entering our eyes into the chemical energy of nerve impulses.

In our brain, they have neurological functions that involve energy conversion and electron transfer. They attract the oxygen necessary for intense chemical activity of brain cells. In adrenal and sex glands, they provide increased chemical activity.

Easily Destroyed

EPA and DHA are even more sensitive to destruction by light, air, and heat than LNA, the 'prima donna' of EFAs. EPA and DHA belong in completely opaque capsules made under conditions that exclude light, air, and heat. Most capsules marketed today contain 'fishy' tasting (partly rancid) oil. Sardines canned in their own (sardine or sild) oil are the only processed source I know of fish oils without rancid taste. The *best* way to eat fish is to get it so fresh it's 'still wiggling', and then prepare and eat it immediately.

Fresh EPA and DHA can be a valuable addition to the human diet. They provide one of the main reasons why traditional Inuit were virtually free of disease of fatty degeneration, even though their diets contained 39% fat providing almost 60% of total calories (of which more than one-tenth was EPA and DHA), but very little fiber.

Fish Farming

Salmon and trout are being raised in tanks or shallow ponds, much like chickens in the chicken coop. Fish in the fish coop are fed commercialized, convenient foods that are not the fresh live krill, copepods, plankton, and algae that feed these fish in nature. Since their fat content depends on what they eat, their fat content is different from that of free-swimming ocean or fresh-water fish. The process of changing fat content in fish has begun, similar to changes that have occurred in beef farming (see Chapter 46, Meats) and egg production (see Chapter 49, Eggs).

Commercial fish foods contain less vitamins A and C, and less w3 fatty acids than the foods that wild fish eat. These three spoilable nutrients are essential to fish,[5] but further shorten the already short shelf life of fish foods. Commercial dry fish foods last only 2 months. Wet refrigerated foods last 3 months.

Experts in fish farming consider farmed salmon to be inferior to fresh ocean fish. Their meat is less firm. The fish are less viable. Sometimes algal blooms kill the entire cooped-up fish school, because the fish are not free to escape these blooms.

Decreased quality of farmed fish is offset by some advantages. Farmed fish

---

[5] W6 fatty acids, which are essential in human nutrition, are not essential to fish. Fish can convert w3 fatty acids, which *are* essential for them, into w6 fatty acids.

can reach consumers within 48 hours. Ocean fish may be dead (on ice) a week or two before the boat comes in. Farmed fish are available fresh all year round, while ocean salmon are fresh only in season, and must be frozen, dried, smoked, or canned the rest of the year.

Market surveys indicate that buyers prefer fresh ocean salmon to fresh farmed salmon, but prefer fresh farmed salmon to frozen ocean salmon. This preference mirrors nutritional quality.

Snake Oil (EPA) and Patent Medicines 56

The term 'snake oil salesman' has, in most people's minds, come to signify the epitome of the charlatan and huckster who peddles worthless nostrums and quack remedies on the basis of unwarranted health claims – the fast talker who preys on the vulnerabilities of the ill, gives false hope, and makes off with their money. The term enjoys particular popularity with those who administer 'professional' drug-oriented medicine, which is gradually being shown to be less noble and more motivated by base vested interest like profit and power than its *public image* suggests to us. (see Chapter 88, The Business and Politics of Health).

Goodness knows there are enough charlatans around, but the snake oil salesman wasn't one. Did you ever wonder about the history of the term? A doctor from San Francisco did, and decided to find out what snake oil consists of. Before I tell that story, I want to trace the history of healing back to its Greek roots.

Two Sides of the Healing Coin
Ancient Greeks followed two lines of thought in healing practices. These two lines of thought survive to the present day.

Hygeia. One line of thought, the head of the healing coin, was the 'natural' approach to healing. It used nutrition, water, air, light, herbs, activity, massage, touch, love, and other natural and non-invasive methods. It attempted to provide the body with the tools it needs to heal itself. Healing was seen as an innate power of our body, and healing took place from within. The point of treatment was to realign the body with nature; to build, rebuild, and strengthen the body so that infections could not take hold; to build up innate resistance to infection and deterioration; and, if infection and deterioration did take hold, to overcome them by supporting the body's natural healing mechanisms with the use of natural substances. This branch of healing was embodied by Hygeia, the Greek goddess of health and beauty.

A remnant of this line of thought survives today as public health and hygiene, which attempts to prevent disease through personal cleanliness, prevention of food and water contamination by pathogenic organisms, sewage treatment, etc.

For the last 50 years or more, the part of Hygeia concerned with building healthy human bodies through food, water, air, light, herbs, activity, etc. was set aside by medicine for political and marketing reasons, and continued to receive attention from only the few people who, in spite of our love affair with machinery, technology, and 'progress', continued to believe in the power of nature. Today, as health is being more clearly defined, health care through natural means is going mainstream because it works, and is therefore good business in a polluted world inhabited by poorly-nourished people.

Aesculapius. The second line of Greek thought used toxic and invasive methods to suppress or treat symptoms, stop infections, poison parts with tar, mercury, and arsenic (and now, synthetic compounds), or simply cut them out. This branch of healing became present-day surgery-, radiation-, and drug-oriented (cut, burn, poison) practices. Aesculapius, the Greek god of medicine, embodied this approach. His staff, with a snake coiled around it, is the symbol of medicine and the official emblem of the American Medical Association (ironic, given their stand on snake oil).

Healers in ancient times used the natural approach for the long term, and resorted to the toxic approach only for the short term, to manage crises. Hippocrates, the 'father of modern medicine' paid attention to both approaches. One of his statements "Let foods be your medicine!" is often quoted, but not yet well understood or widely practiced by the members of a profession that takes his oath.

Early America

Patent medicines. In the 1800s, the Aesculapian method of healing was embodied by sellers of patent medicines. As the name implies, patent medicines were medicines that had been patented. They were substances concocted in the primitive laboratories of the time. Sellers of patent medicines enjoyed a commercial advantage over sellers of natural products because patents confer monopoly rights, prevent competition, protect high markups by manufacturers, and therefore bring good profits – regardless of whether the products benefit health, are useless, or even do harm.

Natural medicines. Natural substances like foods, juices, super-foods, and herbs (and today, vitamins, minerals, oils, and food concentrates) cannot be patented. They therefore lack protection from competition, which drives down price and profit. Snake oil, being a natural product, belonged to the low-price, low-profit category. But many of these natural products had years of traditional use and success to back them, though the reasons for their effectiveness were usually unknown, and the explanations then given for their effectiveness sound strange to us today. They had products that worked, with explanations that didn't. More coherent and sensible explanations had to await the development of modern analytical technology that can identify active principles on the molecular level.

Some healers who developed natural products kept their ingredients secret from others, and passed them on only to their students. This secrecy served two functions. It ensured that formulas and methods were faithfully adhered to (a healing consideration), and it protected their effort and increased the time it would take someone to copy a product and compete (a commercial consideration).

Smear and Innuendo

Natural substances helped improve health in the 1800s, just as they do today, because our body, then as now, is made from foods, water, and air and, then as now, is made for activity that contributes to harmonious living. Natural products provided competition for sellers of patent medicines on the basis of their healing success. Patent medicine salesmen fought this competition by time-tested business tactics – smear and innuendo – that are still alive and well today.

Pharmaceutical companies. Today, makers of patent medicines are known as pharmaceutical companies. Sellers of patent medicines are druggists and doctors trained on an ongoing basis by drug company detail people who introduce an endless parade of new toxic drugs to pharmacists and physicians. Incentives to use drugs, such as gifts, books, and trips, are part of their presentation. Health is not an issue, as long as the drugs are not clearly toxic, carcinogenic, or life-threatening. Side effects (which are toxic reactions by our body to toxic substances) are not only acceptable, but are the rule in drug-oriented medical practice, because all drugs are foreign to the body and therefore all drugs are toxic.

A big scam. By and large, the makers of patent medicines (drug companies) won the commercial contest. They became powerful enough to determine the direction that medicine took, and the courses taught to medical students. Due to their influence, nutrition teaching did not keep pace with nutrition research, but became minimal, ineffective generalities. Drug-related information now fills the doctors' training courses, and medical students and doctors are kept up-to-date with the latest details of drug research information and the newest drugs, which via doctors' prescriptions, translate into product sales and protected profits for pharmaceutical companies. This 'professional' network is one of the greatest marketing success stories in history, but from the viewpoint of health, it is one of history's biggest scams.

Drug companies and the profits generated from the sale of patented drugs are the major driving force behind the turn of medicine away from natural methods to become almost exclusively drug- and crisis-oriented. This history has been documented.

Patent- and drug-oriented medicine is about profit, not health. Drug companies have not been supportive of efforts to clearly define the nature of health, the molecular root cause of diseases, and *natural* approaches to health.

Efforts toward health are driven by curious researchers, sick people searching for *real* solutions, and an educated public demanding natural methods because they know that drugs have failed to cure degenerative conditions including cancer, cardiovascular disease, and many others. For almost three generations, these conditions have been growing into epidemics that now kill 1.5 million people each year in the U.S. alone.

The attention being paid to the newest threat – AIDS – which at this time kills about 50 thousand each year, provides a focus that attracts research grants, and also acts as a smoke screen that hides greater, continuing failures in medicine. AIDS *is* a serious threat, but the attention being paid to new diseases should not blind us to the fact that more affluent people are dying from nutrition-related degenerative diseases than are killed by AIDS *and* all the wars of history. It should not let us forget that what we *really* need to study is the nature of health – that natural biological condition of the human body the enables it to cope effectively with *all* stressors involved in living: cuts, injuries, broken limbs, infectious organisms, the demands of pregnancy, labor, and superior performance, as well as the unsolved new and old disease conditions. The majority of our answers will be found in eating, life-styles, and environmental management that harmonize us within the natural system and align us with our own nature.

Political Moves

The political moves that turned the tide in favor of drug-oriented medicine and forced natural methods into hiding go beyond the scope of this chapter and book. Two accounts that document some of what took place are recorded in Harvey W. Wiley's *History of a Crime Against the Food Law* and Harris Coulter's three volume epic *Divided Legacy: The Conflict Between Homeopathy and the American Medical Association.*

The age-old conflict between healing and profiteering is not likely to go away in the near future. Health takes special care. Profits depend upon speeding up, cutting corners, developing hard-to-copy complexity, painting pretty pictures to make sales, lobbying, and enacting laws that favor the rich and clever rather than the caring and healing personality.

Vindication of Snake Oil

Snake oil originally came from China, where it was used to alleviate inflammation and pain in rheumatoid arthritis, bursitis, and similar conditions. Chinese laborers on section gangs doing the grunt work involved in building the railroad tracks to link North America coast to coast gave it to Europeans with joint pain (bursitis, arthritis). When rubbed on the skin above the pain, snake oil brought relief, so the story goes. Patent medicine men ridiculed the claim.

In 1989, a nutrition-oriented medical doctor from California decided to find out what snake oil contains. He obtained a sample of the oil from San Francisco's Chinatown, had it analyzed, and found that it contains 75% unidentified carrier material, presumably for emulsifying the snake oil and helping to transport it through the skin. It also contains camphor. The remaining 25% of the product is oil from Chinese water snakes, which contains 20% of the important omega 3 derivative eicosapentaenoic acid (EPA) as well as 48% myristic acid (14:0), 10% stearic acid (18:0), 14% oleic acid (18:1w9), and 7% linoleic (18:2w6) plus arachidonic (20:4w6) acids. At 20% EPA, Chinese water snake is the richest known natural source of the parent of series 3 prostaglandins, which inhibit the production of pro-inflammatory series 2 prostaglandins. Like essential fatty acids and their other derivatives, EPA can be absorbed through our skin. Salmon oil, the next-best source of EPA, contains a maximum of only 18% EPA. Other fish oils contain less.

Not all snake oils contain 20% EPA. Rattlesnake oil contains only 8.5% EPA. Other snake oils have not been tested. Here is a worthwhile project for a budding young scientist, which could earn him/her a PhD, and start a new field of research: 'snakeoilology' – the scientific study of snake oils.

But the bottom line is that traditional snake oil is natural and therapeutic. The snake oil salesman is vindicated. The patent medicine salesman can expect a dimmer future.

Protecting the Image

Dr. Richard Kunin, the California doctor, submitted a report of his findings on the ingredients of snake oil to the *New England Journal of Medicine*. They were unwilling to publish it. Might it be more important to keep the image from being tarnished than to disseminate accurate information? If they were wrong about snake oil, what else should we question about the patent medicines-cum-drugs approach?

Evening Primrose, Borage, and Black Currant Oils: GLA 57

The evening primrose *plant* was used for healing by North American natives long before white men took the continent from them. From natives, European explorers learned the healing properties of this common weed. Pilgrims sent the plant back to Europe where, according to one account, it became known as the 'king's cure-all'. The therapeutic value of the *seed oil* of evening primrose is a more recent discovery. It had to await the development of solvent extraction techniques (the

17% oil content of its seeds is rather low for expeller pressing) and modern methods for fatty acid analysis that discovered GLA.

Evening Primrose, Borage, and Black Currant Oils

Evening Primrose oil (EPO) contains 72% linoleic acid (LA, 18:2w6), the essential fatty acid (EFA) that is abundant in commercial seed oils (safflower, sunflower, corn, grape, sesame). Like all other oils, it contains a small amount of non-essential fatty acids (11% oleic acid, 18:1w9; 6% palmitic acid, 16:0; and 2% stearic acid, 18:0). EPO also contains 9% gamma-linolenic acid (GLA, 18:3w6), which is present in only a few other plant seeds.[1] Efamol, the brand on which most of the research was done is unrefined. Most other brands of EPO are refined and deodorized.

Borage oil contains up to 24% GLA, more than twice as much as EPO. It contains about 34% LA, and the rest is saturated and monounsaturated fatty acids, except for about 2.4% erucic acid, long-chain SaFAs, and possibly toxic minor ingredients.

Black currant seed oil contains both EFAs, and up to 18% GLA, as well as 9% of the w3 derivative stearidonic acid (18:4w3), which is not present in other commercial seed oils. Unfortunately this oil is always refined and deodorized.

In comparison, hemp seed oil contains about 2% GLA, and flax, safflower, sunflower, sesame and other common vegetable oils contain no GLA at all.

Gamma-Linolenic Acid (GLA)

GLA results from our body's first biochemical step in transforming the main EFA (LA) into the PG1 family of prostaglandins (see Chapter 58, Prostaglandins). Healthy human cells transform LA into GLA by removing one hydrogen atom each from carbons 12 and 13, and double-bonding these carbons.

Blocks to conversion. But dietary deficiencies and disease conditions may block, slow down, or interfere with the enzyme[2] that catalyzes the conversion of LA to GLA. They include:

- *excess cholesterol,* common in diets rich in meat, eggs, and dairy products;
- *excess saturated and monounsaturated long-chain fatty acids,* which together constitute 85 to 93% of all fatty acids in Western diets;
- *processed vegetable oils,* which make up over 90% of all oil sold to consumers;
- *trans-* fatty acids from margarines, shortenings, shortening oils, and partially hydrogenated vegetable oils;
- *heated oils* from food preparation that involves frying or deep-frying;
- *alcohol,* whose use is widespread;

---

[1] GLA is also found in the seed oils of hemp, several members of the borage family (up to 20% of total fatty acids), in black (18%) and red (12%) currant seed oils, in gooseberry seeds, in poplar seeds, seed oils from several species of the lily family (12-30%), a blue-green alga (21.4%), and several fungi, mosses, and protozoa. Some of these seeds are not edible.

[2] The enzyme is called delta-6-desaturase.

- *aging,* which makes enzymes function less efficiently, and catches up with all of us eventually.
- *zinc deficiency,* which is widespread (zinc is a co-factor in the enzyme catalyzed conversion of LA to GLA);
- common *viral infections,* a result of weak tissues and weak immune systems brought about by poor nutrition;
- *diabetes* and *prediabetic conditions* affect 10 to 20% of the population (from lack of EFAs, excess sugars, excess saturated fatty acids [SaFAs], excess monounsaturated fatty acids, and deficiency of zinc, chromium, and other minerals); and
- high *sugar consumption* – is the rule in the Western diet – which prevents mobilization of EFAs from fat deposits in our body, and interferes with EFAs' work.

In theory, this means that part of the population cannot convert LA to GLA efficiently. Since GLA is available from evening primrose and other seeds, we can take oils containing it, bypass the deficiency or blocked enzyme, and go on to produce the prostaglandins our body needs without making drastic alterations in diet and life-style. Our smartest move would be improved diets and life-style, but supplementation with GLA is better than doing nothing.

Comparing GLA (18:3w6) and LNA (18:3w3)

Before continuing our discussion of GLA-containing oils, let's clear up confusion between GLA (18:3w6) and LNA (18:3w3). Some writers have made no distinction between them, while others have confused the functions of the two, and still others think there is only one linolenic acid, when in fact there are two.

GLA (18:3w6), found in hemp, borage, black currant, and evening primrose oils, is a member of the w6 family of fatty acids, to which the major essential fatty acid (LA, 18:2w6) belongs.

GLA is the precursor of DGLA (20:3w6), the parent of the 'beneficial' prostaglandin PG1 family as well as a precursor of arachidonic acid (20:4w6), and of the 'damaging' prostaglandin PG2 family (see Chapter 58, Prostaglandins).

Contrary to advertising claims, little GLA is found in human mother's milk – nature's exceptional baby food – whereas DGLA *is* present in this precious fluid.

LNA (18:3w3), found in flax, hemp, rape (canola) seed, soybean, walnut, and dark green leaves, is a member of the w3 family, to which EPA (20:5w3) and DHA (22:6w3) also belong. LNA is the second EFA required for human health. Our body cannot make it, and it must therefore be supplied by foods.

GLA and LNA are *almost* identical. Both are fatty acids. Both have 18-carbon atoms in their fatty acid chain. Both have 3 double bonds. Both have double bonds in the w6 and w9 positions. All double bonds of both are methylene interrupted (see Chapter 3, Fatty Acids Overview). Both can be useful in treating degenerative diseases. The shapes of these two fatty acids are quite similar. The only difference between them is the position of one double bond: in GLA, it is between carbons 12 and 13; in LNA, it is between carbons 3 and 4.

Because of their similarities, we should expect GLA and LNA to have several overlapping general functions. But they are also somewhat different. We should therefore expect them to also have unique, specific, individual functions in which they cannot substitute for one another. In clinical practice, we find this to be true.

Studies with Evening Primrose Oil (EPO) Compared to w3s

EPO was extensively tested in double blind trials in hospital settings on several continents for therapeutic effects on an impressive list of diseases, mainly under the stewardship of Dr. David Horrobin, who pioneered its clinical use and markets a brand of EPO. Fish oil w3s have also been tested, both in controlled studies and clinical practice, and flax oil had been used in clinical practice, but has been documented far less extensively in journals than EPO. Evening primrose oil/GLA studies tested the possibility that it might:

- lower blood pressure, lower blood cholesterol level, and lower risk of stroke and heart attack (w3 fatty acids lower blood pressure, platelet stickiness, and cardiovascular risk more effectively);
- normalize fat metabolism in diabetes, and decrease the amount of insulin required by diabetics (w3s do this also);
- prevent liver damage due to alcoholism, hangovers (Europeans traditionally used pickled herring containing w3 fatty acids for this purpose), and withdrawal symptoms after discontinuing the habitual use of alcohol;
- provide adjunctive treatment for schizophrenics, who have low levels of prostaglandin E1, one of several prostaglandins made from w6 fatty acids; when PGE1 was increased by giving EPO, some improvement was noted in those whose disease began less than 5 years ago (w3s have given equal or better results in clinical experience);
- cause weight loss by increasing metabolic rate and fat burn-off (w3s are more effective for this application);
- relieve premenstrual breast pain (mastalgia) and premenstrual syndrome which involves bloating, irritability, and depression, often leading to aggressive behavior; EPO plus vitamins and minerals led to improvement in almost 90% of sufferers (w3s do this for only about 50% of sufferers);
- prevent drying and atrophy of tear and salivary glands (Sjogren's syndrome);
- prevent arthritis in animals, based on the fact that increased levels of prostaglandin E1 prevent arthritis (w3s also help relieve arthritis);
- improve the condition of hair, nails, and skin (w3s do an even better job here);
- improve certain kinds of eczema (w3s also help);
- slow down or stop deterioration in multiple sclerosis, especially if the program is started soon after the initial diagnosis of MS is made (unrefined sunflower oil and w3s have been used with equal effectiveness);
- help treat diabetic neuropathy in Type II diabetes (removal of sugar and SaFAs and addition of w3s also works well); and

- kill cancer cells in tissue culture without harming normal (fibroblast) cells (w3s more effectively inhibit cancer cells in practice).

Continuing Results with EPO and GLA

Good results continue to be obtained in some cases of premenstrual syndrome, atopic eczema, Sjogren's syndrome, and some cases of arthritis. Many of the other conditions for which EPO was originally used are addressed equally well or better with w3 oils.

EPO use might benefit 10 to 25% of the world's affluent population. To provide a comparison, 95% of affluent people lack w3s in their food supply and would benefit from w3 supplementation. EPO has the drawback that it does not supply the missing w3s, and adds to an already existing overload of w6s.

Non-specific effects of EPO, which overlap with the effects of w3s, likely result from the fact that GLA (an w6 derivative) and LNA (the w3 EFA) both contain 3 double bonds and are similar in chemical reactivity. In the absence of w3s in our diet, GLA may pinch-hit for LNA in some of its functions. This phenomenon has been documented for several EFA derivatives.

Problems with EPO

The biggest problem with EPO is that it addresses only half of the EFA conversion problem. If the conversion of w6s (LA to GLA) is blocked, the conversion of w3 (LNA to SDA) is also blocked, because the same enzyme converts both EFAs to derivatives. But EPO contains only w6s, and therefore cannot address the equally important w3 block. Black currant seed oil, on the other hand, contains both w6 and w3 derivatives, and can therefore address the conversion of both EFAs.

To address the conversion problem, EPO must be combined with an oil containing w3 derivatives, such as fish oil. Fish oil by itself will do as good a job alone as when it is mixed with a GLA-containing oil if the *key* problem is w3 deficiency. Blocked conversion of EFAs to derivatives seems to be a problem less often than a lack of w3s in our food supply.

Note: Some people experience worsening of symptoms with EPO, probably due either to solvent residues in the oil – only tiny (homeopathic) doses are required to set off reactions in some people – or because more w6s in a diet *already* too rich in them and too poor in w3s make this imbalance worse.

It is especially critical that EPO not be given without including w3 fatty acids in cancer, because w6s enhance tumor formation and growth, while w3s inhibit tumors. Studies are beginning to show that the conversion of LA to GLA is less often blocked than was first supposed, meaning that most people do make the conversion in their own body., and that w3 deficiency is often the *main* problem. For this reason, the first step in essential fatty acid therapy is to balance w3 and w6 intake by adding w3s to the diet. The *second* step would be to add EFA derivatives and these should also have a balanced ratio of w3s to w6s.

Borage and Black Currant Oils

Less research has been published on borage and black currant seed oils, but some clinicians claim to get good results with them. Like EPO, borage contains only w6s and therefore does only half of the job. Borage oil should therefore be combined with an w3 derivative oil such as fish oil.

Black currant seed oil contains derivatives of both w6 and w3 EFAs, as well as GLA and the equivalent w3 derivative, stearidonic acid (SDA). It can therefore compensate for a block in both w3 and w6 conversion.

Evening primrose, borage, and black currant are usually refined oils. They are usually solvent-extracted as well. Mechanically pressed, fresh, unrefined borage oil from organically grown seeds would be better for health, and is becoming available. Mechanically pressed, refined EPO is also available now.

Co-Factors with EPO, Borage, Black Currant, and Other Oils

Zinc, magnesium, vitamin C, and vitamins B_3 and B_6 must be adequately present in the diet, because they are co-factors in our body's conversion of GLA to prostaglandin E1 (see Chapter 35, Vitamin and Mineral Co-Factors). These co-factors should accompany therapy with all oils, including fish, snake, flax, hemp, and food oils. Once again, we are reminded that human health requires a *complete* program of balanced nutrition.

Biological Engineering

Therapy with oils of evening primrose, borage, and black currant (as well as fish, snake, flax, and hemp) are examples of the use of substances biologically engineered by nature for the control and prevention of diseases and the maintenance of health. Natural healers use knowledge of nutrition and biochemistry to help people heal themselves.

Natural healers were recommending beta-carotene for the prevention of cancer before the medical profession recognized its use. They were recommending vitamin C to strengthen connective tissues, bones, gums, and teeth, for treating cardiovascular disease and cancer, and for fighting viral and bacterial infections before doctors began to take vitamin C seriously. They pioneered the use of vitamin E to prevent cardiovascular disease 40 years before it became fashionable.[3] And now natural healers are also pioneering the importance of oils in human nutrition. Maybe the medical profession should just listen with an open mind, and then try these simple, non-toxic remedies from nature.

---

[3] The brothers Wilfred and Evan Shute who, in the 1950s and 60s, were first to point out the effectiveness of vitamin E to prevent and treat cardiovascular disease in their patients, were written off as crackpots by their own medical colleagues.

Prostaglandins (PGs) **58**

Prostaglandins are extremely powerful. They affect every aspect of our health through their hormone-like effects, and our body makes them from essential fatty acids (EFAs).

History

Prostaglandins were named for the gland from which they were first isolated in 1930 – the prostate gland of sheep. Later, they were also isolated from many other tissues and many other organisms including men, and PGs are now known to be present in all organs, tissues, and cells. The study of prostaglandins is still in its infancy, and is one of the most fascinating areas of fats and oils (lipid) biochemistry.

Description

Functionally, PGs are short-lived, hormone-like chemicals that regulate cellular activities on a moment-to-moment basis. Chemically, PGs are products of enzyme-controlled oxidation of highly unsaturated fatty acids. Our body makes enzymes that oxidize fatty acids in specific ways to make molecules of specific PGs.

The precision of *enzyme-controlled* oxidation reactions stands in stark contrast to *random* oxidation of oils in air, which produces rancid oils instead of hormones. Our body, through enzymes, has remarkably precise control over the outcomes of chemical reactions by guiding them in only the desired direction.

Types of Prostaglandins

Over 30 different PGs have been isolated and identified. Each has different and highly specific functions, and some PGs are stronger in their function than others. Prostaglandins fall into 3 families or series, depending on which fatty acid they were made from. All PGs have 20 carbon atoms, a 5-membered ring, and 2 side chains. They differ in the number of double bonds in the side chain.

Series 1 and 2 prostaglandins come from the w6 family, with the EFA linoleic acid (LA, 18:2w6) as the starting material. Our body changes LA into gamma-linolenic acid (GLA, 18:3w6), then to dihomo-gamma-linolenic acid (DGLA, 20:3w6),[1] and then to arachidonic acid (AA, 20:4w6).[2]

Series 1 prostaglandins are made from DGLA and have 1 double bond in their side chains. Series 2 prostaglandins are made from AA and have 2 double bonds in their side chains. Figure 42 shows the steps by which LA is converted to AA and what one member each of series 1 and 2 prostaglandins look like.

---

[1] DGLA is also found in human breast milk.
[2] AA is also found in meats.

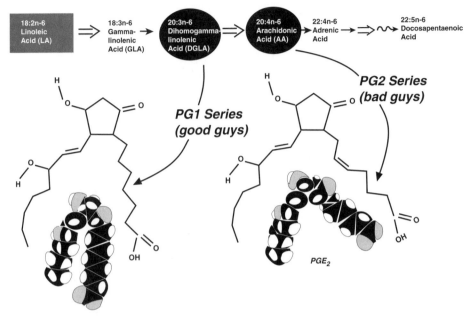

Figure 42. Prostaglandins of the PG1 and PG2 series.

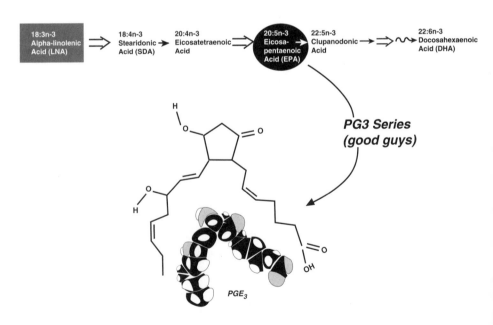

Figure 43. Prostaglandins of the PG3 series.

Series 3 prostaglandins are made from the w3 family, with the EFA alpha-linolenic acid (LNA, 18:3w3) as the starting material. Our body first changes LNA to stearidonic acid (SDA, 18:4w3),[3] then to eicosatetraenoic acid (ETA, 20:4w3), then to eicosapentaenoic acid (EPA, 20:5w3).[4] Series 3 prostaglandins are made from EPA and have 3 double bonds in their side chains. Figure 43 shows the steps by which LNA is converted to EPA, and what one member of series 3 prostaglandins looks like.

Functions of Prostaglandins

Series 1 prostaglandins made from DGLA have been studied in some detail. The most famous member of the series is prostaglandin E1, or PGE1. PGE1 has important functions in several different tissues in our body. It keeps blood platelets from sticking together, and thereby helps prevent heart attacks and strokes caused by blood clots in our arteries. In our kidneys, it helps remove sodium and excess fluid from our body. It is said that each atom of sodium takes 21 molecules of water with it, resulting in increased urine flow (a diuretic effect). PGE1 relaxes blood vessels, improving circulation, lowering blood pressure, and relieving angina. PGE1 may even slow down cholesterol production. It decreases inflammation response, helping to control arthritis. It makes insulin work more effectively, helping diabetics. It improves nerve function, producing a sense of well-being. It regulates calcium metabolism. It improves the functioning of T-cells in our immune system, which destroy foreign molecules and cells. Finally, PGE1 prevents the release of AA from our cell membranes. This is important for the reason given below. PGE1 is one of the 'good guys' among prostaglandins.

Series 2 prostaglandins are made from arachidonic acid (AA). One member, PGI2, acts like PGE1, helping to keep platelets from sticking together. But another member, called PGE2, promotes platelet aggregation, which is the first step in clot formation. PGE2 also induces the kidney to retain salt, leading to water retention and high blood pressure. It also causes inflammation. PGE2 opposes PGE1 functions. It is a 'bad guy' PG in the course of 'civilized', sedentary living, but has survival value under jungle conditions of 'fight or flight'.

PGE1 inhibits the release of AA from cell membranes where AA is stored. As long as AA remains in membranes, it cannot be converted into series 2 prostaglandins.[5] This prevents the bad effects of PGE2 from occurring. The good effect of PGI2 in preventing platelet stickiness is already covered by PGE1 and

---

[3] SDA is also found in seeds of black currants.

[4] EPA is also found in cold water fish oils.

[5] For added protection from the damaging effects of PG2 prostaglandins, the human body converts DGLA (20:3w6) only *slowly* to AA (20:4w6). Since animal products contain AA, however, a high meat diet works against this protection, making people who consume diets rich in animal products more prone to cardiovascular, inflammatory, and kidney diseases.

also by series 3 prostaglandins described below.

Series 3 prostaglandins are made from eicosapentaenoic acid (EPA). Two members of this series, called PGE3 and PGI3, have very weak platelet stickiness (aggregating) effects.

The most powerful effect of PG3s is not so much in their specific action, but in the fact that EPA, their parent, prevents AA from being released from membranes, thereby preventing 'bad' PG2s from being made. EPA is the single most important factor limiting PG2 production, and explains why fish oils can prevent degenerative cardiovascular changes, water retention, and inflammation caused by excessive PG2s (see Chapter 55, Oils from Fish and Seafoods).

Prostaglandins in Health and Disease

Healthy human beings make the prostaglandins they need from EFAs – LA (18:2w6) and LNA (18:3w3) – but nutritional and metabolic conditions can block the ability to convert EFAs into PGs (see Chapter 57, Evening Primrose, Borage, and Black Currant Oils) at the first (delta-6-desaturase) step.[6] In these conditions, oil supplements can bypass the block. Although blocked conversion is probably overstated by those who sell GLA products, supplements of GLA (18:3w6) can bypass the block that prevents series 1 prostaglandins from being made, and oils containing EPA (20:5w3) can bypass the block that prevents series 3 prostaglandins from being made. Under such circumstances, nutritional supplements allow production of PGs by our body to proceed properly, and can help reestablish and maintain health.

PG production from EFAs requires vitamins and minerals that can also be taken as supplements. Vitamins C, B_3, B_6, and the minerals zinc and magnesium are involved. There may be others yet to be identified. The relationship between PGs and health is complex. Research in the field is still in its infancy.

Pharmaceutical preparations of prostaglandin-like substances induce abortions, lower high blood pressure, and decrease platelet stickiness. But this use of PGs, like fixing a wristwatch with a sledgehammer, is extremely crude. Because they are short-lived, much of an injected dose of PGs breaks down before it reaches target tissues. Doses far larger than the body normally produces have to be administered by injection because, added to foods, PGs are destroyed during digestion.

By providing oil supplements – EFAs and EFA derivatives from which PGs are made – our body is given the material it needs to make its own supply of PGs, in the required location, at the required time, and in the required quantities, according to its own internal requirements for health. Doing it nature's way is simpler, and brings better results with no side effects. All we have to do is eat the EFAs or their derivatives.

---

[6] The step blocked in series 1 prostaglandin formation is: LA (18:2w6) to GLA (18:3w6).

The step blocked in series 3 prostaglandin formation is: LNA (18:3w3) to SDA (18:4w3).

Flax: LNA 59

Flax is rapidly becoming a wonder grain of health. Flax is a 'miracle that science forgot' for several generations. It has the potential to help heal and prevent cardio-vascular disease, cancer, diabetes, and many other degenerative conditions.

Old History

Flax may be new to the generation born after the second world war, but its known history is very old, and its use is likely much older. It is one of the oldest known cultivated plants, probably originating in the Orient.

Flax was traditionally grown both for its fiber, which was woven into linen cloth, and for its seeds, which provided w3-rich oils for food (flax oil) and paint (linseed oil), as well as other nutrients and mucilage fiber for normalizing gastro-intestinal function.

According to archaeological authorities on the subject, flax was already being cultivated in Babylon around 5000 BC. Flax seeds and seed pods, wall paintings depicting its cultivation, and cloth made of flax fiber were found in the oldest known Egyptian burial chambers from around 3000 BC. Late stone age archaeological digs in Switzerland dated 3000 to 4000 BC turned up flax seed and flax fiber cloth.

References to the healing properties of flax are found in Greek and Roman writings dating around 650 BC. Hippocrates, in the 5th century BC, mentioned the use of flax to relieve inflamed mucous membranes, and for relieving abdominal pains and diarrhea. Theophrastus (Paracelsus) recommended the use of flax mucilage against coughs. Ancient East Indian scriptures state that in order to reach the highest state of contentment and joy, a yogi must eat flax daily. The Roman writer Tacitus of the 1st century AD praised the virtues of flax in his writings. The 8th century emperor Charlemagne considered flax so important for the health of his subjects that he passed laws and regulations *requiring* its consumption. A 15th century abbess, Hildegard von Bingen, used flax meal in hot compresses to treat both external and internal ailments.

Europeans cultivated flax on a large scale for hundreds of years, to obtain both seeds and fiber. The seeds found many uses in both nutrition and folk medicines used to treat ailments in humans and livestock. Flax oil was so highly regarded in Europe that the hero of Ehm Welk's autobiographical novel from the 1800s exclaims: "Truly, flax oil lubricates our way into eternal life." Mahatma Gandhi once observed: "Wherever flax seed becomes a regular food item among the people, there will be better health."

Recent History

After the second world war, flax was almost forgotten in Europe. Large oil mills chose to press oil seeds inferior in health value but with longer shelf life; the textile industry temporarily went to synthetics; the paint industry turned to manmade drying oils. But flax is making a comeback in all three areas.

Flax grows in every part of the world except the tropics and the arctic. The world's main suppliers are Argentina, India, and the U.S. It is also grown in Canada, and many European countries including Germany, Hungary, France, Holland, Austria, and Poland. It is cultivated in Russia and other former Soviet republics, China, Egypt, and Morocco.

Flax has been used since antiquity to maintain healthy animals. Its uses include:

- correcting digestive disturbances, especially in calves, where losses due to these disturbances can be very high;
- feeding to pregnant cows to make calving easier and to produce healthier calves;
- preventing infectious diseases in cattle, such as hoof-and-mouth, which often took heavy tolls;
- treating respiratory problems in horses (reported by my father, born in 1907);
- improving coats, preventing distemper, improving general health of pets;
- making horses' coats glossy; and show animals' coats full, shiny, and luxuriant; and
- improving the general health and disposition of animals.

The Plant

Flax is an annual plant which, when grown in good soil, may reach a height of 1 meter (3.3 ft), although it usually grows only half that high. It has small, green, pointed (lanceolate) leaves on a tough stalk, and small, deep-blue flowers. Ornamental varieties of flax also exist, with white, gold, and red flowers.

The Latin name for flax is *Linum usitatissimum*. Where my mother grew up, people used to soak flax stalks in shallow ponds for 2 to 3 weeks to rot the flesh off the fibers. They spread out the fibers to dry, then danced on them with rubber boots to break the remaining debris off the dry fibers. The clean fibers were collected and subjected to further processing to make textiles and string. More sophisticated methods are now used, but the principle remains the same. It is the first step in making high-quality cloth called 'linen', its name derived from the Latin name *Linum*. *Usitatissimum* means 'most useful', and the other 'most useful' part of flax is its seed, which is cut and threshed by methods similar to those used to harvest other grains.

The seeds come in golden and brown varieties and can be large or small. Some people prefer golden flax while others find brown flax more useful, but all varieties are nutritious.

Nutrients Contained in Flax

Although their contents vary slightly from year to year and from different growing regions – northern latitudes produce seeds with higher oil and higher w3 content – a sample of 100 grams of seed will give about 35 grams of oil, 26 grams of protein, 14 grams of fiber, 12 grams of mucilage, 4 grams of minerals, and 9 grams of water. It is also the richest known source of lignans (described below), which are rarely found in other seeds.

Whole flax nutrition. If you swallow flax seeds whole, your body will not get the nutrients they contain, because they are protected by a tough seed coat. After the seeds go through you, you could plant them and they would still grow. To break the seed coat and make the nutrients available for digestion, grind whole flax seeds in a small grinder (costing less than $50) or blender cup. In this way, you get the freshest, best-tasting, least spoiled oil possible, plus all of the other nutrients contained in flax. Even better results can be expected from flax if vitamin and mineral intake is optimized.

Note: Take freshly ground flax with plenty of fluid, because its mucilage absorbs 5 times the seed's weight of water. Use from 1 to 6 tablespoons per day: 1 tablespoon of flax contains about 1 teaspoon of oil; 6 tablespoons of flax contain 2 tablespoons of oil.[1]

The use of freshly ground flax seeds can improve digestion, prevent and reverse constipation, stabilize blood glucose levels, improve cardiovascular health, inhibit tumor formation, and bring about many other beneficial effects. Ground flax meal sold in plastic containers in stores is usually rancid and should be avoided.

Oil. The fresh oil of the 'most useful' flax seed is the w3-richest edible oil we know. It has a rich, deep-golden color like fresh, liquid sunshine – which is what it is: sunlight energy stored in bonds between the carbon and hydrogen atoms of which oils are composed, to the tune of 9 Kilocalories per gram. Its aroma is a gentle, pleasant, nutty bouquet. Fresh, it has a light and nutty taste that is delightful, much lighter than that of commercial oils, which have a heavy, 'oily' texture.

People who have tried both fresh and old flax oil sometimes go to great lengths to get it air-shipped fresh. This is because fresh flax oil spoils when exposed to light, oxygen, and heat, and therefore care needs to be taken in pressing, filling, storing, and shipping operations. If this care is not taken, fresh flax oil turns into rancid linseed oil which should be thrown out or used to paint furniture. When someone tells me that they have tried flax oil and don't like its taste, I suspect that they have not tried *fresh* flax oil. Fresh flax oil exposed to light and air loses its fresh taste within a matter of a few days.

Contrary to advertising hype, flax seed is *not* the richest source of *both*

---

[1] If you need to take *more* than 2 tablespoons of oil per day, take up to 6 tablespoons of ground seeds and get the rest from fresh bottled oil.

EFAs. It is a *poor* source of the twice unsaturated linoleic acid (LA, 18:2w6), containing less than 20% LA. Oils containing more LA than flax oil include safflower, sunflower, and sesame oils, but none of these three oils contain LNA.

Flax oil *is* the richest known source of the three times unsaturated alpha-linolenic acid (LNA, 18:3w3), which is necessary for physical health but lacking in the foods most people regularly eat (see Chapter 8, The Healing Essential Fatty Acids). Flax oil contains 45 to 65% LNA (average 55+%). The remainder of the oil is about 18% monounsaturated oleic acid (18:1w9), and about 10% saturated fatty acids (16:0 and 18:0) neither of which are essential, although all oils contain them.

LNA is useful for treating fatty degeneration in cardiovascular disease, cancer, diabetes, and others. Flax oil is a powerful traditional, clinical, and therapeutic tool against these conditions. It is gaining popularity in medical practice, where nutrition-oriented doctors prescribe it for patients to make up for dietary w3 deficiency. To convert LNA to EPA to series 3 prostaglandins, the diet should provide optimum amounts of the conversion co-factors: vitamins B_3, B_6, and C, and the minerals magnesium and zinc.

A unique feature of flax seed is that it may contain a substance resembling prostaglandins that regulate blood pressure, platelet, kidney, immune, and arterial function, inflammatory response, and play important roles in calcium and energy metabolism (see Chapter 58, Prostaglandins).

Fresh, unrefined flax oil contains lecithin and other phospholipids that help emulsify fats and oils for easier digestion, and contribute to physical health. It contains carotene (pro-vitamin A) and vitamin E. These vitamins are necessary to stabilize the oil in both bottle and body. When oil is refined, vitamins and lecithin are removed, and its stability and many health-giving minor components are lost (see Chapter 16, From Seed to Oil).

Flax oil is used in some European suntan and skin oils that nourish the skin with EFAs. Fresh, these preparations are better for our skin than other, more stable commercial preparations, but they will not keep long. The biggest drawback to flax oil as skin or suntan oil is that it oxidizes rapidly on our skin, and then we start smelling like paint. Its short shelf life is the other drawback. It smells horrid when rancid, and the rancidity is masked only poorly by flower essence oils. It also stains clothing, and may collect in seams, from where it cannot be removed once it has dried and hardened.

Lipid researcher Johanna Budwig recommends flax oil for enemas in colon cancer and bowel obstruction. Research in North America is beginning to discover the value of flax oil's LNA in treating cancer. The first papers hinting renewed interest in this direction were presented at the annual Oil Chemists' Meetings in 1984 and 1985. In rats and mice, dietary LNA from linseed oil resulted in fewer tumors, smaller tumors, less metastasis, and longer survival time. Since 1985, dozens of studies have been carried out with flax and flax oil in animals and humans. The results are impressive. Flax is becoming known as the 'wonder grain' of the 1990s.

The drawback of flax oil is that over the long term, it is too rich in w3s. It is the best therapeutic oil for use in making up w3 deficiency. It is useful in cancer treatment, inflammatory conditions, high triglycerides, cardiovascular conditions, diabetes, weight loss, and other degenerative illnesses. Other oils may provide a better balance of EFAs for long-term use (see Chapter 60, Hemp).

Protein. Flax seeds contain high-quality, easily digestible protein that contains all amino acids essential to human health. Essential amino acids lysine, leucine, isoleucine, valine, threonine, methionine, phenylalanine, and tryptophan cannot be made by our body and must therefore be provided by foods. If all essential amino acids are supplied, our body can manufacture from them the other dozen amino acids required to make proteins. If any one or more essential amino acids is missing from our diet, protein deficiency disease develops. The textbook example of protein deficiency disease – kwashiorkor – occurs in African children on a diet of bean protein which is low in the essential amino acid methionine.[2] The children are emaciated, with protruding bellies. The disease is fatal if the diet is not improved.

Flax seeds contain all essential amino acids but, like most vegetable proteins, are low in both lysine and methionine. Flax seed contains histidine and arginine, which are essential for infants. Flax seed is low in cysteine which is essential for *premature* infants. Lysine, methionine, and cysteine are abundant in fish, chicken, and other animal proteins, or can be taken as powdered supplements of lysine, methionine, and N-acetyl cysteine.

Fiber. A lot has been written about fiber. It keeps our digestive tract from getting clogged with mucus, toxic materials, and metabolic wastes. It keeps our colon swept and moving. Fiber is necessary for intestine and colon health. It feeds and maintains a healthy intestinal flora made up of friendly little bacteria and yeasts that make some of our vitamins and protect us from unfriendly intestinal 'bugs'. A healthy colon minimizes release of toxins back into our blood. Healthy blood means that we may live long enough to reach a wise (or foolish) old age.

Fiber also lowers blood cholesterol, because it prevents cholesterol and bile acids from being reabsorbed into our body from our intestine. Cholesterol and bile acids attach to fiber, and are carried out of our body into the toilet with solid wastes. Fiber also softens stools, prevents constipation, and maintains regularity. Flax is an excellent source of fiber.

Mucilage. Its 12% content of mucilage makes flax seeds the best natural

---

[2] Beans are low in methionine, but rich in lysine. Most grains, on the other hand, are low in lysine and rich in methionine. Beans and grains together supply a better balance of all essential amino acids than either one alone. Their complementary nature is the basis of Mexican bean-and-grain dishes.

laxative available. This soft, water-soluble kind of fiber soothes and protects the delicate stomach and intestinal lining, prevents irritation, and keeps the contents moving smoothly along. It absorbs water and swells to about 20 times its dry volume (therefore, 5 times the volume of the flax being eaten, as fluid, should accompany its consumption). Stools don't become hard and dry. Considering that about 30% of the North American adults have constipation, flax could offer a great service here. It has no side effects. This alone makes it the laxative of choice.

Flax mucilage also has the ability to buffer excess acid. This makes it ideal for people with acid or sensitive stomachs, ulcers, and inflammatory conditions of any part of the intestine.

Mucilage from flax lowers elevated cholesterol by preventing reabsorption of bile acids, and decreases absorption of cholesterol from foods, increasing the amount of cholesterol excreted.

Mucilage helps stabilize and modulate blood glucose, which is useful in diabetes and hypoglycemia. Mucilage is perfect food for beneficial bacteria in our colon, helping them keep bad intestinal 'bugs' under control.

Minerals. According to one analysis, 100 grams (3.3 ounces) of flax seeds contain the following amounts of minerals (in grams):

potassium	0.74	sodium	0.046
phosphorus	0.70	chlorine	0.043
magnesium	0.38	iron	0.0077
calcium	0.21	zinc	0.0057
sulphur	0.21		

Flax seeds also contain trace amounts of manganese, silicon, copper, fluorine, nickel, cobalt, iodine, molybdenum, and chromium. The only essential trace minerals not listed are selenium and vanadium. Their absence may be flax seed's flaw, but it's more likely that the laboratory chemist did not test for these more recently discovered trace minerals.

Vitamins. Besides this array of minerals, flax seeds also contain fat-soluble vitamins E and carotene. It also contains water-soluble vitamins B_1, B_2, and C, but is low in vitamins B_3 and B_6.

Lignans. Lignans are cyclic molecules with anti-viral, anti-fungal, anti-bacterial, and anti-cancer properties. Flax contains 100 times the quantity of lignans as the next best source, which is wheat bran. Their richness in lignans makes flax seeds useful for treating viral, fungal and bacterial infections, as well as cancer. Lignans must be differentiated from lignins, which are a kind of insoluble fiber.

Two percent of the lignans found in flax seeds end up in flax oil; the other 98% remain in the seed meal. As a result, freshly ground flax seed has some advantages over the oil, providing the freshest possible oil, as well as mucilage and fiber, other nutrients, and lignans. Six to eight tablespoons of seed is a daily maximum, because flax seeds absorb about 5 times their volume of water. **Note:** Take freshly-ground flax seed with five time its volume of fluid.

Beware of a marketing gimmick that offers 'lignan flax oil'. This is simply crude flax oil as it comes out of the press. The 'mud' it contains is fine seed material. The manufacturer simply did not let this fine seed material settle out of the oil. Because such oil takes less work to make, it should be *cheaper* than clear oil. 'Lignan flax oil' provides only about 90% as much oil, the remaining 10% being the seed 'mud' settled from the oil. If you want lignans, use freshly ground seeds, which are far cheaper and contain far more lignans.

Uses for Flax Seeds

Flax is excellent food, because it contains a good part of a complete diet. Its components are used to treat many ailments which, if flax were a regular part of the diet, would not occur in the first place.

Flax seeds provide good nutrition in the form of protein, oil containing lecithin, phytosterols, and other valuable minor ingredients, minerals, vitamins, soluble and insoluble fiber, and lignans.

A flax seed placed inside the eyelid soothes inflammation and helps lessen pain if sharp grit gets into an eye, and it also helps move the grit into the corner of the eye, from where it can be easily removed.

The *mucilage* part of the seed soothes our digestive tract. Whole or freshly ground seeds are used in digestive, eliminative, toxic diseases of the stomach, intestines, and colon, which include inflammation of stomach (gastritis), intestinal tract (ileitis), or colon (colitis, diverticulitis). Taken with fluids, flax mucilage alleviates constipation, increasing stool bulk and softness, and speeding up stool movement out of our body, and preventing toxin buildup in our bowel. Stools smell less foul, our liver is relieved of toxic stress, and our breath sweetens. According to Bernard Jensen, one of the best-known natural healers alive today, many degenerative diseases start in our colon through the toxic effects of constipation. In Europe, flax is guaranteed to cure constipation within 3 days. Externally, hot compresses of flax swelled with hot water draw toxins, and soothe and heal boils, bruises, and other skin afflictions.

Flax mucilage is a natural, non-toxic hair-setting gel.

A handful of flax seeds will plug small leaks in car and tractor radiators.

Fiber present in flax seed is also good food for feeding friendly bacteria in our intestinal tract, and helps them keep disease-causing organisms under control.

According to East Indian medicine, flax creates heat. In Western terms, flax increases metabolic rate. It stimulates oxidation by which energy is produced, which we experience as warmth. Flax enhances all life processes, because all our life processes depend on energy production.

Uses for Flax Oil

Flax oil has been used both clinically and in self-responsible health care for hundreds of years in Europe and for about 10 years in North America.

Flax oil reverses conditions caused by deficiency of alpha-linolenic acid. It is beneficial in treatment programs against all major degenerative conditions, including cancer, cardiovascular disease, diabetes, multiple sclerosis, arthritis, premenstrual syndrome, overweight, and many more.

Specifically, the oil has been used to lower high blood pressure and high serum triglycerides. It is used to make platelets less sticky through its conversion to eicosapentaenoic acid (EPA, 20:5w3) and series 3 prostaglandins (PG3s). Through PG3s, flax oil can help decrease inflammation, help reduce water retention (edema), and enhance some functions of the immune system. In some people, flax oil lowers cholesterol.

Compared to corn oil, flax oil has been shown in animals to produce fewer tumors, smaller tumors, less metastasis, and longer survival time. In mice, linseed oil (the paint grade oil from flax) produced fewer tumors in tumor-prone mice than did safflower, corn, lard, and fish oils. In clinical practice in Europe and North America, flax oil had been used with some success as the only oil allowed in natural treatments of cancer and AIDS.

Flax oil lowers the amount of insulin required by diabetics, which brings them one step closer to health. It has been found to be helpful in some cases of rheumatoid and osteoarthritis, as well as lupus. It is useful in some cases of premenstrual syndrome and conditions that involve edema. The oil can make some pregnancies less eventful, make deliveries easier, and produce healthier offspring.

The oil is very helpful for treating dry skin, dandruff, sun-sensitive skin, and even eczema and psoriasis. It also helps relieve some cases of asthma and allergies. Flax oil often improves liver function, metabolism of calcium and other minerals, fights infections such as staphylococcus and malaria, and contains ingredients with anti-viral, anti-fungal and antibacterial properties.

Donald Rudin, a physician and medical researcher, showed that flax oil can improve the behavior of schizophrenics and juvenile delinquents who fail to respond to counseling, and effectively treats some cases of depression. It can also improve visual function, color perception, and mental acuity in some older people. It often improves symptoms of multiple sclerosis. In many people, it brings on a feeling of calmness.

The oil shortens the time necessary for fatigued muscles to recover after exertion, and shortens healing time for bruises, sprains, and other injuries. It increases energy, stamina, and the feeling of vitality, and makes skin soft, hair shiny, and nails strong.

While some of these effects of flax oil *are* documented in the scientific research literature, many are not (yet). Properly made fresh flax oil, or balanced blends containing it, ought to become part of the intake of virtually the entire population.

Remember, however, that antioxidants are necessary to prevent its deterioration, that vitamins B_3, B_6, and C, and the minerals magnesium and zinc are necessary to make prostaglandins, and that health is possible only if a complete, balanced program containing all the essential nutrients is used. Flax oil is a useful therapeutic oil, but it is not a magic bullet that can act alone without help. In this sense, the seed is better that the oil, and the seed enriched with antioxidants, vitamins, and minerals is even better.

Research Interest

Since the original publication of this book in 1986, and a meeting of the Flax Council in Winnipeg in March of 1988 where I made several bold statements to both the general meeting and the private board meeting about the potential of flax to prevent and treat cancer, cardiovascular disease, and diabetes, many experimental studies have been carried out on flax grain, and some on its oil. Some of the recent human nutrition and health studies with flax were funded by the Flax Council.

Research on flax is now well under way. The value of flax, one of the wonder grains of the world, will be 'newly discovered' by researchers in the next few years. But their work will simply confirm and give better scientific explanations for its curative properties, which have been known since antiquity.

Hemp: LA, LNA, & GLA 60

WARNING: Hemp seeds and hemp oil contain traces of THC, which show up in urine drug tests and may result in the loss of jobs requiring mandatory drug screens.

Hemp is the twin of flax, and they share a long history. They are two of the oldest known plants to be grown by humanity. Both were cultivated for their fiber and for the nutrients contained in their seeds.

The fiber from flax was used to make linen. The fiber from hemp was used to make canvas and rope. The oil of both was used both as edible oil and as paint. The seeds of both provided a rich source of nutrients. The seeds and oils of both twins – flax and hemp – support good health.

Hemp Plants

Hemp is one of the sturdiest plants known to us. It can grow to a height of 10 feet or more in a year, and its roots penetrate equally deep into the ground. Hemp roots draw minerals buried deep in the soil up to the surface. As a result, they enrich the soils on which they grow, and require little fertilizer.

Another unique feature of hemp is that most pests leave it alone, and therefore it can be grown without pesticides. Hemp has been used as companion plants to cabbage and other vegetables to protect them from pests.

As a result of its innate sturdiness, hemp fits the requirements for 'organic cultivation' – which is recommended for growing foods most conducive to healthy eating – without special growing methods having to be instituted, compliance having to be confirmed and verified, or cheating becoming necessary to save an organic crop from infestation.

Hemp is one of the fastest growing plants on the planet. It has been recommended as a way to slow down and reverse the 'greenhouse effect' resulting from carbon dioxide released by our massive burning of fossil fuels. Hemp 'fixes' this carbon dioxide and turns it into oxygen and fiber more quickly than most other green plants, including grasses and trees. Environmentalists hold out great hope for this aspect of hemp's usefulness.

Hemp Fiber

Linen is used for tablecloths and clothing. Canvas, the most durable natural fiber known, was used to make sails for ships, canvas tents, and even the uppers for canvas shoes. The word 'canvas' is derived from *Cannabis,* which is the Latin name for hemp.

Hemp was also used to make rope used by the navy. It is durable and does not stretch, which is important for rope used to fasten sails. If the rope stretches (as does one made from synthetics like nylon), the sails move too much, which is inefficient at best and can be disastrous in a storm.

Hemp cloth was also used to make textiles that are more durable than linen and that, properly worked, are softer than cotton.

Hemp fiber was also used to make extremely durable paper (the first and second drafts of the U.S. Declaration of Independence were printed on hemp paper), excellent for archival material that must last for many years.

Hemp produces high-quality cellulose for making pulp and paper products. Because of its rapid growth, it is estimated to provide about 4 times more cellulose over 20 years than an equivalent acreage of trees.

Using modern methods, hemp fiber can also be used to make building materials and lumber as durable as, and at a fraction of the cost of, wood pilfered from our dwindling old-growth forests.

Hemp was a common farm crop in North America until the 1930s. Thomas Jefferson and George Washington were hemp farmers. A 1942 film (now available on video) made by the U.S. Department of Agriculture and called 'Hemp for Victory', documents the commercial value of hemp.

Hemp Seeds

Hemp seeds were used for food. While flax seeds were thought of as therapeutic and used to treat several conditions, hemp seeds were used nutritionally with less fanfare. In Russia, for instance, hemp seeds were ground into a delicious hemp seed butter containing protein, oil, minerals, vitamins, and fiber, and far superior to peanut butter in nutritional value. They are less likely than peanuts to contain carcinogenic aflatoxins. On the downside, hemp seed butter has a shorter shelf-life than peanut butter, and must be fresh unless it is specially protected against spoilage.

Hemp seeds contain about 3% soluble fiber and 27% insoluble fiber. Hemp seeds are green, rich in chlorophyll, and rich in magnesium, potassium, sulphur, and other key elements. Ground hemp seeds are somewhat more stable than ground flax, but also deteriorate relatively rapidly.

Hemp Seed Oil

Like linseed oil, hemp seed oil was used in paint because it, too, is rich in essential fatty acids (EFAs) that react with oxygen and then dry in a thin film. The oil covers wood and other materials with an extremely strong coat that protects these materials from wear by wind, water, salt water, and sunlight, and slows down the deterioration of materials exposed to the elements. Hemp seed oil was also used in lamps before electricity was harnessed for producing light.

The history of hemp seed oil in food use is similar to that of flax. The oil was used in food preparation. It had to be obtained fresh and used within a week or two before the invention of special manufacturing methods and refrigeration. Hemp oil is more difficult to make than flax oil because it is much harder on machinery.

But hemp seed oil appears to be one of nature's reasonably balanced EFA oils. It contains both EFAs in proportions suitable for long-term use, and also contains GLA.

Hemp seed is difficult to obtain. It must be imported from China, India, or Europe where it is grown without the use of pesticides, and must be fumigated to prevent the import of foreign pests that it might carry. Since the fumigants are volatile, they evaporate. Tests show no detectible residues at the limit of detection, 50 parts per billion. In order to grow hemp under 'organic' guidelines, it would have to be grown locally.

In spite of all its virtues and commercial potential, hemp is illegal to grow in North America. Hemp *oil* is legal. *Steamed* hemp seeds are legal. Hemp *fiber,* *cloth,* and *rope* are legal. Sproutable seeds are illegal because they could be used to grow hemp, some strains of which contain the drug tetrahydrocannabinol (THC) in their leaves and flowers.

Unfortunately, hemp seeds split when they are steamed, resulting in some oxidation of its oil. Instead of a peroxide value (PV) – a measure of the degree of rancidity of an oil – of 0.1 to 0.5 which is attained in careful pressings, the PV of hemp oil goes up to about 6 or 7 – another good reason for legalizing the seed. The PV is safe and does not ruin its taste. For comparison, flax oil with a PV of 2 or 3 tastes bad; the PV of virgin olive oil is about 20; the PV of unrefined corn oil may be as high as 40 to 60.

By legalizing the seed, the quality of the oil could be improved. As health becomes more important to citizens, those who make our laws will eventually legalize hemp. Strains of hemp containing very little THC are available. These strains can be used to exploit the commercial aspects of hemp without having to embrace any of its controversial drug aspects.

A Modern Conspiracy?

According to an account documented in Jack Herer's 1991 book *The Emperor Wears No Clothes – Hemp and the Marijuana Conspiracy*, DuPont in 1937 patented new (sulfate/sulfite) processes for making paper from wood. They were also involved in synthetics, munitions, and processing cellulose. They hoped that synthetic fibers would replace natural fibers. The newspaper giant Hearst had interests in timber and paper. New technology had put hemp in a position to replace wood (cellulose) as raw material for paper. According to Herer, these two industrial giants set out on a disinformation campaign. They hired someone to travel around the country to give hemp a bad name. They renamed the well-known and useful hemp plant (which had been grown in the U.S. by thousands of farmers for almost two centuries) 'marijuana', the 'killer weed from Mexico'. They combined anti-Mexican racist images from the war between Mexico and the U.S. with their anti-hemp propaganda to create a negative public perception of hemp. They invented undocumented, unsupported claims that its use leads to criminal activity.[1] Hearst used its newspaper chain to mobilize public opinion against hemp. Their business interests and political clout prevailed over truth, and laws were enacted to entrench their vested industry interests.

Hemp became illegal. Its drug properties were blown completely out of proportion. Its commercial value for food, clothing, paper, tents, shoes, rope, and building materials was completely ignored. The vested interests behind the killer weed image duped an entire continent for a whole generation for private gain.

A Reasonably Balanced Oil

One day in 1990, I got a call from a lady in Los Angeles. She noted that I had made

---

[1] Closer to the truth is the observation that people 'stoned' on hemp are too relaxed to engage in criminal activities that require planning, organization, and focused thinking. Research confirms that 'stoned' people make poor criminals. The only consistently observed change is *psychological:* 'stoned' people become less driven and more laid back. Judging from the effects of drivenness on personal, political, and environmental landscapes, this effect could almost be argued to be beneficial.

reference to the food use of hemp seed in Russia in my book. We had an interview. Since I thought that hemp was illegal, I was uninterested in it. A few months later, someone sent me the very interesting fatty acid profile of hemp seed oil.

While flax oil is useful for treating degenerative diseases, it is too w3-rich (about 4 times as much w3 as w6) to be used exclusively in the long term. One can develop w6 deficiency by using *only* flax oil for too long. While it took me about 2 years to end up with thin, papery-feeling skin that dried out and cracked easily, w6 deficiency could develop in as short a time as 10 to 16 months of *exclusive* use of flax oil.

Knowing this, I began to look at producing a *balanced* w6-w3 oil blend. But other matters intervened, and before I finished designing my balanced blend, the fatty acid profile of hemp seed oil arrived in the mail.

Hemp seed oil can be used over the long term to maintain a healthy EFA balance without leading to either EFA deficiency or imbalance. This is because it contains w6 and w3 EFAs in a better long-term balance: 3 to 1. In addition, it contains almost 2% GLA, the w6 derivative that is a key active ingredient in evening primrose and borage oils. The samples of hemp seed oil that we tested contained about 57% LA (18:2w6), 19% LNA (18:3w3), and 1.7% GLA (18:3w6). Like the fatty acid profile of all natural oils, that of hemp oil will vary, depending on the strain, location, latitude, and weather conditions of the year the plants were grown.

Hemp seeds and hemp oil produce no 'high' in humans or animals. They contain very small amounts of THC, unless the seeds have been contaminated. A good reason for growing hemp seeds locally is that one can then dry, clean, and supervise the process properly to prevent this contamination.

Hemp seed oil tastes like sunflower oil. It is green in color due to its content of magnesium-containing chlorophyll. Most people that sampled hemp oil preferred its taste over the taste of flax oil.

Hemp seed oil is good for all food uses except frying and deep-frying. Like flax oil, its twin, hemp seed oil needs to be refrigerated or frozen to prevent deterioration, and must be shielded from light and oxygen to prevent rancidity.

Oil Blends

Between flax oil, with 4 times as much w3 as w6 (too rich in w3), and w6-rich oils, the best balanced of which is hemp oil with 3 times as much w6 as w3, there is a wide gap in which there are no natural oils. Yet EFA-rich oils with the greatest health potential fit into this gap. W3-rich flax oil and w6-rich oils can be blended to balance EFAs and best support human EFA needs and optimum health. In practice, we get our best results with a w3:w6 ratio of 2:1. This ratio can be obtained by adding w6-rich sunflower and sesame oils to flax oil. The 2:1 ratio and the above oils are used to make Udo's Choice Oil Blend.

61 *Exotic Oils*

A few exotic oils from other parts of the world are worth naming. Some of these oils contain both w3 and w6 essential fatty acids, and have therapeutic potential. Another is EFA-poor, but has therapeutic value due to its minor components.

Kukui (Candlenut)

The kukui nut tree grows only in tropical climates: Hawaii and the Pacific Islands to New Zealand. It is the state tree of Hawaii, where it has a long traditional history of use as a source of therapeutic agents and of skin oil. Its oil is protected from light and oxygen by being surrounded by an extremely dense, hard, pitch-black shell. Hawaiian princesses used kukui nut oil to protect their skin from sun and salt, and to keep it soft and beautiful. Hawaiians used the flesh from the nut for medicinal purposes. Among other things, it loosens stools.

The nut is so rich in oil that it burns. The name 'candlenut', given to it by Western explorers, derives from the fact that many nuts skewered in rows on sticks could be lit and used as torches to light up the night or explore caves.

The shell, drilled from both ends with the nut meat poked out, was made into pitch-black, polished ornamental necklaces.

Candlenut oil contains about 40% w6 LA (18:2w6) and 29% w3 LNA (18:3w3). It is the richest source of w3 fatty acids for dwellers of tropical isles where local fish contain little, if any, w3 fatty acids.

Chia Seeds

In the desert of New Mexico, natives eat chia seeds. These tiny seeds contain about 40% LA and 30% LNA. Their essential fatty acids (EFAs) are protected from light and air in the same way as the EFAs in flax, with a brown seed coat, which is further covered with water-absorbing mucilage like that which covers flax seeds. Chia seeds provide a well-protected source of w3 and w6 EFAs in the hot desert climate.

Psyllium Seeds

Psyllium seeds also contain about 40% LA and 30% LNA. In India and Middle Eastern countries, the whole seed is used for food.

We import only the husks from India. These are a source of water-soluble fiber, but contain no oil. Psyllium husks swell to 20 times their volume with water. They are used to prevent and alleviate constipation. The most nutritious part of the seed stays in the countries that grow it.

Other W3/W6 Seeds?

No doubt there are other w3/w6 EFA-containing seeds. Knowing the importance of these two fatty acids to human biology, it is likely that every part of the globe has a source of them.

In the tropics, we expect sources of w3 and w6 oils to be more heavily protected from light and oxygen than in temperate climates, where protection would have to be better than in arctic climates. Future explorations will likely discover sources of both EFAs in traditional foods around the world.

Neem Oil

Pressed from the seeds of a tree grown in lowland tropical areas, neem oil has remarkable properties that reside in its minor components (see Chapter 54, Virgin Olive Oils). Its fatty acid profile is unremarkable, consisting mainly of saturated and monounsaturated fatty acids (see Table D7). Neem oil's minor components, which are also found in neem leaves and bark, are useful in diverse applications of which the following are the main ones:

- *Skin and hair care:* Used in soaps, shampoos, and skin creams, neem oil kills viruses, fungi, and bacteria such as wart, pox, hepatitis, athlete's foot, ringworm, candida, staph, and salmonella.
- *Oral hygiene:* Used in toothpaste, neem oil inhibits gum inflammation (pyorrhea), receding gums, mouth ulcers, and tooth decay. Neem sticks are used as toothbrushes by people in areas where it grows.
- *Pest control:* Applied in the home, it repels house flies, and fleas; applied to the skin, neem oil acts as an insect repellent; it keeps mosquitoes, fleas, and sandflies (no-seeums) from biting; applied to plants as a systemic pesticide, it keeps insects as diverse as fruit flies, flour beetles, gypsy moths, weevils, fire ants, cabbage loopers, and leafminers from feeding, and disrupts the development of insects like thrips, cockroaches, and potato beetles that do feed on such plants, sterilizing, deforming, or killing them; neem also kills snails, slugs, viruses, fungi, and bacteria, and inhibits aflatoxin production by fungi; applied to soil, neem leaves and seed cake protect plant roots from nematodes and insects, as well as making soils more fertile by preventing soil bacteria from wasting nitrogen.
- *Veterinary medicine:* Neem oil can be used to treat intestinal parasites, including roundworms, tapeworms, nematodes, and insects such as biting flies, lice ticks, fleas, and tropical skin parasites. It also helps in genital tract infections.
- *Human skin, blood, lymph, and intestinal parasite control:* Neem holds out promise in all of these parasite-caused conditions. Its toxicity appears to be low. It has been used traditionally for a long, long time, but more testing is still being done.
- *Birth control:* Neem may provide the basis for morning-after birth control, spermicides, and 6-month reversible sterility preparations. These applications,

based on traditional uses, are just beginning to be researched.

Never underestimate the power of minor ingredients present in natural, unrefined seed oils!

62 *Oil & Protein Work Together*

Essential fatty acids (EFAs) do not act alone. EFA-rich oil and protein belong together in our body, and are found together in whole foods. A balance of good oil and good protein is necessary for a healthy body. Evidence from both experience and laboratory links oils with proteins in nutrition. Personal observations can verify their interdependence.

Everyday, Common Observations

Dry skin. The human skin is made largely of collagen, which is protein. On a diet low in fats, or for other nutritional reasons, our skin may become dry, flaky, and hard. What do we do with such skin? We oil it. The kinds of oil that work best are those that our skin absorbs – oils containing EFAs that it can use for nourishment. To a smaller extent, skin also absorbs monounsaturated oleic acid. Saturated fatty acids are poorly absorbed. Non-natural, artificial mineral oil and petroleum jelly are not absorbed at all, providing only a protective coat.

Infant eczema. When they are weaned from mother's breast, some young children get an eczema-like skin condition over many parts of their body, because they change from mother's milk containing 8% or more of its fatty acids as EFAs to a diet of baby foods and dairy containing ample protein but little or no EFAs. This rash can be eliminated by rubbing oil containing EFAs on these children's skin. Their skin absorbs the oil and transports it throughout their body.

Skin and cosmetic creams consist of an oil base, with other substances added to give smooth texture, fragrance, and other desirable external properties.

Manufacturers of common skin products prefer to use oils that will not spoil. These products can protect the skin against the drying effects of sun, wind, and rain by covering it, but do not actively build healthy skin because they largely lack the spoilable EFAs necessary for skin health.

Better types of skin creams nourish the protein skin with EFAs. The best ones *do* really work, and *do* contain EFAs. Sesame oil is most often used because it has the best resistance to spoilage. Since EFAs spoil rapidly, EFA-rich skin preparations have a short shelf-life (six months maximum), and therefore cost more. They make skin supple and soft, and help slow down the development of lines, wrinkles, and dryness as we age.

The use of w3 fatty acids would shorten shelf-life to a month. As a result, w3s should not be used in cosmetics and skin creams without special preparatory and protective processes. Some manufacturers use just enough to make a label claim but not enough to bring benefit to the skin of consumers – a small amount of w3s can go rancid without detection. Some newer preparations contain more w3s, but then the product goes, and smells, rancid very quickly, making it unsuitable for commercial trade, which requires longer shelf-life. Neither method is good for our skin. The best way to get skin-beautifying w3 EFAs to our skin is to eat fresh w3-rich foods. Then our skin becomes velvety and smooth without the use of expensive creams and lotions. Our *best* 'cosmetics' are fresh, edible ones, which oil our skin from within.

Many people who begin to use better edible oils are amazed at the difference in their skin. They find that their skin feels creamy, supple, soft, and lovely to touch. Hard skin, greasy pores, 'zits', bumps, and acne disappear. These are the most obvious changes that many people notice on using good oils along with balanced nutrition. They also get an enhanced feeling of well-being.

Leather is collagen protein that was once living skin. To keep leather soft, we must oil it. When water from snow or rain draws out the oil, the leather hardens. The same holds true for us. Our skin – living leather – must be oiled to remain soft. During baths and showers, even too much hot water removes softening oils from our skin, drying and hardening it thereby, perhaps also making it itchy.

Diet. Many people on high protein diets suffer from constipation. Athletes know that protein powders build muscle, but also constipates them, and they avoid fat, which has a bad reputation in this age of muscle and protein consciousness. Most of the constipated 30% of our population can be relieved by simply including stool-softening oils containing EFAs. Flax oil has this stool-softening effect. By changing the type and amount of oil in the diet, we can obtain the precise stool consistency we want. An oil enema relieves constipation and gives the smoothest move in town.[1] Try it! Drinking more water and eating more fiber-rich foods also help relieve constipation.

Problem skin. When labor, detergents, soaps, or solvents dry and crack the skin on our hands, we use oils to soften it again. The skin proteins of our hands need to be oiled to stay supple and soft. Oils also speed healing processes.

People with dry skin, eczema, and psoriasis, and also older folk and those with arthritis, find that their skin gets dry and rough, and skin conditions worsen in winter and from soap. They discover that it is better for their skin to use soap only on the hairy parts of their body. Soap emulsifies and removes oils, leaving the skin's proteins oil-less. Organic solvents, household cleaners, and gasoline-like products also remove oils from our hands, leaving them chapped, hard, dry, and

---

[1] Oils also have widespread industrial applications as lubricants.

prone to cracking.

Equally good advice is to eat more EFA-containing oils to replenish, from the inside, our body's own supply with which to oil our skin.

Lips. We treat chapped lips with an oil-based chapstick or oil-based lip gloss. When the oil on our lips is licked or washed off, our lips dry and crack.

Early Scientific Evidence

According to her own account, lipid researcher Johanna Budwig (see Chapter 63, Budwig, Flax Oil, and Protein) succeeded where several giants in research had failed. Here is her version of the history of combining oil and protein.

Hints. Scientific evidence linking oil and protein in nutrition goes back many years, and includes work carried out by some of the best scientists of their time. Liebig in 1842, Pflueger in 1875, and Hoppe-Seyler in 1876 had shown a clear connection between oil and protein nutrition on one hand, and oxygen uptake and biological oxidation in tissues on the other hand.

In 1888, Lebedow showed that if starving dogs are given either protein or fat alone, they die even faster than if they receive no food at all (that is, continue to be starved). However, if they receive good protein and good fat *together,* they recover quickly from starvation. Good protein was protein rich in sulphur-containing amino acids (methionine and cysteine), which includes all animal proteins: dairy, beef, chicken, fish, shellfish, and egg, as well as soybean (especially soft tofu).

Most plant proteins are low in sulphur amino acids, but can be improved by using garlic, onions, or a supplement of N-acetyl cysteine or methionine. Plant proteins are also low in lysine, which can also be taken as a supplement. 'Good' fat in this experiment was fresh flax oil, which is the richest source of w3 essential fatty acids. 'Bad' fats were animal fats high in saturated fatty acids.

In 1899, Rosenfeld showed that the consumption of animal fats high in saturated and low in EFAs causes obesity and fatty degeneration of inner organs.

At the time that the above experiments were carried out, the difference between saturated fatty acids and EFAs had not yet been discovered. Nevertheless, the observations are in line with what we now know about the effects of EFAs and SaFAs on animal and human health.

The essentiality of EFAs was not known until 1930. That year, researchers Burr and Burr discovered EFAs and showed that if protein is given to animals deficient in EFAs, the animals die very quickly.

In 1902, Rosenfeld showed that a high-carbohydrate, low protein diet results in fat deposition. So does a high-carbohydrate, high-protein diet. But when 'good' fats are added, less fat deposition occurs and better food utilization and energy production take place. In other words, 'good' fats help one stay slim. Contrary to popular opinion, not all fats make us fat.

The biological reasons behind these observations took longer to work out, but are now better understood:

1. Fats are digested slowly and prevent hunger from recurring for as long as 5 to 8 hours after a meal, whereas proteins and carbohydrates are digested in 2 to 5 hours and hunger recurs much sooner, encouraging overeating.
2. EFAs increase metabolic rate and help mobilize and burn excess saturated fats.
3. Our body loses its craving for food when its need for EFAs is satisfied.

Our hunger mechanism shuts off only when the nutrient needs of our body are fulfilled. A poor diet lacking essential substances fails to still hunger, leading to overeating and weight gain.

More findings. Several other researchers obtained results in their experiments that consistently showed that protein and oil belong together in nutrition and work together in our body. They are also found together in natural foods: whole seeds, nuts, eggs, meat, membranes, fish, etc. This is because oils and proteins are the main structural components of all living organisms.

Sensitivity to toxins increases if oil and protein are not given together, or in the right proportions. Researchers also found that too much protein causes disease. If oil is withdrawn from such a diet, disease from too much protein is worsened. Most modern diets contain too much protein and not enough of the 'good', w3 EFA-rich oils.

In intensely active tissues, increased amounts of sulphur-rich protein are found, paralleled by increased concentrations of EFAs.

In Italy where, according to Budwig, flax oil consumption was high, sulphur-containing proteins effectively treated severe liver disease, skin afflictions, eclampsia[2] of pregnancy, and other toxic conditions. These proteins also revived patients from anesthesia. In the U.S., where flax oil was not commonly consumed and the w3 EFA content of the diet was generally low, the same proteins failed in these medical applications, to the surprise and dismay of doctors. The combination of the right oil with proteins is important in these clinical applications.

By the 1920s, the synergistic (cooperative) action of sulphur-rich protein and fatty substances in the body was already firmly established, though the identity of the fatty substances was still unknown.

Nobel prize-winning scientists. By 1911, Thorsten Thunberg knew of the importance of sulphur-rich (animal) proteins, and knew that these proteins work in combination with a functional partner in biological systems. He searched for, but was unable to isolate that partner, because techniques necessary for isolating and identifying EFAs had not yet been invented.

In 1920, Meyerhof found that a fatty acid called linoleic acid (now, but not then, known to be essential) and sulphur-rich proteins work together to help fatigued muscle recover rapidly from exercise and exertion. He failed recognize the

---

[2] Eclampsia (toxemia of pregnancy) is a convulsive disorder occurring near the end of pregnancy, a serious toxic condition which endangers the life of both mother and child.

significance of this finding.

In 1924, Szent-Gyorgyi discovered that the system of sulphur-rich protein and linoleic acid takes up oxygen. He lacked the biochemical techniques to prove the identity of the components of this system conclusively.

In 1926, Otto Warburg showed that a fatty substance was required to restart oxidation when it was low, as is the case in cancer and other degenerative conditions. He didn't know which substance it was, and tested several different fatty acids including saturated butyric acid (4:0) and monounsaturated oleic acid (18:1w9) (see Chapter 3, Fatty Acids Overview). He was surprised and disappointed that the expected increase in oxidation did not take place. For some reason, it did not dawn on him that linoleic acid (18:2w6) might do the trick, although he was familiar with this substance.

All four of the above Nobelists missed the solution they were so close to. They turned their attention to other scientific questions of their time, and the question about oil and protein that they had asked and almost answered was shelved for years.

With increasing specialization, scientists developed tunnel vision. Protein scientists studied proteins in detail. Oil chemists studied oils. Both fields grew enormously, especially protein biochemistry. Proteins and oils, which are partners that belong together in our body, became separated in researchers' minds.

63 *Budwig, Flax Oil, & Protein*

Johanna Budwig, a German researcher, did the lion's share of the early work on flax oil and its therapeutic uses in the early 1950s. Her account of historical, biological, and therapeutic perspectives was a part of my early inspiration write this book.

Having studied chemistry, and being familiar with physics, biochemistry, pharmacology, and medicine, Budwig recognized the logjam in research that had stopped previous scientists. A lack of techniques for separating and accurately identifying different fatty components present in a mixture of biological material meant that problems involving fat metabolism could be identified only on autopsy after the patient had died.

Technical Breakthrough

She developed techniques in paper chromatography that seem crude now, but were a step forward then. Night after night she and co-workers sat in the laboratory, systematically testing different substances under different conditions of temperature, concentration, and acidity in different solvents. Her techniques were the first to separate and identify fats from a drop of blood. The earlier scientists' leads could now be followed. Pieces of an unsolved puzzle began to fall into place.

Clinical Application

Blood samples from healthy and sick people were systematically analyzed, and the findings tabulated. According to her, blood samples from people with cancer, diabetes, and some kinds of liver disease (a frequent forerunner of cancer) consistently lacked linoleic acid (LA, 18:2w6). They lacked LA-containing phospholipids necessary to develop and maintain integrity of cell membranes. They lacked a blood lipoprotein now known as fatty acid-carrying albumin.

This information and her conclusions (which follow) are not yet widely documented by other researchers or papers. Lack of phospholipids provided her with a way to explain the fact that cancer cells often have multiple sets of chromosomes (polyploidy). The genetic material divides, but the cell membranes (made of phospholipids containing LA) can't be made due to a lack of the material (LA) from which they are made. Cell division remains incomplete.

Lipoproteins, which contain linoleic acid combined with sulphur-rich protein, are missing from the blood. She found instead a yellow-green protein substance which, when LA and sulphur-rich protein are added, makes the yellow-green color disappear, and the red blood pigment hemoglobin appear. This explains anemia, lack of oxygen, and lack of energy in cancer. The blood's oxygen carrier (hemoglobin) is low; the blood can't carry enough oxygen; the process which produces energy for life functions is stifled. Oxygen is lacking due to lack of hemoglobin. Lack of LA prevents hemoglobin from being made.

It appeared to her, she says, that cancer, diabetes, and some liver diseases involve deficiency of EFAs. These must be provided in the diet. The human body cannot make them. Their absence from our body results from a diet deficient in EFAs. She claims that blood from people with other diseases did not show this severe deficiency and that healthy people's blood always contained EFAs. If cancer is a deficiency disease brought on by lack of EFAs, she reasoned, a diet high in EFAs should alleviate at least some cancer patients' problems.

It is not clear from her account of her work why flax oil, which is a rich source of LNA but a relatively poor source of LA, helps cancer patients, when her research showed that *LA* was the missing EFA. Whatever the reason for this discrepancy in her story, flax oil and LNA do in practice inhibit tumor growth and are useful in the natural treatment of cancer. *Excess* LA from refined, antioxidant-poor oils, on the other hand, helps promote tumor growth (even though some LA is essential for health). LA-rich oils and *all* oils except unrefined, fresh flax oil are forbidden in natural nutritional cancer treatments.

Combining Oil and Protein

Based on the old information about oil and protein working together, Budwig fed terminal cancer patients a mixture of skim milk protein[1] (a sulphur-containing protein), and flax oil in the ratio of 20 parts by weight skim milk protein, 8 parts fresh flax oil, and 5 parts milk (to liquefy the mixture and make it easier to work with), and monitored their blood changes.

She claims that the yellow-green pigment slowly disappeared; red blood pigment reappeared; phospholipids returned; lipoproteins reappeared; tumors receded and disappeared; anemia was alleviated; energy increased and vitality returned; some patients recovered. Concurrently, other symptoms of cancer also disappeared. To get healthy required three to five years of whole foods, carrot juice, some herbs, lots of flax, flax oil, flax oil compresses, and even flax oil enemas. Disappearance of tumors is not the end of the toxicity present throughout the body, which must be reversed (see Chapter 80, Cancer).

Note: For most people, healthy or cancerous, lack of sulphur-containing proteins is not a problem because most of us eat plenty of protein,[2] but most people do lack w3s. Therefore w3-containing oils need to be brought into the protein-laden body. Natural treatments of cancer other than Budwig's are lower in protein. In addition, other nutritional factors: minerals, vitamins, fiber, digestive enzymes, hydrochloric acid and friendly bacteria must *all* be normalized. Allergy-causing foods must be eliminated. With a properly managed program of whole foods, juices, and supplements, some people have completely cured themselves of cancer and its toxicity within two years of strict healthy living (compared to three to five years on Budwig's program).

Further Findings and Claims
Budwig claims that she demonstrated that:
- lipoproteins in all biochemically active tissues (plants' buds, liver, brain, glands, skin) always contain highly unsaturated fatty acids and sulphur-rich proteins, and the association between these two substances can be broken by oxygen from the air;
- anesthetics and many drugs including barbiturates, sleeping pills, and painkillers separate highly unsaturated fatty acids from their normal association with sulphur-containing protein;
- blood lipoproteins migrate into our skin where they break into their components: LA and sulphur-containing proteins. Usually, LA is conserved and oleic

---

[1] Skim milk protein is prepared by souring skim milk with acidophilus (yogurt) culture, then dripping off the whey. The white protein remainder, which is smooth in texture because it has not been 'curded' by heat, is also called kwark.

[2] Protein deficiency occurs in some elderly people living alone, poor and destitute (street people), and physically and mentally handicapped people who are unable to care for themselves. Attention must be given to ensure these people receive adequate protein as well as adequate oils.

acid is secreted to oil our skin, but if the diet contains plenty of LA, LA also appears in our skin's oils;

- LA reacts with sulphur-containing proteins to form a new product with new properties. This product is water-soluble (unlike linoleic acid) and attracts oxygen from the air (today, we call fat-protein associations 'lipoproteins');

- hard carcinoma tumors can be dissolved by cysteine or insulin (both of which contain sulphur groups) and LA (18:2w6), or by horse serum, which is high in both LNA (18:3w3) and organically bound sulphur; and

- substances isolated from soft tumors contain polymerized fats of marine origin. Such substances are formed when highly unsaturated fish and whale oils, used to make margarines, are subjected to high temperatures.

As government spokesperson for the use of fats and fat (lipid) products in health and nutrition at the time, she made public statements to that effect.

Conflict of Interests

Dr. Budwig found herself in the midst of conflict. The head of the institute where she worked (who was reverentially nicknamed the 'pope of fats and oils' by his contemporaries) held patents for hydrogenation processes that produce the toxic polymers she claims to have found in tumors, and had financial interests in margarine. One can only speculate that he feared that Budwig would destroy margarine sales, his profits, and his reputation. She claims that he tried to bribe her with an offer of money and ownership of a drug store if she promised not to further publicize her findings. Refusing his bribe, she says he threatened her, then denied her access to laboratory facilities. When she tried to find another institute in which to continue her research, she says she found her way blocked by an industry-wide conspiracy against her, and she could neither continue her research nor publish her discoveries in research journals, after being excommunicated by the 'pope of fats and oils'. She copyrighted her work and published it in the form of a book.

It is difficult to judge from 40 years ago how much of this story is true. She insists that she should have been awarded a Nobel prize for her work, but was deprived of the recognition due her by the margarine politics that she claims dominates the Nobel Committee. She says the margarine industry tried to destroy her legally and financially.

Consultation

Dr. Budwig began a consultation practice, to apply her ideas and methods to cancer cases doctors had given up as hopeless. She recommends against surgery, radiation, or drugs. She says that one must choose between toxic and natural treatments, and that one should not expect good results from combining them. Her treatments are strictly nutritional. They use a lot of flax oil and dairy protein. The diet she strictly imposes on patients includes plenty of carrot juice, fresh greens, whole grains (especially buckwheat), flax oil, skim milk protein, nuts, and a few herbs. She recommends rainbow trout because of its high content of w3 fatty acids. She refuses to use supplements, on principle.

She considers her protocol to be a return to the way we should have been eating in order not to get sick in the first place. Once sick, a return to her way of eating supplies the materials needed for repair and rebuilding.

Dr. Budwig claims to have successfully treated cancer (colon, brain, lung, stomach, breast, lymph, liver, melanoma, and leukemia), cardiovascular disease, diabetes, acne and other skin conditions, weak vision and hearing, constipation, sterility, dry skin, menstrual problems (cramps, foul odors, breast pain), glandular atrophy, fatty liver and other liver complaints, gallstones, pancreatic malfunction, kidney degeneration, blood disorders, anoxia, arthritic conditions, childhood diseases such as mumps, measles, and swollen tonsils, immune deficiency, and low vitality.

Pioneering Personalities

Pioneers are a special breed of people. They take the world as it exists and begin to transform it into what it could become. It requires confidence in one's unique perception, vision, or hunch (which detractors call madness), the courage of one's convictions (which detractors call stubbornness), perseverance, persistence, and 'stick-to-itiveness' (which detractors call pigheadedness), and confidence in one's ability to succeed (which detractors call arrogance).

Pioneers always face resistance: from those not sharing their convictions, those whose beliefs are being challenged, those with a financial interest in maintaining the status quo, and those who would steal their work. They have to have personalities able to deal with this resistance.

Those who do not share a pioneer's understanding or vision must first be made to see. This is one of the pioneer's tasks. To expect support *before* having convinced others, just because one is convinced, is an unrealistic expectation that leads to failure and bitterness.

Perspective. If you hold a dime very close to your eye, it blots out the whole world. Ideas can also do that. Narrowly focused on a new idea or invention, one can lose perspective. Pioneers may think that others *should* see what is obvious to them only because *they've* dwelled on it. Absorbed in the beauty of their ideas and their effort, it can be disappointing and painful to get no credit for insights and accomplishments.

Pioneers often have difficult personalities. It goes with the territory of pioneering in at least two ways. In pursuing a hunch, they spend many hours alone and socially isolated. In addition, their personal quirks and neuroses may have led them to such isolated pursuits in the first place. A great need for recognition, one such neurosis, leads to feeling deprived when that recognition is not forthcoming.

Feedback

People who return from consultations with Dr. Budwig (she does not treat or run a clinic) report that they find her both expensive and rude; that she refuses to answer their questions, demands total obedience, shouts, slams doors, has even kicked some people out, blames all failures on non-compliance, appears to be open neither to possibilities other than her own nor to improvements in her method, refuses to acknowledge the possibility of allergy to dairy products (even though she herself is constantly clearing a phlegm-laden throat, a common symptom of allergy to dairy), and spends much of her consultation time on her own agenda – lamenting persecution and deprivation of deserved recognition by the scientific world.

All of this might be excused if her results were *truly* outstanding. She *has* documented a few successes in her writing, but more thorough and effective programs with a more solid foundation in human biology are now available, programs that bring positive clinical results in a shorter time.

But Johanna Budwig *does* deserve credit for pioneering, during the early 1950s, the use of flax oil in nutritional therapy, contributions to our understanding of the partnership of oil and protein, and research in other lipid-related topics.

Flax and Oil Blend Recipes **64**

With Help from Thelma Ruck-Keene

It is quite simple to use flax or a balanced oil blend in our foods. Although these oils may be new to you, you can use them like other oils that you already know. If you use them in your foods, they can help you enjoy better health and a longer life.

Simply substitute flax and or a blend for other oils in food preparation, with the exception that these oils are damaged by heat and you should not use them for frying, deep-frying, or other high-heat uses. They are great in salads and other cold dishes such as tabouleh, homus (mixed 50:50 with olive oil), protein shakes, and marinated vegetables. They can be mixed with skim milk yogurt, or with butter to make a softer, more nutritious spread. Flax and oil blends can be used on hot vegetables, in hot cereals, on pasta (it may be mixed with olive oil for taste), in mashed potatoes, on hot corn, and on toast, added just before eating. Flax and oil blends can be used in bread – the inside of bread is protected from light and oxygen, and is steamed during the baking process at about 105°C or 221°F, a safe temperature for the oil – except that the oil in the crust is burned brown along with the flour.

Why Use Flax or Perfected Oil Blends?

The need to incorporate flax or w3-rich oil blends into our foods arises from poor oil and food choices that have particularly taken hold in affluent Western societies. Overemphasis on protein-rich foods and the removal or over-processing of easily spoilable w3 oils from our food supply underlies this need. As the w3-richest food available to us, flax oil most easily redresses this nutritional imbalance between proteins in our foods and good oils.

Caution: Remember that exclusive reliance on flax oil for all our oil needs can bring about w6 deficiency after a year or two, so don't become fanatic about this oil. Once your body has had its w3 supply replenished and you are healthy, consume a better balanced oil blend in place of flax oil.

Note: Use fresh flax or oil blend straight from the refrigerator, and make sure each bottle is used within three to six weeks after opening. A stock of oil can be kept frozen solid in a freezer, where it will remain fresh for over a year.

The suggestions in this chapter on how to use flax and other oils are suitable for all readers (eaters).

Special Needs for Degenerative Conditions?

Those having degenerative conditions may benefit from taking larger quantities of oil, and can use flax oil to begin with. While 1 teaspoon to 2 tablespoons per day of flax oil are appropriate for healthy people, those suffering from degenerative conditions may benefit from taking 3 to 5 tablespoons per day of the oil. In extreme cases such as terminal cancer, people like Dr. Budwig recommend up to 7 or 8 tablespoons per day of flax oil plus 6 to 8 tablespoons per day of freshly ground flax seeds. An enrichment with *all* minerals and vitamins (from whole foods, juices, or supplements) should accompany this much oil and seed.

A flax oil-protein mixture can be used both by people with degenerative conditions and by people who are healthy, if allergies to the protein used are not an issue. If allergies exist, balanced proteins that do not produce allergies must be selected.

Minimum Daily Amount

1 teaspoon to 2 tablespoons of flax oil (or more, as desired). After about 6 months, you can begin to use other fresh, unrefined oils as well.

Take the oil plain (it tastes good, rather nutty when fresh), use it in salad dressings, mix it with yogurt, or incorporate it into other foods.

Salad Dressing for One

    1/2 tablespoon of apple cider vinegar or lemon juice
        (a dash of vinegar in the lemon spices up the taste)

1 tablespoon of flax, blend, or other oil

Vary this liquid dressing by adding one, or combining some of the following: Dijon mustard, crushed garlic, cayenne (for hotness), a dash of honey or maple syrup (for sweetness). A source of more moderate sweetness is brown rice syrup, to be found in natural food stores.

Mix herbs and/or spices with the liquid dressing. Try adding one herb (basil, tarragon, marjoram, rosemary, dill); then combine thyme and tarragon, marjoram and basil, oregano and . . . whatever you fancy. Play with it.

Use herbal rather than plain salt. Herbal salt has less sodium and more potassium as well as additional minerals. Extra potassium can be helpful in healing.

An interesting combination for a one-person salad is:

1 tablespoon flax or balanced oil blend
1 teaspoon nutritional yeast
1/2 teaspoon powdered fenugreek
1/2 tablespoon sunflower seeds
A sprinkle of herbal salt (omit if you are trying to reverse degeneration)

The golden rule for salad dressing is simple: if you want a really good, nutritious one, make your own. Store-bought dressings simply don't compare, are always the same, are never quite as fresh, must use stable (and therefore less nutritious) oils, and cannot measure up to an interesting, homemade dressing that uses fresh flax (or hemp) oil with additions of specially selected ingredients.

Powdered mineral and vitamin supplements are also valuable. Not everyone can resist the occasional temptation of low-nutrient junk food; supplements boost the missing nutrients.

Salad Ingredients

For the absolute beginner, remember that salad ingredients comprise whatever vegetables (and appropriate fruit) are in season and that the dishes need to please the eye as well as the stomach. Art is not just for hanging framed on walls. Don't be afraid to try anything once – if it turns out *really* awful, recycle it!

So with an eye to color combinations, make use of lettuce, spinach, and parsley for green; sliced red sweet peppers, tomatoes, and grated carrots for lively reds. Furthermore, tickle your tastebuds with additions such as sliced young zucchini, mushrooms, chopped apple, flowerets of broccoli, or cauliflower.

For a change, try marinating raw vegetables (except leafy ones like lettuce and spinach) in an oil blend dressing with added herbs and spices. This is a delicious alternative to the usual green salad. Suitable vegetables are mushrooms, green (and red) onions, cucumbers, tomatoes, sweet peppers, cauliflower, and broccoli.

You can also try mixing the marinade with lightly steamed root vegetables such as carrots and potatoes as well as green beans, cauliflower, and broccoli. Pour the marinade on the vegetables while still hot, and refrigerate until ready to serve.

Raw and steamed vegetables can be mixed together with the marinade. This salad keeps well in the fridge for several days, but is most nutritious when eaten fresh. It can be served on a base of leafy greens.

A simple marinade. To the basic oil blend dressing, add small amounts of several herbs. Choose from fresh or dried marjoram, thyme, basil, dill, tarragon, or oregano, and include a clove of crushed garlic, chopped parsley, and a sprinkle of herbal salt.

Oil-Protein Mixture

This mixture makes a nutritious base for use at any meal. The following is for readers without dairy allergies:

> 20 measures (spoons, cups, or buckets) skim milk yogurt. This contains about 6% protein.
> 2-3 measures fresh oil blend
> Mix ingredients together until oil is no longer visible. That's all there is to it.

Allergies?

Readers with dairy allergies can use tofu, adding onions or garlic to enrich tofu with sulphur. People allergic to both dairy and soy can use proteins from almonds and other nuts and seeds, but also need additional lysine and sulphur (the latter can come from a supplement of the amino acid N-acetyl cysteine).

Oil-Protein Mixture for All Meals

Breakfast. To the basic oil-protein paste, add a little honey, maple syrup, or organic brown rice syrup. This makes a tasty, nutritious breakfast that stays with you all morning. Ground flax or hemp seeds stirred into the paste give a nutty flavor and are super-nutritious, as are sunflower seeds and all kinds of nuts (chopped or lightly ground in the blender).

Add chopped fruit to the mixture, or serve the oil-protein mixture as an accompaniment to prepared fruit.

Lunch and supper: main dishes. Remember that the more vegetables are eaten raw, the better. For people with chewing problems, don't think food must be cooked to make it chewable; just use a blender or a juicer. Fresh, raw food is preferable, particularly for elderly people, because nutrient (vitamin and mineral) requirements increase with age. Cooking destroys a part of the vitamins in foods, and leaches minerals.

This is where the oil-protein mixture comes in handy, enlivening and enriching vegetables and fruit. Chop, slice, or blend onions, parsley, carrots, garlic, green onions, and green and red peppers. On hot summer days, adding chopped cucumbers and fresh mint leaves to the mixture is deliciously cooling.

An old traditional recipe, one national dish in Silesia simply combines a flax oil-dairy protein mixture with potatoes. Try mixing green onions into the oil-protein mixture.

You can improve a *mayonnaise-like* dressing from the oil-protein mixture by adding judicious amounts of the following:

apple cider vinegar, lemon, tamari, or soy sauce will make the oil-protein mixture more liquid;
dijon mustard, cayenne, paprika, or horseradish add a lively touch;
try selecting different herbs and/or spices to taste;
sprinkle in a little herb salt, (not for patients) and perhaps a pinch of yeast.

Lunch and supper: desserts. Fresh fruit and nuts with added sweetener have already been suggested. For variety, flavor the oil-protein mixture with carob chips or powder, vanilla, cinnamon, cloves, cardamom, powdered ginger, chopped mint, rosemary, etc. Certain herbs or spices enhance particular fruits: apples go well with rosemary or cloves; ginger complements pears.

In your experiments with natural flavors, be guided by your tastebuds, and perhaps a bit of cookery-book research. Above all, enjoy the adventure. Preparing and serving meals is an expression of love. The best meals are those that come joyfully from our hearts, expressed in artful dishes based on sober reasoning about natural ingredients that support human health.

Budwig's Flax Oil-Coconut Fat Spread
250 grams (1/2 pound) of coconut fat
100 grams of fresh flax oil

Heat the coconut fat to boiling point. While this is heating, put the flax oil in the freezer. When the coconut fat boils (160°C [320°F]), add sliced garlic or onions and let them sizzle, but take them out before they turn brown, and remove the pan from the burner.

Let the coconut oil cool, but before it hardens, pour the coconut oil into the cold flax oil and mix. Return the mixture to the freezer and leave until hardened.

If a softer product is desired, add more flax oil; increase the amount of coconut fat for a harder texture.

If you hate the taste of onions and garlic (which are good for you!) sulphur can be incorporated by adding oats, peppers, or buckwheat. According to Budwig, these foods provide organic sulphur, which protects essential fatty acids (EFAs) from destruction by oxygen; they also provide our body with sulphur for antioxidant functions and, usefully, sulphur protects flax oil so the spread keeps longer.

Budwig's flax oil-coconut fat spread contains no cholesterol and no *trans-*

fatty acids. It contains about 25% EFAs.

Caution: Budwig's spread contains lots of tropical fats. The use of tropical fats received much negative press in North America over the past few years (see Chapter 52, Tropical Fats). Research indicates that processed tropical fats increase blood fats (triglycerides) and cholesterol, considered risk factors for cardiovascular disease (CVD). Hardened tropical fats also make platelets more sticky, another risk factor for CVD. Natural tropical oils do not appear to have these negative effects.

Truly fresh and undamaged coconut fat does not cause CVD problems. Damage done during processing is once again a key concern in our food supply. Dipping bread in olive oil is a tradition in Italy, Spain, and other Mediterranean countries. It's a good choice for people in other parts of the world as well.

65 *Medium-Chain Triglycerides* (MCTs)

Medium-chain triglycerides (MCTs) are an industrial invention with some therapeutic benefits. They do not exist in nature in the concentrated form in which we obtain them from bottles. They are triglycerides whose fatty acids are saturated, and have medium-chain lengths (6 to 12 carbons; mainly 8 and 10).

The raw material for making MCTs is tropical oil. MCTs can be separated from coconut and palm kernel oils by clipping fatty acids off glycerol (hydrolysis) followed by separating medium-chain fatty acids from long-chain fatty acids in the fatty acid mixture (fractionation), and then reconnecting the medium-chain fatty acids to glycerol (reesterification) (see Chapter 23, Fractionation and Transesterification). MCTs have lost the minor components of the coconut from which they are made.

MCTs are a by-product of fractionation used to separate lauric and myristic acid-rich fractions from these oils for use in margarines.

Unique Properties

MCTs have unique properties. With relatively shorter fatty acid chains, they are more water-soluble than long-chain (16, 18 and even longer carbon chain) saturated fatty acids. This means that the fat-digesting lipase enzymes are able to digest them rapidly. They require less lecithin and bile salts for digestion. Instead of having to be transported by chylomicrons in our lymphatics, their fatty acids are absorbed directly into veins, and are transported to all parts of our body by albumin proteins.

MCTs pass through membranes easily, are transported and metabolized quickly, and are not stored as fat deposits. Being made of saturated fatty acids, MCTs are stable. On the other hand, they provide no EFAs.

MCTs are useful in conditions where fat malabsorption is a problem, or in conditions where liver function is impaired.

Athletes use MCTs – about one tablespoon – as a source of energy before workouts. The oil has a light coconut flavor, but can produce an uncomfortable scratchy sensation at the back of the throat. More than 2 tablespoons may produce stomach discomfort.

Limits of Usefulness

MCTs are sometimes used for weight loss. This application is neither necessary nor more than minimally helpful. Fiber-rich natural foods – supplemented with minerals, vitamins, and w3 EFAs; increased activity; and counseling to deal with beliefs that underlie a weight problem are more likely to benefit (see Chapter 74, Overweight and Constipation).

An excess of MCTs can have negative effects: one effect is ketosis; another effect is that an excess ties up albumin protein that is necessary for other transport functions in our blood, such as carrying vitamin E, amino acids, and other substances.

Finally, MCTs contain neither EFAs nor other essential nutrients. They are not a required part of a natural diet. Like other refined, concentrated substances, MCTs are useful only for a limited number of special applications.

Alkylglycerols **66**

Remember stories about tuna being contaminated by mercury? That story scared many people away from eating open ocean fish. The part of the story that was not included in this 'scare' is that these fish also contain substances (alkylglycerols) that remove mercury from their body. When we eat fish, alkylglycerols also remove mercury from *our* body.

When we talk about mercury contamination, we must distinguish between metallic mercury, which is less toxic and passes through our body, and methylmercury, an organically-bound, more toxic form that produced deformity and mental deficiency in children of Japanese women who ate fish contaminated by industrial effluents containing large amounts of the organic form of mercury in Minamata Bay, Japan. Another contamination of water by the more toxic form of mercury poisoned Natives near Hudson Bay in Canada.

Chelating Agents

Alkylglycerols are unique in that they are *oil-based* chelating agents. They 'grab' and remove mercury from human tissues. They also decrease the risk of cancer.

Alkylglycerols are different from fats, oils, and membranes in several ways. They are not sources of EFAs. Their fatty acids are saturated or monounsaturated, 16 and 18 carbons long. The way these are bonded to glycerol is different, too. Instead of ester bonds, they are linked to glycerol by ether bonds. They contain no phosphate groups, lecithin, choline, or inositol.

To be fair, alkylglycerols are not the only chelating agent that can remove mercury from our tissues. Sulphur compounds in garlic, as well as vitamin C and ethylene diamine tetraacetic acid (EDTA of chelation therapy fame) also remove heavy metals from our system, but all of these are water-soluble chelating agents. Nor are alkylglycerols alone in decreasing cancer risk. Here, vitamin C, EDTA, w3 fatty acids, iodine, niacin, potassium, magnesium, antioxidants, fiber, and enzymes also play powerful roles.

Products

Alkylglycerols are made by our body. They are present in both mother's milk and bone marrow. Not much is known about the range of their normal biological functions, but their presence and non-toxic nature is established.

Alkylglycerol products in commercial trade originate in Sweden, made from shark livers, the richest source of these unusual fatty substances. They are sold in capsules after undergoing extensive refining to remove triglycerides and phospholipids, and to concentrate the fraction of shark's liver oil that is alkylglycerols.

Less common and more esoteric than fats, oils, and EFAs, alkylglycerols may nevertheless provide health benefits.

67 *Oils and Sunshine – Light and Health*

It is difficult to resist the temptation to prescribe a single diet for everyone – you know, the one that works for the person who wrote the book. Many so-called 'experts' do just that and, in so doing, mislead many people.

Optimum nutrient requirements for health are individual and different (see

Chapter 36, Individuality). Optimum fat and optimum essential fatty acid (EFA) requirements also vary widely between individuals. In part, fat and EFA requirements are also climactically determined. If 'expert' advice does not work for you, your body lets you know, and the 'expert' is wrong. Each of us must learn to listen to the real expert: our own body.

Much controversy exists about how much fat a diet should contain. Has man always been a hunter eating meats high in animal fats? Were humans' ancestors fruit and vegetable eating monkeys? Is humanity's natural diet made up of complex carbohydrates mainly derived from greens and grains? About the only thing common to all traditional diets of the past is that they ate whole, unrefined, locally grown, seasonally harvested, pesticide-free foods.

Different Strokes

Natural diets of traditional people living in different areas indicate that human digestion is versatile, and adapts to subsist on foods that grow in the location, climate, and environment to which (our food) plants and animals became adapted.

Far North. For instance, Inuit living in the far North traditionally consumed diets high in meats from fish, marine mammals, and arctic wildlife. Their diet contained few vegetables and little fiber. They ate large quantities of fat, especially fats rich in very highly unsaturated w3 fatty acids. Fats supplied almost 60% of their calories. Yet Inuit on this diet were free of cancer, heart attacks, blood clot (embolism) strokes, arthritis, multiple sclerosis, diabetes, appendicitis, colitis, gallstones, dental cavities, and acne.[1] When Inuit changed from their traditional high-fat diet to a Western diet (lower in total fat, but higher in saturated and monounsaturated fatty acids [SaFAs and MUFAs], and altered fats), their incidence of degenerative diseases increased. *Lowering* fat intake to 40% of calories *increased* their degenerative problems. This is attributable to the difference between healing and killing fats.

Temperate. People in temperate regions have a diet of vegetables and grains, or of vegetables and lean meats from wild animals that they manage to chase down, because that's what nature provided.

Later, agriculture and domestication of animals resulted in both less activity and greater SaFA content in temperate diets.

Added to that are the more recent industrial innovations: removal of essential nutrients and production of altered molecules by processing.

Tropics. In tropical areas, the natural diet comes close to fresh vegetable and fruit popularized by monkeys (gorillas in Africa, arboreal equatorial chimpanzees, and orangutans in Borneo). This diet is low in fats and rich in minerals, vitamins

---

[1] Inuit *did* suffer burst blood vessel strokes most likely due to lack of vitamins C and E in their diet, and osteoporosis due to a diet extremely high in protein, which leaches calcium from bones.

(especially vitamin C), and fiber. The fats found in the cell membranes of green plants are rich in EFAs. High-fat diets do not sit well in tropical climates. Some additional fats come from seeds.

Individuality. But even in each climactic region, individuals differ markedly from one another in their nutrient needs for health. The optimum diet for each of us has to be individually determined. Need for EFAs may vary by a factor of 10 or more between individuals.

Seasonality. Seasonally too, there is a shift in food consumption, based on sunshine and warmth, at least in temperate regions. In winter, our consumption naturally turns more toward northern diets, and in summer, it turns more toward tropical diets.

When people from any part of the earth consume foods high in animal products from domesticated, fattened beef and pork, they set themselves up for the degenerative conditions that did not afflict traditional northern, tropical, or temperate dwellers on their traditional diets.[2]

Therapy. A program of vegetables, grains, and exercise, with fat intake of 10% of calories or less reverses many degenerative conditions brought on by a beef and pork diet, but is *too* lean for long-term health for most people.

Oil and Sunshine

Sunlight is related to fats. Excessive sunlight destroys unsaturated fatty acids, and causes skin spots, free radical-induced oxidation, and skin cancer. The more highly unsaturated a fatty acid, the more sensitive it is to destruction by light. The more of it we consume, the more antioxidant protection we need.

Geography. As we go from the poles to the equator, double bonds in fatty acids decrease from five and six to three, then two, then one, and then zero. As light intensity increases, double bonds decrease.

In wonderful adaptation to the sunlight present in an area, we find that in *polar areas* with the least sunlight, wild animals carry the most highly unsaturated, sunlight-storing, energy-rich w3 fatty acids (20:5w3 and 22:6w3) in their tissues. Humans living in polar areas and eating the wild creatures that live there also carry these fatty acids. If they eat foods grown further south, they thrive less well. Because there is so little sunlight, the highly unsaturated fatty acids cause few problems for Inuit and Northern Natives.

As we leave the poles and move into *temperate zones,* we find that foods growing wild contain less of the above, but contain two and three times unsaturated (18:2w6 and 18:3w3) EFAs instead. These are less sensitive to destruction by light than five and six times unsaturated, but are still very delicate.

Seeds of a plant growing further north contain more oil and more highly

---

[2] Modern Inuit, on modern diets: white sugar, white flour, alcohol, canned foods, and refined oils, are prone to all the degenerative conditions of white man.

unsaturated EFAs than seeds of the same type of plant growing further south.

By the time we get to the sun-drenched *Mediterranean* where it is warm, olive and almond oils containing mostly monounsaturated (18:1w9) fatty acids are the common, natural oils.

In the *tropics,* we find coconut and palm oils, containing mostly saturated (12:0, 14:0, 16:0) fatty acids.

Anatomy. Animals and humans contain saturated, monounsaturated, essential (2 and 3 times unsaturated), and highly unsaturated (5 and 6 times) fatty acids within their tissues. The most highly unsaturated fatty acids are concentrated in inner organs such as our brain, adrenal, and reproductive glands, protected from direct light by being located deep within our body out of the reach of sunlight.

In our retinas, highly unsaturated fatty acids serve special functions in vision. Here, they are exposed to indirect light; exposure to direct sunlight (looking at the sun) destroys the fatty acids and other tissues, blinding us.

The oils in our skin are exposed to direct sunlight. They consist mostly of monounsaturated (and saturated) fatty acids, which best resist destruction by light.

Northern (Polar) Exposure. Essential and even more highly unsaturated w3 fatty acids store a great deal of readily usable sunlight in their chemical bonds (*cis*- methylene interrupted, *pi*- double bonds). In sunless polar winters, these provide our body with stored 'sunlight' energy from within.

Traditional Inuit did not get depressed and suicidal during winters of total darkness. Their diet of fish and marine animals provided large quantities of EPA (20:5w3) and DHA (22:6w3), the 'liquid' sunshine of oils stored within these animals. Europeans wintering north of the Arctic Circle or in Antarctica on Western diets rich in SaFAs (16:0 and 18:0), suffer winter blues – neurotic, psychotic, and suicidal tendencies – and often have to be flown out to 'see the light.' EPA and DHA are required for brain cells and synapse functions. In winter, SaFA-fed brains become depleted of EPA and DHA. Depressed brain function leads to behavioral depression.

Budwig (see Chapter 63, Budwig, Flax Oil, and Protein) claims that the eyes and skin of healthy people absorb sunlight and store its energy in chemical bonds for future (or immediate) use. She claims that EFAs must be present for this absorption of sunlight to take place. SaFAs and MUFAs cannot substitute for EFAs in this function, and the excessive quantities of SaFAs and MUFAs present in 'modern' diets may interfere with this function of EFAs.

Science. Budwig has proposed a theory of light absorption through human skin, quoting principles established by Nobel prize-winning researchers in physics, chemistry, and biology. Controlled studies to confirm or refute her theory are virtually non-existent at this time.

The physical properties of light waves, pi-electrons, and double bonds in EFAs make such a relationship plausible. The wavelengths of sunlight vibrate at the same frequency as (resonate with) pi-electrons in double bonds; these electrons can therefore capture light energy. EFAs do absorb light (they are part of photosynthesis, by which plants absorb sunlight) and are chemically sensitive to light. They also react with oxygen. A part of EFA function in brain and other active tissues is to attract oxygen, enabling these tissues to produce the energy necessary to be active.

Lack of oxygen in tissues lowers their metabolic rate and depresses cell functions. Low tissue oxygen and depressed cell function are common to many degenerative diseases, and low tissue oxygen can be used to induce cancer. Only a 35% decrease from normal is required. Discovered by Nobel prize winner Otto Warburg, this has been known since the 1920s.

Finally, according to Budwig, EFAs react with sulphur-containing proteins. EFAs and sulphur-rich proteins form an association within which the sunlight energy stored in foods is released, oscillates, and dances. Their association attracts the oxygen needed to keep the dance of life energy going.

Light and Health

We are creatures of the sun. Our history on this planet is one of exposure to full spectrum sunlight, including ultraviolet (UV) rays. Ozone has always blocked out a percentage of these rays and allowed some of them to pass down to us. The thickness of the ozone layer has always fluctuated, being thinner in some years than in others.

Only in the last few years has sunlight been painted as our enemy. If we hide from the sun, we become more likely to get osteoporosis. If 'expert' advice to avoid the sun is followed, expect osteoporosis to increase in the next 20 years from lack of exposure to sunlight.

If we *overexpose* to the sun, we can burn and get skin cancer, especially if we burn repeatedly. There is a middle road of moderation.

Healers who work with light find that full-spectrum light as well as UV rays are beneficial to health. Artificial lights like incandescent and especially fluorescent lack important wavelengths, oscillate (60 cycles per second) in ways that are stressful to our eyes, and lead to degenerative conditions including hyperactivity, hormonal imbalances, and even cancer. Light therapy can be helpful in the treatment of diseases and the reestablishment of health.

Recommended Light Exposure

At least one hour each day of open-air, unfiltered sunlight is recommended for health. The sun does not have to be shining directly on our skin. Indirect sunlight is acceptable, but it should not be filtered through glass or glasses that block UV rays.

Don't trust the 'experts' too much. They have an annoying tendency to generalize from the limited to the infinite. There is some truth to what they find, but their information must be kept in context. Have more faith in the natural system than in the test tube. The sun has been around much longer than the experts. A little knowledge is a dangerous thing.

Enjoy the sun. Don't burn. Be observant. Learn. Keep your intake of essential nutrients optimal. Let your cells use these nutrients to do what they know how to do. Have faith in the wisdom of your cells. And enjoy a life in harmony with the natural system within which you live.

Conclusions

Light is vital to human health. Sunlight, including UV, has beneficial effects on our eyes, brain, skin, and glands, and helps to keep us healthy, provided that we avoid sunburn. Artificial lights, on the other hand, lack certain wavelengths present in natural (sun) light, and can lead to disease.

Sunlight and highly unsaturated oils complement each other. Each can substitute for the other to some extent, although both are necessary. Their partnership explains why diets in different latitudes may be drastically different in fat content and fat type, yet be health-giving and life-sustaining for the people living in the area where these foods are naturally found.

Every region of the globe gets at least a little light, and every area grows organisms that contain at least some EFAs. The more light there is, the less EFAs seem to be needed. The less light there is, the more these fatty acids appear to be necessary in the diet (and the more unsaturated they must be).

If an Inuit ate only fruits and vegetables during Arctic winter, he would starve. If a Samoan ate the Inuit's protein and marine oils diet under a hot tropical sun, he would suffer. Each, in his place and on his native diet, thrives.

Balanced Nutrition and Life-Style 68

There's more to health than just an oil change. There's more to it than just eating right. Health is more than just physical. Let us make a few general points about oils, proteins, carbohydrates, and essential nutrients, and then touch on a few other areas involved in health.

The major *structural* components of our body are **good oils** that supply balanced amounts of both essential fatty acids (EFAs), and **complete proteins** that supply balanced amounts of all essential amino acids. They must be provided by a wholesome diet. To remain healthy, we need enough protein and fat to build, repair, and replace cell structures. An adequate amount is 10 to 12% of calories as whole food proteins. Athletes in both muscle building and aerobic training need more. Body builders need still more to build huge (protein) muscles. An optimal amount of oil for most people is 15 to 20% of calories as fresh, unrefined oils, with one-third of that as w6s (LA and its derivatives) and one-fifth to one-ninth as w3s (LNA and its derivatives).

Protein and oil, found together in membranes, play the key roles in forming the structures of our cells and tissues. These structures provide the framework and scaffolding – the stage – upon which the energy made available for life functions plays out the drama of our life. Like points on spark plugs, protein and oil form associations between which the spark of life – life's energy – sizzles and dances.

Good oils are systematically destroyed by commercial processing methods because the EFAs contained in good oils spoil easily during processing, storage, and food preparation if care is not taken (see Chapter 28, Making Oils with Human Health in Mind).

Although both oils and proteins can also be used for fuel, they do not burn 'clean', producing ketones and ammonia, respectively, which can have toxic effects in liver, kidneys, and brain. **Complex carbohydrates** provide *clean-burning fuel*. In most diets they should make up 68 to 75% of calories, and come from fresh, fiber-rich leaf and root vegetables, and from whole grains.

Major Components of Nutrition

EFAs are major essential nutrients (only oxygen, water, and glucose are required in larger daily amounts). Deficiencies of EFAs result in *major* health problems.

Calcium, potassium, magnesium, sulphur (from protein), sodium, and chloride are other major essential nutrients. All are required in quantities smaller than our requirement of EFAs. Among vitamins, only vitamin C might have an optimum of more than 3 grams per day.

Optimum for LA may be about 11 grams per day (5% of daily calories); optimum for LNA may be about 4.5 grams per day (2% of daily calories), but varies from person to person. There are about 5 grams in a teaspoon, 14 grams in a tablespoon, and 28 grams (2 tablespoons) in an ounce.

Minor Components

The remaining vitamins and minerals, though just as essential for physical health as major components, fulfill their functions in much smaller concentrations. Carotene, vitamin E, the B-complex vitamins, chromium, selenium, iodine, and zinc are especially important in helping EFAs fulfill their functions, but all other minor nutrients must be present for physical health. For optimum health, wholesome nutrition providing optimum amounts of *all* essential nutrients is necessary.

Our nutrient requirements were developed within the natural system over the course of millions of years of natural evolution and fetal development, and are now built into our genetic material. We are arrogant to think that we can just replace the requirements for our own health, set by nature's meticulous work over million of years, with our half-baked notions based on nothing more than the convenience of a long shelf-life. White sugar, white flour, 'white' (refined) fats and oils require removing essential nutrients that are nature's gift to our health. We undertake food processing as though these actions had no consequences. Some of the changes in nutrient content produced by processing are outlined in Chapter 13.

We have been hoodwinked into thinking that only the poor eat whole, natural foods in their natural state. Many people consciously or subconsciously believe that eating 'white' has more class, which we can therefore attain without effort by eating these 'white', deficient foods.

Nutritious Foods

Fresh root and leafy green vegetables, nuts, seeds, whole grains, and fruits, plus herbs and spices, are the basis of wholesome nutrient-dense, health-sustaining nutrition. From the perspective of health, the extra effort required to obtain foods that are garden-fresh, sun-ripened, organic, in season, locally grown on rich soils, and grown without body-foreign, poisonous pesticides and artificial fertilizers, is worth making.

Artificial fertilizers are not 'evil', as some proponents of 'natural' food growing practices indicate. They *are* deficient. A plant takes 20 minerals from the soil, and we put back only 3 to 6. We flush the rest, as digested food remains – human wastes – down the toilet, into our rivers, and out to the ocean. Down the toilet goes our topsoil, our minerals, and our organic plant materials, to become mud on the bottom of the ocean.

Fertilizers are often high in nitrogen, which 'drives' plants to suck up extra water (producing vegetables with edema), but not extra nutrients. Composting is recommended over artificial fertilizer, because good composting returns to soils *all* the minerals that plants take out and supports the development of beneficial soil bacteria, organic matter (humus), and earthworms that aerate and loosen soils.

Raw Foods

In theory, the more of our food that is consumed in its natural, raw state, the higher the content of essential nutrients will be in our diet, and the healthier we will be. However, there are limits to raw foods consumption. Raw potatoes are nutrient-rich, but most people find them unpalatable. Raw beans contain a protein factor, phaseolin, which causes indigestion. This is inactivated when beans are sprouted, and destroyed when they are cooked. Raw egg whites contain avidin, a protein which, if you consume 29 or more raw eggs at one sitting, interferes with the absorption of the vitamin biotin. Cooking destroys avidin.

More recently, our import of raw vegetables from hot climates like Mexico has brought with it an import of intestinal parasites. These are destroyed by cooking foods. They also underscore one reason for growing foods locally.

How much raw? Opinions among researchers and health advocates also differ on how much raw food we should eat. They range from one extreme – 'everything raw' – through 80% raw, to 50% raw, to the other extreme – 'makes no difference'. Research from the 1950s in Europe suggests that eating cooked (or dead) food sets off a defense reaction in the tissues of stomach and digestive tract. This reaction, similar to what we find in infections and around tumors, involves accumulations of white blood cells, swelling, fever-like increase of stomach and intestinal tissue temperature, and tiredness after eating a meal. This reaction also takes place when half of the food eaten is raw with the cooked part eaten first. When raw foods are eaten first, however, this reaction does not take place.

This is because raw foods contain enzymes that help digest these foods and whatever else we eat. Our digestive glands need to secrete fewer enzymes to do the work of digestion. When foods are cooked, these enzymes – being protein – are destroyed (denatured). Our digestive system must then produce more digestive enzymes, increasing its workload, and wearing it out faster.

It is surprising how much better we start to feel when we eat more raw foods or their fresh juices. Carrots and dark green, leafy vegetables are especially good for us. Onions and garlic are the richest vegetarian sources of sulphur. Sauerkraut, yogurt, and other homemade lactic acid-fermented foods retain their enzymes, provide friendly bacteria for intestinal health, and are easy to digest.[1] Whole (sprouted) grains, raw milk, sunflower seeds, and raw nuts all contain enzymes.

Flax is excellent for digestive functions. It should be ground or dry blended not more than 15 minutes before eating, as it spoils rapidly once the seeds are opened to air (if it is ground or blended wet, it gets very sticky and slimy). Flax swells to 5 times its dry volume by soaking up water, so ample liquid should accompany its consumption. Ground flax meal sold in plastic containers in stores is usually rancid and should be avoided.

Avoid Deficient Foods

Sugars, refined starches, commercial white flour, white flour pasta, white rice, 'white' fat, and processed oils cannot support health and should be avoided.

Whole-wheat bread is not made with whole wheat. 'Whole-wheat flour' is white flour with a little bran added back, but is deficient in minerals, vitamins, and EFAs, and therefore cannot support our health. Whole-grain breads should be made from whole grains.

In Europe, many people acquire a grain mill and buy organically grown whole grain by the sack-full from a farmer whose growing practices they know

---

[1] Commercial sources of these foods are usually pasteurized, killing enzymes and friendly bacteria, and are often soured by acids rather than lactic acid bacteria. Commercially quicker and cheaper, such foods are nutritionally less valuable.

and trust, grind their own flour just before baking, and make great-tasting fresh bread. Grain mills are reasonable in price, and thus affordable. Unfortunately, oil mills need parts that can withstand several tons of pressure, and there are no household mills on the market because they would cost several thousand dollars.

Margarines and shortenings should be completely avoided. Non-dairy creamers and hard fats (except a bit of butter) are not recommended for sedentary people – loggers and others performing heavy physical labor may be able to metabolize saturated fatty acids adequately. Processed oils and products containing them (mayonnaise, dressings, etc.) are not recommended. Roasted, salted seeds and nuts may be very old. Roasting and salting mask rancid tastes.

Sausages and other processed meats contain cancer-causing preservatives like nitrites (vitamin C blocks nitrite toxicity), fillers like refined starch, and saturated fats, all of which fail to supply minerals and vitamins necessary for biochemical functions in our body.

Nutrient Enrichment

Since most of our foods are not garden-fresh, sun-ripened, organic, in season, and locally grown, and since we live in an environment polluted with lead, cadmium, smoke, carbon monoxide, plastics, pesticides, and other toxins (and if we smoke, drink alcohol, and use toxic recreational or pharmaceutical drugs), we will likely benefit if we enrich the best-balanced, fresh, whole foods diet we can get with fresh juices, super-foods, food concentrates, or high-quality vitamin and mineral supplements.

Good supplement preparations provide 200 micrograms (mcg) per day each of chromium and selenium. They should contain more than the recommended (minimum) daily amount (RDA) of vitamins, but usually contain less than optimal vitamins C and E, so additional amounts of these might be wise. An optimum daily amount of vitamin C is usually between 2 and 10 grams, and for vitamin E is between 400 and 800 IU for most people. **Note:** People with rheumatic heart disease may not tolerate more than 150 to 200 IU of vitamin E per day.

A large body of clinical evidence attests to the value of nutrient enrichment in the treatment of diseases. The results are extremely exciting and encouraging.

The value of clean water, fresh air, and sunshine cannot be overemphasized. While we don't *eat* them, they *are* food for our body. All are essential for health.

Sunshine and Flax Oil

According to lipid researcher Dr. Budwig, when flax oil (or both EFAs in their natural state) is a regular part of our diet, the presence of EFAs in our skin acts as an 'antenna' that absorbs photons of sunlight energy into our body, and transfers this energy to chemical bonds for future use in biochemical reactions. Light absorption and photosynthesis (synthesis of molecules by light), according to her, are not limited to plants. She is not alone in making this claim. Healers who work with light have come to similar conclusions.

She claims that cancer patients who lack these oils in their skin may become 'allergic' to the sun. It burns them, makes them nauseous, dizzy, faint. Within a few days of adding flax oil to their foods, such patients may be able to sit in the sun and enjoy it without problems, and the sun may even help heal their cancer. According to her, sun-caused skin cancers result from deficiency of the necessary oils.[2] She recommends EFA-containing oils to be used both in diets and on skin. She even extols the virtues of flax oil enemas. **Caution:** The oil is so smooth that you may inadvertently 'oil your underwear' when you think you're just going to pass a little gas.

Wavelengths. Bugwig has also worked with ruby red (6,900 angstroms) laser light, and claims this wavelength is absorbed by pi-electrons of double bonds in EFA-containing oils, is most appropriate to biological systems, and helps cure cancer. Controlled mainstream research has yet to provide proof.

The energy of x-rays, gamma rays, and other forms of 'hard' *radiation* is far too intense for biological systems. It destroys the delicate pi-electron systems of double bonds in EFAs and their more highly unsaturated derivatives. Hard radiation also damages vitamins, proteins, and molecules containing double bonds. It produces free radicals by the billions, changes molecules, and is extremely destructive to health. One should not expect to cure cancer with rays known to cause cancer.

Food irradiation, if carried out on a large scale, would become the greatest disaster to human health yet invented by industry. It destroys essential and other nutrients, produces billions of free radicals and produces toxic chemical compounds in foods – toxins that are not found in nature. Our body is not well equipped to deal with them. That's why they make us sick and kill us. A radiation dose of 500 to 1000 rads kills a human adult as a result of the chemical changes it produces in the molecules of our cells. To irradiate foods, 100,000 to 20,000,000 rads are used. We then *eat* the results of the chemical mess they make.

Researchers knew the destructive effects of irradiation on molecules long before irradiation was considered for use on our foods. The industry that wants to market food irradiation technology attempts to whitewash this research. Don't buy it. And demand clear identification of irradiated foods, spices, and ingredients, so that you retain your right to choose.

Activity and Rest

Along with a wholesome diet, activity is absolutely necessary for health. Our body is made for activity. It *must* deteriorate if it remains inactive, no matter how well we feed it. Play, exercise, or be active while having fun. The fun is as important as

---

[2] Vitamins C and E, carotene, selenium, zinc, oils, and herbs like aloe vera all help prevent sunburn. They also heal burned skin.

the exercise. Chase the chickens around the barnyard. Climb trees, mountains, and stairs. Bounce on the bed. Swim in lakes or rivers, canoe, raft, toboggan, ski, chase balls, bounce on a mini-trampoline. Laugh.[3] Dance. Stretch. Do yoga or Kung Fu. Do whatever activity you enjoy or can learn to enjoy!

To be healthy, we must balance our times of activity with times of relaxation, rest, and inner quiet.

Faith and Trust

Finally, we need to deepen our faith and trust in life, love it more, get closer to it, get to know it better. Faith in life, gratitude for life, and enjoyment of life are healing. Faith in life is of *key* importance because it makes the challenges of wholesome living in a complex, often confusing, sometimes contradictory, usually hectic, and occasionally unbearably stupid, corrupt, and hateful world easier and worth the effort.

---

[3] Laughter is such an effective form of exercise that it has been called 'inner jogging'!

Fats and Fates

Fats and Degenerative Diseases
(Plus Kids, Athletes, Pets, and Politics)

This section chronicles the changes in our consumption of fats, oils, and cholesterol since 1900, and what they mean to our health. We then outline the use of lipids and other nutrients in the natural treatment of degenerative diseases, including cardiovascular disease, cancer, diabetes, allergies, and quite a few others.

There are chapters on the importance of fats in infant nutrition, the use of fats to improve athletic performance, and the use of fats to keep pets healthy. We end with a look at the effect of vested interests and politics on availability of natural health care, and also what we can do for ourselves.

Not all health problems or degenerative conditions can be reversed by natural (or other) means. Defective genes affect a small part (less than one percent) of the population. Old age will eventually come upon us all.

In this section, we look at some of the main factors that must be considered in order to reverse degenerative conditions that *can* be reversed by natural means. Individuals may also require individual attention that takes their specific food and life-style habits into account. *Reversible* degenerative conditions affect the majority of affluent populations, around the world.

Effects of Killer Fats on Health

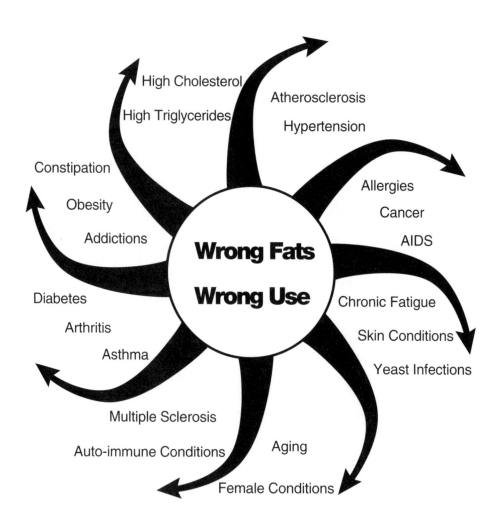

Changes in Fat Consumption and Degenerative Disease 69

If degenerative diseases are due to our use of fats and cholesterol, we should see a relation between fat consumption and these diseases. Let's look at changes and trends in fat consumption during this century, and see if we can find such a correlation.

Fat Consumption – Raw Data

Between 1910 and 1980, many changes took place in the kinds and amounts of fats and oils that people ate.

Total consumption of all fats increased by 35%. Our total fat consumption rose from 32% of daily calories to 42%. Fat consumption in an increasingly large, fitness-conscious part of the population is slowly declining. The average daily fat consumption in Western countries ranges between 140 and 170 grams (5 and 6 ounces) per person.[1]

Fats and oils (shortening, margarine, refined salad and cooking oils) account for 57%, dairy products account for 7%, and meat, poultry and fish account for 31% of the total increase in our fat consumption.

In 1911, the first shortening made by hydrogenating oils appeared on supermarket shelves. The average intake of *trans-* fatty acids in hydrogenated products rose from zero in 1910 to close to 10% of all fats we consume today, or between 10 and 15 grams (0.5 ounce) per person per day.

Our vegetable fat consumption increased from 21 to 70 grams per day, while our consumption of animal fat decreased slightly, from 104 to 99 grams per day.

Our consumption of beef increased, while that of pork, especially since 1947, decreased. Poultry consumption rose, and poultry fat content increased. The use of fish remained essentially stable, and the use of other meats diminished.

Our use of butter declined to 1/5 of its 1910 level, while our use of margarine increased by 9 times. The use of lard went down to about 1/5 of its former

---

[1] The U.S. tops this list

level, while the use of vegetable shortenings almost doubled in the same time span. Our consumption of edible beef fat went up 2.5 times. Our consumption of salad and cooking oils increased by about 12 times.

Consumption of whole milk is less than 1/2 of its level in 1910, consumption of cream is less than 1/3 of its 1910 level, but cheese consumption has almost tripled, ice cream and frozen desserts consumption has increased 5 times, and low-fat milk consumption has increased by a factor of 3.

Our annual consumption of sugar rose from 15 pounds per person in 1815 to about 90 pounds in 1910, about 120 pounds in 1980, and about 135 pounds today. Cholesterol intake from foods has remained essentially constant during the last 70 years.

Our consumption of saturated fatty acids increased 16%, consumption of oleic acid (18:1w9) went up by 33%, and consumption of linoleic acid (LA, 18:2w6) increased by 170%.

The consumption of w3s (LNA, EPA, DHA) decreased to 1/6 of its level in 1850, while w6 (LA, AA) consumption doubled during that time, resulting in widespread w3 deficiency and serious w3:w6 imbalance.

Men consume more fat than women, but not a lot more.

Fat Consumption – Technology

Fat consumption figures are based on the fatty acid content of oil sources in their natural state. They cannot give accurate correlations between LA nutrition and disease trends, for instance, because these figures fail to show how much LA was altered into *trans-* fatty acids, other breakdown products, or saturated fatty acids (SaFAs), or how much LA was denatured by processing and frying. They also neglect decreases in vitamin and mineral co-factors required for LA metabolism.

Between 1900 and 1980, many processed products, deficient in essential fatty acids (EFAs), vitamins, and minerals, were introduced into the marketplace. At the same time, our consumption of fiber decreased. White flour consumption was rare until about 1800, but refining methods improved after 1880, and especially after 1900.

Nutrient- and natural co-factor-rich (unrefined) oils became rare in this time period. The only unrefined oil that remained on the market was the group of 'virgin' olive oils. But even olive oil is available refined now, and the undiscerning customer might lose out on the last unrefined oil in mass markets.

Fat Consumption – Interpretations

Cholesterol cannot be the *primary* cause of cardiovascular disease (CVD), because our cholesterol consumption has remained about the same in the last 100 years, while CVD has skyrocketed. *Trans-* fatty acids and altered vegetable fats deserve suspicion. Sugars deserve suspicion. Processed foods lacking minerals and vitamins deserve suspicion.

Butter is not to blame for increased fatty degeneration, because our consumption of butter has decreased, while fatty degeneration has increased.

Total fat intake may be exceeding our body's capacity for fat metabolism.

Degenerative Disease

In 1900, cancer killed 1 person in 30. In 1980, it killed 1 person in 5. Today, it kills 1 person in 4.

At the turn of the century, cardiovascular disease accounted for 1 death in 7. In 1980, it accounted for 1 death in 2. Today, it still kills more than 1 person in 3. The recent decrease in cardiovascular deaths may be partly due to better post-heart attack management with high-tech medical methods but, as Pauling (see Chapter 71, Is the Cholesterol Theory Wrong?) points out, it is more likely that the main factor reversing CVD deaths is the fact that about 100 million Americans take nutritional supplements (especially vitamin C).

Diabetes rose at a similar rate, and other diseases of fatty degeneration, like multiple sclerosis and liver and kidney degeneration, also increased rapidly.

Degenerative Diseases 70

Fats and degenerative diseases are correlated, but present theories, on which treatment of degenerative diseases are based, fail to give us the practical improvements that we would expect if they were correct.

Degeneration

Degeneration is deterioration of physical health due to deterioration of structure and/or function of organs, tissues, and cells, based in changes on the molecular level. Deterioration of structure ('de-struction') of organs, tissues, and cells leads to deterioration of their functions, because structure determines function. For instance, heat changes the shape of protein molecules, which is why a liquid raw egg becomes hard when it is boiled. Changes in the structure of egg proteins due to heat completely change the functional potential of the egg. Boiled eggs don't hatch.

The roots of physical and functional degeneration, which we call 'degenerative conditions' or 'degenerative diseases', must ultimately be found on the molecular level. Molecular changes *always* result in changes in both structure and function of cells, tissues, and organs.

Degeneration, except when due to genetic mutations, must result from one or both of two general causes:

1. Malnutrition – mainly deficiency of essential substances, but also imbalance and excess of natural substances – which renders our body unable to carry out necessary biochemical functions;

2. Internal Pollution – the presence of toxic (poisonous) substances that interfere with necessary normal biochemical functions.

As a result of either or both of these causes, biochemical reactions required for living are slowed down, blocked, or side-tracked.

Between health – characterized by an optimum molecular mix that makes optimally structured and functioning cells, tissues, organs, and body possible – and death, where our body, organs, tissues, cells, and subcellular molecular structures come apart ('de-struct' or 'dis-integrate') completely, there is a wide range of possible suboptimal, deficient structure and functioning, which determine varying degrees of 'de-generation'.

Diagnosis. Prolonged suboptimal molecular mix results in progressive deterioration of structure and functioning from its natural, biological state. Unidentifiable as full-blown diseases at first, such deterioration continues to worsen with time, giving rise to increasingly noticeable, but still vague, feelings of malaise – tiredness, aches, lack of energy, etc. After weeks, months, or years, worsening degeneration results in a structural and functional state that has deteriorated far enough for a diagnosing physician to identify its signs and symptoms as those of a condition for which he has learned a name. Perhaps he or she calls it cardiovascular disease, or cancer, or diabetes. Unaware of the long developmental history of the now named, visible condition, untrained in molecular biology, normal biochemical function, and nutrition, and lacking precise tests for changes at the molecular level, doctors consider these conditions to be of 'unknown cause' and, since their cause is unknown, their cure is also unknown. It follows that interventions into these conditions consist of *symptomatic* treatments rather than *curative* ones. To date medical interventions into degenerative conditions do not consider their molecular nutritional origins.

Fatty Degeneration

Fatty degeneration involves a lack or imbalance of essential fatty acids (EFAs), the presence of altered (toxic) fatty materials (such as *trans-* fatty acids, oxidized fatty acids, double bond-shifted fatty acids, cross-linked fatty acids, otherwise altered fatty acids, fat-derived polymers, and fat oxidation products), and/or an excess of non-essential fatty materials (fats, oils, cholesterol) in places or quantities in which they are not normally found.

Most of the common degenerative diseases, including cardiovascular disease, cancer, diabetes, obesity, multiple sclerosis, premenstrual syndrome, arthritis, fatty deposits in inner organs, and even some behavioral problems, involve fatty degeneration.

Common Causes

If we picture health as the center of a bull's-eye, then all degenerative conditions are departures from its center – departures from the nutrient richness and balance that the center of that bull's-eye denotes. Degenerative conditions not specifically based in genetic mutations are *always* a matter of malnutrition and/or internal pollution (poisoning).

More specifically, common underlying factors in these degenerative conditions include an inadequate supply of w3 EFAs, lack of fiber, lack of essential minerals and vitamins, excess saturated fatty acids, hard fats and sugars, excess toxic, altered fatty acids such as those listed above, and fatty acid oxidation products. Figure 44 illustrates some sources of fatty degeneration in summary form.

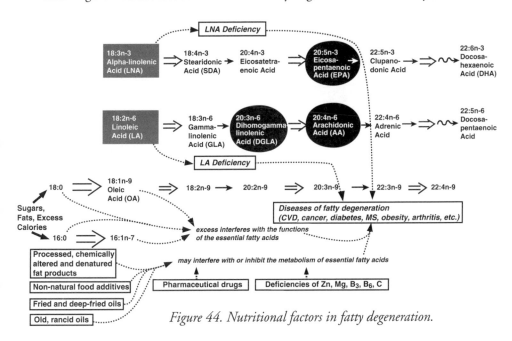

Figure 44. Nutritional factors in fatty degeneration.

The consumption of refined, processed, nutrient-impoverished foods whose EFAs have been systematically destroyed, removed, or altered during processing brings about physical degeneration and degenerative diseases.

Personal choices – self-responsible primary health care. The choice to consume or to purchase deficient foods offered to us by producers, processors, and manufacturers lies with us. We need not buy and eat these foods. Amid a jungle of deficient and toxic foods, we can still find fresh vegetables, whole grains, fruit, nuts, seeds, and fish. In addition, we can find sources of nutrient enrichment: fresh juices, super foods, food concentrates, and supplements of minerals, vitamins, essential amino acids, EFAs, fiber, friendly bacteria, and digestive enzymes.

Some people manage to live free of the fear of acquiring degenerative diseases. Their protection lies in self-responsible primary health care through:

- learning and practicing biologically sound food, water, air, and light choices;
- life-styles in harmony with human nature's biological requirements for activity, rest, social harmony, fun, and harmony with nature; and
- avoidance of undue toxic influences.

There are also people who, having become ill with degenerative diseases through their neglect of self-responsible primary health care have found within themselves the will and wisdom to stop, search, learn, and change – and their body's inherent biochemical healing genius has healed them.

In a world filled with many beneficial (plus) and many toxic (minus) factors, we can choose to maximize our plusses and minimize our minuses.

Differences

The underlying causes for degenerative diseases are not all the same. Keeping with our analogy of the bull's-eye, we can depart from its center of health in many different directions.

Nutritional influences. More specifically, different nutritional deficiencies (or toxic effects) come into play. Deficiency of zinc will cause degeneration in a different way than deficiency of vitamin C or chromium, but all deficiencies cause degeneration and disease. That is why different members of the degenerative family also show differences in their symptoms and treatment.

For instance, adult onset diabetes can be helped with supplements of EFAs, chromium, and zinc, and the avoidance of white sugar, saturated and monounsaturated fats, and altered fatty acids.

In cardiovascular disease, some key factors in addition to w3 and w6 essential fatty acids include vitamin C, active forms of cysteine (N-acetyl cysteine), vitamin B_3 (niacin), carnitine, lysine, and proline, as well as magnesium, co-enzyme $Q_{10,}$ and others.

In cancer, vitamin B_3, potassium, iodine, hydrochloric acid, digestive enzymes, and other substances are helpful in addition to w3 EFAs, as well as antioxidant vitamins C and E, carotene, sulphur, and selenium.

Asthma, arthritis, and auto-immune conditions like multiple sclerosis usually have underlying allergies that need to be addressed. Allergies may also be forerunners of cancer, juvenile onset diabetes, and other chronic illnesses.

Genetic influences. Individual genetic differences determine in part what kind of degenerative disease a person might get. Each person has stronger and weaker organs. The latter are more easily affected by nutrient deficiencies and/or poisons (toxicity). Individuals also differ genetically in what constitutes an optimum daily requirement of each different nutrient that is necessary for that individual's optimum health. Finally, factors such as environmental conditions, existing diseases or presence of their agents, different drugs that people take, life-style and habit factors such as use of alcohol and cigarettes, fresh air and sunshine, exercise, joy, belief systems, and faith all determine how well a body copes with living in a world full of challenges and stress.

Is the Cholesterol Theory Wrong? 71

Heart attacks and strokes are two leading causes of death among affluent people. They accounted for 31% of all deaths in 1987, kill about 650,000 people in the U.S. each year,[1] kill them prematurely, and cost about $60 billion in treatments and lost work time (*U.S. Surgeon General's Report on Nutrition and Health,* 1988). Nutrition plays a major role in both.

Cardiovascular disease (CVD) affects two-thirds of the affluent around the world and kills about 45% of them. The cholesterol theory and treatments based on it are failing too many of us. We need to take a closer look at this theory.

Cholesterol Theory

For 40 years, elevated serum (or blood) cholesterol levels have been blamed for fatal diseases of our heart and arteries (cardiovascular diseases or CVD), which include heart attack, pulmonary and other embolism, peripheral arterial disease, stroke, high blood pressure, heart failure, and kidney failure. According to the cholesterol theory, high total cholesterol and high low-density lipoprotein (LDL) levels predispose us to CVD. Many studies to support this theory have been carried out. All are open to other interpretations.

The average total cholesterol level for Americans is 220 mg/dl. At 240 mg/dl, the death rate from CVD is four times higher than average; at 260 mg/dl, it is six times the average rate. People in poor countries, who live on simpler diets containing whole grains, vegetables, and little food of animal origin, have total cholesterol levels in the 120 to 160 mg/dl range, and CVD is rare.

Strict vegetarians die from CVD only one-quarter as often as average Americans. Furthermore, CVD was rare before 1900. During the first and second world wars, when less animal products and more grains and vegetables were eaten, the CVD death rate fell dramatically. From this evidence, it looks like high cholesterol levels predispose us to CVD, and low cholesterol protects us. Foods containing cholesterol are blamed, along with the cholesterol they contain.

---

[1] As a comparison, the Vietnam war cost 57,000 U.S. lives over 13 years – less than 4400 each year.

A Theory with Many Flaws

The cholesterol theory has many flaws. Doctors have had little success in preventing and curing cardiovascular disease with treatments based on this theory.

Prediction. They can neither predict accurately which individual will fall prey to this epidemic nor when, because risk factors are statistically rather than individually defined. One report claims that 40% of fatal heart attacks and strokes[2] were the first (and only) indication of cardiovascular disease, and that there were no early warning signs to either victim or doctor.

Consumption. There are other flaws. Cholesterol consumption in North America has remained about constant since 1900, while cardiovascular disease increased greatly between then and now. As we look back in time, fat consumption was lower. Sugar consumption was lower. Intake of minerals and vitamins was higher on diets containing more vegetables and whole grains and less meat.

War time. During two world wars, people ate more vegetables, less margarines and shortenings, and consumed the grains fed to meat animals before, between, and after these wars. Although fat and cholesterol consumption was lower, the consumption of minerals, vitamins, essential fatty acids (EFAs), and fiber were higher. Protein and sugar consumption were also lower during these wars. All of these factors – not cholesterol alone – have to be considered as possible reasons for the decrease in cardiovascular and other degenerative conditions during these two wars.

Stress was (presumably) higher during war-time as well, resulting in increased cholesterol production which, if the cholesterol theory was correct, should have increased incidence of CVD.

Compensation. Dietary cholesterol increases blood cholesterol levels in only about 30% of the population. The rest of us are not greatly affected by dietary cholesterol because our liver compensates for *increased* dietary cholesterol by making less.

Food traditions. Greenland Inuit who eat a traditional diet high in meat, fats, and cholesterol, have little atherosclerosis. Cancer, diabetes, arthritis, and other degenerative diseases are also rare on this diet. African tribes that eat a diet high in meat, dairy products, and blood are also free of CVD.

The dentist Weston Price travelled around the globe in the 1930s, examined many different traditional diets, and discovered that *all* traditional diets maintained the health of the local people. But within a single generation of introducing white sugar and white flour (through trade with white men), incidence of degeneration of teeth (decay), dental arches, and bones of natives around the world was as high as ours. He pointed to white sugar and white flour as the sources of their physical degeneration. We now recognize the importance of lack

---

[2] According to this report, 20% die within 60 minutes of the onset of symptoms; another 20% die a little slower, but as a consequence of their first heart attack.

of vitamins, minerals, w3 EFAs, fiber, enzymes, and antioxidants in both sugar and white flour, and should also add nutrient-poor 'white' processed oils and hydrogenated and other altered fatty acids to *our* list.

Failure in practice. The worst flaw in the cholesterol theory is its failures when practically applied. Cholesterol reduction programs through drugs fail to decrease death rates, and *increase* (statistical) incidence of cancer and suicide. Out of the frying pan, into the fire. *Nutritional* programs for cholesterol reduction do more than *just* decrease cholesterol. They also improve cardiovascular health.

Other theories to explain the cause of cardiovascular disease have gathered momentum and followers, and also bring better results.

Triglyceride and Sugar Theories

Triglycerides. The triglyceride (TG) theory is based on discovering that correlation between blood TG levels (see Chapter 9, Triglyceride Fats) and CVD is as good as that between CVD and cholesterol levels. TG levels increase with increasing intake of refined sugars, refined starches, excess calories, and hard, non-essential fats. Increased use of these in our diets parallels the increase in CVD since 1900 (while intake of cholesterol has remained constant).

The conclusion reached by researchers who favor the triglyceride theory is that whatever increases TG levels will increase our risk of CVD. Besides sugars, fats, excess calories, and obesity, lack of exercise increases TG levels, because excess calories that turn to fat are not worked off. Certain toxins and drugs also increase TG levels. These, according to the triglyceride theory, would also increase cardiovascular risk.

Sugar. British researcher John Yudkin blames sugar for the meteoric rise in cardiovascular disease. Sugar consumption is one of the quickest ways to increase TGs, because our body turns sugar into fats to protect itself from the toxic effects of excess sugar. Sugar also increases oxidation damage, cross-links proteins, inhibits immune functions, and interferes with the transport of vitamin C. All of these actions of sugar can affect the development of cardiovascular and other degenerative diseases.

Decreased consumption of refined sugars and non-essential fatty acids prevents and helps reverse CVD and other degenerative conditions. It also increases vigor and longevity.[3] These observations lend weight to triglyceride and sugar theories.

Oxidation Theory

Recent discoveries show that *oxidized* cholesterol, as well as *oxidized* fatty acids in TGs, damage arterial walls, leading to CVD. If this is true, we must ask why cho-

---

[3] When sugar is cut from their diet, rats live almost twice as long as when their diet contains it. The addition of chromium increases rats' life span by 33%.

lesterol and fatty acids in our bloodstream become oxidized. A large part of the answer is that when antioxidants (AOs), which prevent this oxidation from occurring, are lacking in foods due to poor choices or processing, then lipids and cholesterol are attacked by oxygen. More importantly, how do we prevent or reverse their oxidation? There are several steps we can take:

- increase our intake of AO nutrients, such as vitamins C and E, carotene, selenium, and sulphur, because antioxidants (AOs) prevent oxidation of cholesterol and fatty acids by becoming oxidized themselves into forms that are less damaging than oxidized cholesterol and TGs.
- limit intake of sugar, to prevent interference with the transport of the key AO present in our body, namely vitamin C.
- avoid the formation of free radicals by lowering intake of toxic substances and drugs that form free radicals in our body. Chlorine is one such molecule, but there are many others, such as air pollutants and heavy metals.
- avoid aged foods containing cholesterol (animal products), or fats. Aged, stored, scrambled, mixed, or whipped foods contain increased amounts of oxidized fat and cholesterol molecules and decreased amount of the AOs that prevent their oxidation and protect our arteries. Fresh foods do not present this problem.

Deficiency Theory

The deficiency theory suggests that deficiencies of vitamins and minerals (including AOs), fiber, and EFAs (that are necessary for the metabolism of cholesterol and fats in our body but are systematically removed from our foods, or altered by processing methods that came into widespread use since just before 1900) are the key causes of degenerative diseases, including CVD. Refined sugars, refined oils, and refined starches are all deficient in minerals, vitamins, EFAs, fiber, enzymes, and AOs.

The finding that increased intake of vitamins, minerals, EFAs, and fiber can lower cholesterol and TG levels in our blood lends weight to the deficiency theory.

A Comprehensive (Vitamin C) Theory

Drs. Rath and Pauling recently proposed a unified theory for the cause and cure of human cardiovascular disease. They suggest that its primary cause is deficiency of vitamin C, leading to the deposition of repair proteins – apo(a) and fibrinogen/fibrin – in arteries.

Vitamin C is necessary to to form the proteins – collagen and elastin, that make our arteries strong. Vitamin C is also the strongest AO normally present in our body, and it also recharges other AOs such as vitamin E, carotene, and sulphydryl groups. When there is not enough vitamin C in our diet, its level in our blood decreases, leading to a mild (subclinical) scurvy. Under condition of vitamin C deficiency, arteries weaken, bleeding into tissue spaces increases, and oxidation of fats and cholesterol increases.

To protect itself, our body increases its production of healing proteins. These thicken our arteries, thereby protecting us from bleeding into tissue spaces. But thickened arteries also slow down blood flow. In the short term, thickened arteries protect us from the lethal effects of vitamin C deficiency. In the long term, thickened arteries may become blocked and kill us.

A steady optimum intake of vitamin C will reverse and prevent atherosclerosis. Other nutrients that help prevent arterial damage and thickening include niacin and sulphur-containing N-acetyl cysteine. Carnitine, lysine, and proline are helpful in peripheral arterial disease, but vitamin C holds the key.

The beauty of this theory is that it explains *all* of the observations in cardiovascular disease research. The cholesterol theory does not do this. The vitamin C theory is also consistent with the observations that led to the other theories of the cause of cardiovascular disease. Sugar interferes with vitamin C activity. Interference with vitamin C activity increases oxidation of both cholesterol and triglycerides. Lack of vitamin C fits the deficiency theory.

Pauling notes that the decrease in deaths due to cardiovascular diseases from 50% down to 43.8% of all deaths in North America since the 1970s coincides with increased use of vitamin C. In countries where vitamin C use did not increase, deaths due to CVD did not decrease, but remained the same.

Lowering Cholesterol and Blood Fats

If you still believe the old theory that high cholesterol levels lead to CVD, you will want to to know how to lower (or normalize) high cholesterol levels safely. These methods not only lower cholesterol intake and production, but also increase antioxidant and micronutrient intake. For 99.8% (499 out of every 500 individuals) only nutritional changes are required to lower cholesterol. The remaining 1 person in 500 has a genetic problem, but will also benefit from improved nutrition.

Decreased intake of animal products and increased intake of plant foods lowers cholesterol levels of some people. A cholesterol level of 260 mg/dl can come down by as much as 100 mg/dl in one month on a strict vegetarian diet. Such a diet increases vitamin, mineral, AO, fiber, and EFA intake, and lowers hard and altered fat intake. Conversely, 2 quarts per day of whole milk (low in several minerals and vitamins, low in EFAs, completely lacking in fiber, and high in milk sugar (lactose), hard fats, and cholesterol) can *raise* some people's cholesterol level from 180 mg/dl to 400 mg/dl in less than 2 months.

Excess body fat increases blood cholesterol and triglyceride levels. Losing weight lowers both cholesterol and TG levels.

Refined sugars and starches (such as white flour, white rice, pasta), and refined or altered fats and oils raise cholesterol levels. A return to natural, complex, high-fiber carbohydrates and natural, unrefined fats and oils lowers cholesterol. Removing refined (especially sugar-containing) foods from our menu is surprisingly effective in lowering cholesterol and TG levels.

Smoking raises cholesterol levels. So does coffee. Quitting reverses the trend.

Abstinence from food lowers cholesterol level. This is not recommended, since fasting burns up proteins rapidly (our body consumes its muscle tissue for energy), and someone deficient in minerals and vitamins could die during a fast that is improperly carried out.

Vitamin C, niacin (B₃), zinc, magnesium, chromium, selenium, iodine, and fiber can lower cholesterol levels. Fresh, natural, highly unsaturated oils from fish (the Inuit secret to good health) or flax, and several herbs can also lower cholesterol levels.

Exercise lowers cholesterol and blood fat levels. The extra fats burn-off as fuel for physical activity.

Stress increases cholesterol levels. A sunny disposition, inner peace, laughter (the ripe old ages of Bob Hope and George Burns might be an indication that laughter is also good for longevity), and freedom from fear, anxiety, worry, and depression also lower cholesterol levels.

A word of caution. Lower cholesterol levels statistically increase deaths from cancer. It has been suggested that cancer results from deficiency of AOs (especially vitamin E and carotene, which are carried to our cells with cholesterol and fats by LDL). Decrease fats and LDL cholesterol, and less of these oil-soluble anti-cancer AOs get to our cells. It has therefore been recommended that before embarking on a cholesterol-lowering diet, one should load up on carotene and vitamin E for two weeks to stock up one's cells' supplies.

Intake of other AOs (especially vitamin C) and of all essential substances (minerals, vitamins, EFAs, and fiber) should be enhanced by adopting an improved nutritional program before a cholesterol-lowering program is begun. With these measures, a drug-based cholesterol-lowering program will be completely unnecessary for 99.8% of the population.

Increasing Protective HDL Cholesterol

We can increase our 'protective' high-density lipoprotein (HDL), which carries cholesterol to our liver for removal, by indulging in delicacies like garlic, onions, brewer's yeast, ginseng, fish, lecithin, chromium, and vitamins C and E.

HDL also increases through aerobic exercise, which also increases cardiovascular fitness. Walking, dancing, swimming, running, cycling, laughing, and any other activity that brings out beads of perspiration and is prolonged, qualifies.

Reversing Atherosclerosis

Can atherosclerosis be reversed? The medical profession claimed for years that atherosclerosis is irreversible and, at best, could only be arrested by the drugs prescribed by them. We, and they now know better. It makes sense that life's energy within us, which powered the building of our entire body out of a handful of dust, three buckets of water, lots of thin air, and a spark of light, and which maintains our body and repairs injuries by sophisticated, meticulous, precise, beautifully controlled and organized molecule-by-molecule methods, can also repair arterial damage and remove deposits if given the materials and conditions it needs to do so.

Pritikin. Nathan Pritikin, using dietary manipulation and exercise – a low-calorie, low-fat, high-complex carbohydrate diet and a lot of walking (but no vitamin or mineral supplements), succeeded in rehabilitating many cases of severe arterial disease. Of course, he did not section the arteries of his still living subjects, so the evidence is indirect. Such work has, however, been done in monkeys. On a natural, unrefined diet without vitamin or mineral supplements, atherosclerosis was decreased from 90% occluded arteries to 60% occluded. The change took almost four years. No exercise was included in the monkey experiment.

Pritikin himself proved that reversal of atherosclerosis is possible in humans. Starting with almost completely obstructed arteries in his 40s, he died with clean arteries in his 60s. Autopsy examination revealed arteries usually found in young adults. He used no supplements.

Fatty acids. One report in medical literature describes a man who increased the content in his diet of the essential linoleic acid (LA, 18:2w6) to over half (54%) of total fat consumed (he made safflower oil two-thirds of his fat calories). He was able to resume a normal walking and working life within less than one year after being wheelchair-bound because of almost completely obstructed leg arteries. He used no supplements.

Minerals and vitamins. Doctors using an orthomolecular approach – large ('mega') doses of vitamins and minerals (see Chapter 37, Orthomolecular Nutrition) – claim successes in treating all aspects of CVD. Although their clinical case reports are individual histories rather than double-blind, placebo-controlled studies, their results are consistent enough to warrant large, controlled studies carried out according to these doctors' protocols.

Chelation therapy. Doctors may also employ *chelation therapy.* Although the method is not sanctioned by conservative drug and high-tech-oriented medical associations, this simple, inexpensive method appears to bring impressive reversals of atherosclerosis in some patients after a series of treatments. Without a change in food habits and/or life-style, however, arteries will gradually plug up again for the same reasons that plugged them in the first place.

For the long term, our best treatment for preventing and reversing cardiovascular conditions consists of food habits and life-styles in line with human requirements for health, which are dictated by human biology and must therefore be nutritional, natural, and orthomolecular (see Chapter 89, Recommendations for Health).

72 *Cardiovascular Disease* (CVD)

Cardiovascular disease is our number one killer, ending 44% of all U.S. lives (almost one million individuals) each year. Their cost in treatments and lost productivity is over $80 billion each year. Yet it is one of the degenerative conditions that responds most readily to improvements in nutrition and life-style.

Deposits of fatty and other materials in heart and arteries (atherosclerosis) provide one example of fatty degeneration. The deposits contain cholesterol, calcium, hard fats, and oxidized fatty material, as well as adhesive repair proteins such as apo(a) and fibrinogen. Arterial deposits also contain unsaturated fatty acids. Highly unsaturated, natural essential fatty acids (EFAs) keep saturated fatty acids dispersed, by preventing them from aggregating. They are also necessary to transport cholesterol. In this function, EFAs are first hooked up (esterified) with cholesterol.

Atherosclerotic arteries lose their elasticity and become narrowed. Blood pressure increases, leading to heart and kidney failure, which thus are also conditions of fatty degeneration.

Elevated levels of oxidized cholesterol and triglycerides (TGs) often precede atherosclerosis. They result from excessive dietary intake of cholesterol, fats, and sugars; lack of activity; toxins in foods, water, and air; and lack of an adequate supply of vitamins and minerals needed to prevent oxidative damage, keep arteries strong, and metabolize sugars, fats, and cholesterol properly.

Bad Genes?

Rarely, genetic factors alone produce high levels of TGs (in less than 5 per 1000 people) or cholesterol (1 in 500 people). This means that most of us cannot blame our genes for high blood fats. We must therefore look to our habits for their elevation, and can lower blood fats by changes in nutrition and life-style. And even the few unfortunate souls who are genetically predisposed to high cholesterol and TGs will benefit from improved nutrition and better life-style.

Environmental Factors

Fat and cholesterol nutrition. The primary factors that lead to high blood TGs and cholesterol are found in the way we eat: 30% of the population is subject to increasing cholesterol levels by eating cholesterol-rich foods; the other 70% of the population is immune to dietary cholesterol, because their liver makes less cholesterol if they eat more, and makes more cholesterol if they eat less. If eating cholesterol-containing, land-animal food products increases your cholesterol level, you are one in 30% and should limit your intake of these foods. Fish and seafoods do not raise cholesterol or TGs.

Antioxidants. More important than fat and cholesterol intake are antioxidants (AOs) like vitamins C and E, carotene, the mineral selenium, and sulphur. These prevent TGs and cholesterol from oxidizing. Oxidized fats damage arteries, starting the process of atherosclerosis. Once this process has taken place and arteries have become narrowed, hard fats and cholesterol that make platelets more sticky and increase the risk of heart attack, stroke, or plugged artery (embolism). These dietary fats and refined sugars (which our body turns into hard fats) should be avoided. Water-soluble fiber and mucilage should be taken to help remove excess cholesterol from our body. W3 fatty acids should be increased, to make platelets less sticky. AOs should be taken to prevent arterial damage and reverse atherosclerotic deposits that resulted from their absence.

Vitamin C is especially important, but others are also necessary. Studies indicate that 500 to 1000 mg of vitamin C as supplement each day extend life by six years. More vitamin C (3 to 14 grams/day may be an optimum amount for normal adults) might extend life even further.

Under disease conditions, 40 grams/day or even more may be optimal, and up to 200 grams/day have been used clinically with benefit and without serious side effects. The main side effect is loosened stools (the 'bowel tolerance level'). Just below that level is the optimum therapeutic dose. Bowel tolerance varies with our state of health, and increases during illness. If 6 grams/day is bowel tolerance when a person is 'normally' healthy, it may increase to 40 grams/day during hepatitis or mononucleosis, and up to 150 grams/day during certain types of flu.

Other essential nutrients also help keep cholesterol and TGs down. *Copper* deficiency increases cholesterol levels. *Chromium* decreases cholesterol in 50% of those with elevated levels. Chromium also prevents fat deposition, building lean muscle mass instead. *W3 and w6 fatty acids* lower cholesterol levels in some individuals. W3 fatty acids lower elevated TGs substantially, and increase energy levels by increasing metabolic rate. Chromium, *zinc,* EFAs, and copper are involved in the function of insulin, which prevents sugars and starches from turning into hard fats that produce sticky platelets.

Magnesium is necessary for many enzyme functions, especially in energy production throughout our body. It is helpful in both prevention of and recovery from heart attacks. Heart attack patients often have low magnesium levels. Magnesium helps prevent arterial spasm, one possible trigger of heart attacks. *Potassium* is important for heart function, muscle strength, and cellular enzymes.

Niacin lowers our liver's production of very low-density lipoproteins (VLDL) and thereby helps to keep blood fats low. It increases cell metabolism, which 'burns' more glucose, preventing sugars and starches from turning into fats. Research has shown that consistent supplementation with niacin can add two years to a person's life.

Carnitine helps transport fats into our cells' 'furnaces' (mitochondria) that convert fats into energy. *Lysine* and *proline* and vitamin C are necessary to build strong arteries. *Coenzyme Q₁₀* is also beneficial to the health of our heart and arteries. *Orotic acid* in yogurt and milk block cholesterol production.

Garlic lowers TGs, slightly lowers cholesterol, and decreases platelet stickiness. *Hawthorn* contains flavonoids beneficial to heart function.

Stress (life-style). Stress results in the production of adrenaline, which increases oxidation rate and produces free radicals that can damage arteries.

Chronic stress increases the body's production of cholesterol, which serves as the building material for stress hormones (corticosteroids) made by our adrenal glands. But stress also increases the body's fat-burning mechanisms.

Stress reduction, which decreases cholesterol production, depends on external changes in life-style (avoidance of stress-inducing situations) and internal changes in belief systems (changing the way we perceive external situations; learning not to be bothered by some of the things that now bother us; and letting the outside world remain outside).

Allergens create internal stress and may increase cholesterol production. Simple sugars elevate internal cholesterol – producing stress. They also increase the production of saturated fatty acid-containing TGs (hard fats).

Toxins. High cholesterol and TGs may also result from toxic environmental chemicals and drugs that interfere with normal metabolism. Simple sugars should be considered toxic. Coffee, cola, and tobacco smoke and other toxins also increase cholesterol production. Avoidance of toxic substances including drugs, pesticides, heavy metals, and sugars is the best way to avoid their effects on our heart and arteries.

Detoxification can help rid our body of toxins. Vitamin C, sulphur-containing compounds, alkylglycerols (in shark liver oil) and chelating chemicals help remove toxins, as well as increased water intake, increased dietary fiber, and increased sweating through exercise or saunas.

Non-Toxicity of Cholesterol and Triglycerides

It has recently been shown that cholesterol is not the villain it was previously thought to be. People with the genetic trait known as familial hypercholesterolemia have extremely high cholesterol levels, but some of these people carry on quite well in spite of it. Closer examination reveals that total cholesterol levels, low-density lipoproteins (LDL) (the so-called 'bad') cholesterol levels, or TG levels are not the key risk factors. They only worsen cardiovascular conditions that have other *primary* causes.

Strong risk factors include:
- oxidized TGs and cholesterol present in our bloodstream, which damage the inner walls of our arteries. Oxidation occurs when levels of AOs, especially vitamin C, are too low; people with high blood levels of cholesterol and TGs, and also good levels of AOs, remain healthy;
- refined sugar, which damages health in many ways;

- high blood levels of the sticky repair proteins apo(a) and fibrinogen, which thicken arteries to protect us from vitamin C deficiency-induced weakened arterial walls and tissue bleeding; and
- toxic substances that damage arterial linings.

These strong risk factors are united by a key primary risk factor which, according to Rath and Pauling, is the main cause of human cardiovascular disease: deficiency of vitamin C. Vitamin C deficiency induces our liver to produce apo(a), allows oxidation to damage fats which then damage arteries, makes detoxification of toxic substances less effective, and allows sugars to do damage.

Glucose and vitamin C share a common transport mechanism. As a result, excess glucose interferes with the transport of vitamin C across membranes, preventing vitamin C from carrying out its functions.

Conclusions

In the final analysis, a complete program of balanced nutrition consisting of whole foods that emphasize fresh vegetables, fresh fruit, whole grains, and fish, and contains optimum quantities of all essential nutrients, fiber, and friendly bacteria is also the best prescription for cardiovascular health. Foods, water, and air should be free of toxic materials. Life-style should be free of unnecessary stress.

Such a program can be enriched with AOs (especially vitamin C) that protect fats from oxidative destruction, remove toxins from our body, prevent damage to our arteries, and prevent repair proteins from becoming overactive. The main benefit of such a program is improved human health, and a fringe benefit of such a program is normalized TG and cholesterol levels.

Such a program could abolish cardiovascular disease as the number one killer within a few years.

Diabetes 73

Juvenile onset (irreversible, Type I) diabetes is an auto-immune disease in which our immune system destroys insulin-producing cells in our pancreas (islets of Langerhans). It is discussed with other auto-immune diseases (see Chapter 82, Auto-Immune Conditions).

Adult onset (reversible, Type II) diabetes is a dangerous condition that affects about 6% of the population, and accounts for 1.8% of all deaths (about 38,000 individuals) in the U.S. each year, costing about $15 billion annually. Pre-diabetic low (hypoglycemic) and high (hyperglycemic) blood sugar conditions affect about 20% of the population. They result from consuming too much hard fat, refined sugar and starch, and too few vitamins and minerals. They are often accompanied by cardiovascular complications, which cause another 95,000 deaths each year among diabetics. Blindness, blocked circulation of the extremities (leading to gangrene), and heart attacks, all resulting from impaired circulation, are symptoms of fatty degeneration. Diabetes is one of the easiest of 'incurable' diseases to cure, and even easier to prevent.

In part, diabetics suffer from functional essential fatty acid (EFA) deficiency. High sugar levels make EFAs present in fat tissues unavailable to our body. The old name for diabetes was sugar diabetes, in honor of its connection with sugar – high sugar consumption, high blood sugar, and sugar in the urine. EFAs given to diabetics have an insulin-sparing effect, indicating that the effectiveness of insulin depends on them. In fact, dietary w3 fatty acids decrease the amount of insulin needed by diabetics.

Silly Advice. Some 'experts' have suggested that w3 fatty acids should not be used by diabetics because they make insulin too effective (a diabetic then needs to inject less insulin and the usual insulin injection could bring blood sugar too low, resulting in symptoms of hypoglycemia). This silly suggestion ignores the fact that lowering a diabetic's need for injected insulin constitutes healing. If insulin requirement decreases to zero, diabetes is cured. That would be the goal, perhaps not for those who depend on the patient's sickness for their income, but certainly for the patient who wants to get well.

Note: To avoid low blood sugar, insulin requirement should be monitored closely and injections decreased as w3 supplementation decreases the need for injected insulin.

Other Nutrients

In addition to EFAs *(especially w3s), chromium* is vital to insulin action on our cell membranes. Without chromium, insulin cannot attach to cell receptors to do its job of moving sugars into our cells. According to some researchers, chromium deficiency affects over 80% of affluent populations. Chromium also helps build lean body mass, preventing the deposition of flabby fat. In its active form, known as the Glucose Tolerance Factor (GTF), chromium is bound with several molecules of *niacin* (B$_3$) and *glutathione.* This is probably the most beneficial form in which to supplement this important mineral. Yeast provides small quantities of GTF. Chromium picolinate and chromium poly-nicotinate (ChroMate) are the most commonly used concentrated sources. ChroMate, a combination of chromium and vitamin B$_3$, has been patented as a cholesterol-lowering agent, because it effectively performs that function in 50% of those with elevated cholesterol levels.

Insulin, which is a protein hormone, also cannot act without *zinc,* a mineral involved in at least 80 different enzyme reaction in our body. Zinc deficiency is common, estimated at 30% or more of the population. Up to 80% or more of growing children, adolescents, pregnant women, and the elderly get less than the recommended amount of zinc.

More recently, *copper* has also been implicated in diabetes. According to the U.S. Department of Agriculture figures, about 85% of the population gets less copper than recommended.

Fiber such as that found in okra, flax, and psyllium helps stabilize blood sugar by slowing down the rate at which it is absorbed from our intestinal tract.

Cinnamon is one herb that can also be helpful to diabetics.

The key roles that the above substances play in glucose metabolism make them particularly useful in treating reversible diabetes. However, we should remember that a complete program of whole food, clean water, fresh air, and sunlight that provides optimum quantities of all 50 essential substances, as well as the avoidance of toxic influences, are necessary to reach our ultimate goal of optimum human health, even when treating diabetes and other nutrition-based degenerative diseases.

Overweight and Constipation 74

Both overweight and constipation are dangerous to health, and both can easily be improved by natural methods.

Obesity

About 30% of affluent people are overweight, and 10% are obese. Both are forms of fatty degeneration. Both increase our risk of cardiovascular disease, cancer, and diabetes. Low metabolic rate, excess fats in fat depots and organs, and low tissue content of essential fatty acids all occur together. Refined sugars and starches containing too many calories and too little fiber turn into saturated (hard) fats. Refined sugars, starches, and oils lack the vitamins and minerals necessary for their own metabolism.

W3 fatty acids, which increase metabolic rate, can be used for weight loss. One woman in California lost 80 pounds of excess fat by adding 3 tablespoons per day of fresh flax oil to her dietary program. She had been eating relatively nutritious foods for some time, without effect. The addition of the flax oil was the missing key for her. Weight watchers may find it hard to believe, but here is a 'fat' (actually, an oil) that can *make fats burn more rapidly*. The story illustrates the importance of knowing the difference between killing and healing fats. The right kind of fat can help you lose weight.

W3 fatty acids help in weight loss in three major ways:
1. W3s serve as building materials for series 3 prostaglandins (see Chapter 58, Prostaglandins), some of which help our kidneys get rid of excess water held in tissues. The excess weight of some overweight people is largely retained

water (edema). W3s help dump this water.

2. W3s increase metabolic rate, oxidation rate, and energy production. This effect begins to show up when 3 or more tablespoons of flax oil per day are used.[1] When metabolic rate goes up, more fat and glucose are burned. Less fat deposition takes place. This increased production of energy is the opposite of what happens when we fast or diet on calorie-restricted programs. The latter decrease our metabolic rate, and lead us to put on weight even on a small intake of food. There is some evidence that obesity is the result of gross over-eating in only about 10% of cases. The other 90% are lacking exercise and choosing foods lacking important essential nutrients.

3. W3s help us lose weight because with increased energy levels, we feel more like being active. This is a special bonus, because activity makes us feel good, builds lean body (muscle) mass, makes us healthier, increases our metabolic rate, and resets our fat thermostat to a lower level, helping make weight loss permanent.

Chromium and carnitine. In addition to w3s, chromium helps build lean body mass and increases energy levels in the 80% of the population that is deficient in this mineral. Carnitine helps transport fatty acids into the mitochondria in our cells where they are burned to produce energy.

Iodine increases metabolic rate. Its richest source in our foods is kelp, other seaweeds, and seafoods. Iodine can also be supplemented. **Caution:** Supplementation with iodine requires supervision, because too much iodine can be toxic. Supervised iodine supplementation should be undertaken when iodine levels, body temperature, and metabolic rate are lower than normal.

Potassium helps increase energy level and muscle strength. It is often replaced by sodium in processed foods. Sodium weakens muscles and leads to water retention, increasing body weight.

Minerals and vitamins. A full spectrum of minerals and vitamins can help normalize the presence in our tissues of these essential nutrients required for optimum metabolism.

Fiber provides bulk that prevents the over-assimilation of calories from our intestines.

The stimulant herb *ephedra* is often used to increase metabolic rate for burn-off.

Avoid sugars! Sweet fruits contain a lot of sugar and should be eaten only in moderation. Concentrated foods – meats, cheese, eggs – must be decreased because they contain too many calories and not enough fiber. Fiber-rich vegetables should be emphasized.

Counseling. Some people also require counseling, because their eating

---

[1] In human studies, when more than 12.5 to 15% of daily calories were LNA, metabolic rate increased measurably.

habits are based on belief systems out of line with the biological function of eating – to replenish the essential nutrients and energy required by our tissues. Eating can become a substitute for friendship, a way of passing time, a way to distance oneself from other people (in our society, most people don't like fat people) or serve other social functions out of line with nature's reasons for having us eat. There are other ways of fulfilling these functions, ways that are less damaging to health than obesity.

Constipation

Thirty percent of our adult population is chronically constipated. Constipation leads to many other problems: hemorrhoids, varicose veins, toxin reabsorption, bad breath, liver damage, and even aneurisms from straining. Most constipation has one of three nutritional causes that can be addressed by nutritional means.

Too much protein – too little oil. High-protein diets tend to constipate. Athletes who take high-protein powder drinks often discover this unpleasant fact. Oils soften protein-hardened stools. They work in opposition to protein's tendency to constipate. The addition of essential fatty acid-containing oils to a protein shake usually takes care of the constipation problem caused by excess protein without adding fattening fats.

Too little fiber. Fiber, which absorbs water and provides bulk to our stools, can prevent and reverse constipation. All kinds of fiber help do this, but the best kinds are found in okra, psyllium, and flax. The mucilage found in these foods not only absorbs many times its volume of water, but also soothes our intestinal tract, makes stools slippery, and makes bowel movements easy. Pectins and gums are other types of helpful soluble fiber.

On the other hand, wheat bran contains a harsher kind of insoluble fiber. While it helps prevent constipation by adding bulk to our stools, excess of this kind of fiber can irritate delicate linings of our intestinal tract, which can be counterproductive. Cellulose, hemi-cellulose, and lignin are other kinds of harsher insoluble fiber.

Too little water. If we drink too little water, our body drags the water it needs out of our intestinal tract. Our stools then become drier, harder, and more compact. The obvious solution is to drink more liquids. Water, herbal teas, soups, and broths are the best beverages. Juices may contain too much sugar. Tea and coffee contain stimulants that are not recommended for health. Alcohol contains water, but also dehydrates our cells. Pure H_2O is the magic ingredient in all liquids. No additives are needed to make it effective. The water that best supports our health has been filtered to remove chlorine, 'bugs', and other impurities.

75 Skin Conditions, Tanning Lotions, and Ozone

This chapter is not just for teenagers, models, and actors – those especially concerned with how they look. Beautiful skin is for everyone. It is one external manifestation of an internally healthy body. Oils can help children and adults with skin conditions (including sunburns). Most skin problems can be prevented and reversed.

Healthy teenagers have 'zit'-less skin. Hard and altered fats in cheese, pizza, ice cream, french fries, and hamburgers produce acne, as does sugar in drinks, ice cream, and junk foods. Too much sweet fruit can also result in acne. Allergies to dairy products and wheat also affect skin.

Acne, blackheads, whiteheads, 'bumpy' skin, some kinds of eczema, 'greasy' skin, and dry skin all involve fatty degeneration. Improvements in nutrition can help all of these skin conditions.

Acne results from consuming fats that associate poorly with proteins, an excess of hard fats (such as those found in beef, lamb, pork, butter, and cheese) that will not flow, and too little of the liquid, freely flowing, essential fatty acid- (EFA-) containing oils. Chemically altered fats including margarines and shortenings belong to the list. Hard fats and (hard) protein debris clog narrow pores and channels in our skin, and invite infection by bacteria who feast on the mess.[1]

Soaps and skin creams containing neem oil, whose minor ingredients have antiseptic properties can help keep pores from becoming infected.

Liquid, freely flowing, *EFA-containing* oils are required for healthy skin. W3s make skin soft and velvety. They should be consumed rather than used topically. Put on our skin from outside, some absorption takes place, but most of the oil becomes rancid (we smell like paint), and permanently stains clothing and hardens in seams. Hardened flax or hemp oil in clothing cannot be washed out. The best way to oil our skin is from inside, using liquid, flowing, unrefined w3 and w6 oils in foods.

Teenage diets often lack several other essential nutrients as well. Main deficiencies include *vitamin A, vitamin E,* and *zinc.* Zinc deserves special attention. When boys become sexually active, they often become zinc-deficient, because semen is zinc-rich. Increased zinc loss through sexual activity must be balanced by increased zinc intake. Teenagers usually give sex, but not zinc, a lot of attention.

Chromium and detoxifying *fiber* also help improve skin conditions. *Sweating* produces glowing skin by freeing the facial skin of toxins and improving circula-

---

[1] Zits are gourmet food for these bacteria!

tion. *Cold water* also works by improving circulation.

Avoidance of toxins helps skin condition, because our body uses our skin as one avenue for ridding itself of toxins which, on their way out, can cause skin reactions.

Fresh foods – especially vegetables – are recommended. Whole grains like brown rice, buckwheat, oats, barley, and millet are good sources of carbohydrates. Proteins such as fish and soybeans (tofu) are recommended. Freshly pressed vegetable juice, and a well-balanced mineral-vitamin supplement may also be helpful.

When nutritional deficiencies are normalized and toxins removed from the body, acne disappears. It is not an inevitable teenage condition.

Skin rash. Skin rashes often result from an allergic response to one or more specific substances. Here, the offending food, toxic chemical, metal, or clothing material must be removed from diet or contact with skin.

Blackheads and whiteheads. These are similar. Fats that are unable to flow clog pores. Blackheads result when sunshine and air react with these fats and with pigments they carry, changing their color. Whiteheads remain white because they remain protected from air and therefore do not change color.

Bumpy skin. Bumps on the skin are most often found on the backs of our upper arms. These respond well to better oils and to supplementation with carotene and vitamin A. They may also be due to allergies, especially to dairy products. Some healers call them 'milk bumps'.

Eczema. Eczema can result from two major causes: allergic reaction to food or environmental allergens, and lack of EFAs. To treat the former, the offending food factor or environmental allergen must be identified and avoided (see Chapter 77, Allergies). To treat the latter, EFA-rich oils must be provided. Flax and hemp (seed or oil) provide w3s. Soybean, walnut, safflower, sunflower, and sesame oils provide mainly w6s. Virgin olive oil is an unrefined, unheated source of unsaturated fatty acids. Eczema often responds well to treatment with neem oil-containing skin creams. It also gives excellent results when used topically on psoriasis, and on dandruff when included in shampoo formulations.

Dry skin. Human skin becomes drier with age. The condition is usually worse in winter than in summer as cold weather causes oils to flow less freely. This condition is easy to clear up by using an oil that flows easily. Such an oil must be rich in EFAs, especially w3s. EFA-rich oils continue to flow easily even in cold weather. Obviously, oils that flow only with difficulty when the weather is warm, flow even more poorly when our skin becomes cold due to environmental influences.

'Greasy' skin. The term 'greaser' is derived in part from using grease on the hair, but also from the greasy, light-reflecting forehead often seen on street people eating junk foods rich in sugars (which the body turns into saturated fatty acids) and hard fats, which tend to stick together. On our forehead, they form a film of fat that feels slippery and reflects light.

This 'greasy' look disappears when we replace sugars and hard fats with EFA-rich oils. EFA-rich oils make skin feel and look velvety instead of 'greasy', because their molecules spread out away from each other (disperse) rather than sticking together, and therefore do not produce the 'greaser' forehead streak.

Beautiful Skin

Beautiful skin requires EFAs. Skin properly nourished with EFAs is smoother, feels softer, shows less of the above conditions, is infected less easily, and looks radiant. It also ages more slowly and remains wrinkle-free longer.

Other nutritional factors that help make skin beautiful include vitamin A, zinc, silicon, sulphur, vitamin E, and vitamin C. Saunas, exercise, and cold water make skin glow by removing toxins and improving circulation. Herbs such as rosemary, camomile, aloe vera and peppermint are helpful, and neem oil both protects skin and kills virus, fungus, and bacterial infections.

While the entire nutritional program is important to healthy skin, EFAs hold a main key to skin that is pleasant to look at, beautiful to photograph, and silky to touch.

Tanning Lotions

An excellent tanning lotion can be made by mixing equal parts of coconut, almond (or walnut), and flax oils, with added vitamin E and aloe vera. It protects skin from burning and produces a golden tan. Oils absorb ultraviolet (UV) rays. Remember to avoid contact with clothing. The stains it causes may be permanent. Substances such as PABA, the most commonly used ingredient for protection from UV in suntan creams and lotions, will also stain clothing. PABA also interferes with vitamin D production.

In choosing a suntan lotion, be aware that there are rumors suggesting that some contain chemicals that may become carcinogenic when exposed to UV.

Skin Protection and Repair

Protect your skin from damage due to overexposure to sunlight in three ways:

1. Nutrition. A skin-protecting nutritional program must include:
- fresh, unrefined, EFA-rich oils, which oil our skin from within;
- carotene, which migrates to the skin and increases its exposure time before burning;
- vitamin E, which helps prevent free radicals generated by UV rays in our skin from doing damage;
- vitamin C, which is an antioxidant, recharges vitamins E and carotene, and also prevents skin damage due to UV-generated free radicals;
- selenium, an antioxidant and another free radical neutralizer;
- zinc, which is involved in enzyme function and tissue repair;
- sulphur, is an antioxidant and is also used in the formation of new tissues; and

348

- vitamin A, which is necessary for skin growth.

2. External application of the above nutrients also protects and heals skin.

3. 'Conscious living' (practicing self-awareness), which means paying attention to your exposure to healing but potentially also burning rays, learning the limits to your body's exposure to the sun, and covering up when that limit has been reached. Since the full effect of UV on the skin takes several hours to develop, don't stay in the sun until your skin is red. That could become a horrendous sunburn. Start with short exposures and build up exposure time gradually.

Some sun is good for health, too much is damaging. How much sun is right for you depends on your individual makeup, and can only be discovered through your own observation. With good nutrition and a bit of awareness, we can develop a golden tan without skin lotions most of the time.

Repair. Zinc, selenium, and vitamins C and E help to heal sun-damaged skin, both when taken internally and when used externally.

Carotene taken internally, in quantities large enough to color the skin, protects skin against sunburn. Vitamin A helps grow new skin. Aloe Vera applied to sunburnt skin soothes and helps heal.

A Note on Ozone

Ozone is nature's original sunscreen for planet Earth. It blocks some of the UV rays that come from the sun, but also allows some UV rays to pass.

The thickness of the ozone layer has always fluctuated naturally from year to year. Also, the ozone layer is always thinner at the poles and thicker at the equator, and UV rays are always less intense at the poles and more intense at the equator.

Overexposure to UV has always burned human skin. Thus we have always needed to practice care to prevent sunburn.

Industrial products have further thinned the ozone layer. Less ozone in the atmosphere means that we could burn more easily, as more UV will reach the earth. This means that exposure time before burning has been shortened and, to prevent sunburns, we need to exercise even greater care today than people did in years gone by.

Ozone for Healing

Ozone in smog can damage human lungs. But ozone also has beneficial applications. It is an excellent anti-viral, anti-fungal, and anti-bacterial agent. As such, it can be used to sterilize swimming pools. Even more exciting, ozone sterilizes blood contaminated with the AIDS or hepatitis viruses within a few minutes. Ozone has been thoroughly tested by the Canadian army as one way to ensure a clean blood supply for wounded soldiers. It has also been used to clean the blood of AIDS patients. Their blood is withdrawn, treated with ozone, and reinjected. It prolongs survival time, but does not *cure* AIDS.

76 *Female Conditions*

This chapter deals with premenstrual syndrome and fibrocystic breast disease, which have nutritional causes involving fats and other substances, and respond well to improvements in nutrition. Fibroid tumors and endometriosis are more difficult. Cancers of breasts, ovaries, and uterus will be discussed in Chapter 80.

Premenstrual Syndrome (PMS)

PMS includes symptoms of cramps before periods, breast pain, water retention, extreme mood swings, and behavioral difficulties.

PMS has a strong component of fatty degeneration. Some women find relief with evening primrose oil supplements. Others get equally good results with flax oil or fish oils. The treatment depends on the exact nature of the fatty problem. The beneficial effect of essential fatty acids (EFAs) and EFA derivatives on PMS are related to their effects on prostaglandin production. Along with EFAs, PMS treatment should include vitamins B_3, B_6, and C, and the minerals magnesium and zinc. Vitamin E may also be helpful. Increased potassium and decreased table salt may help decrease water retention. Calcium and vitamin D may also help.

On the other side of the equation, it is important to avoid sugar, hard fats, *trans-* fatty acids, and other altered, toxic, fat-related products that alter prostaglandin production. Margarines and shortenings should be avoided. Fats from land animals (beef, pork, mutton, dairy) should be minimized. Allergies to common foods may also be involved. These must be treated.

A complete program of whole foods and supplements is helpful. PMS was *not* ordained by God to be the lot of women. Like other degenerative conditions, it is the biological result of unbiological habits: malnutrition and internal pollution, and responds to nutrification and detoxification. To enjoy the gift of life, we must live in line with our genetically and biologically determined nature.

Fibrocystic Breast Disease (FBD)

EFAs – especially w3s – and vitamin E are helpful in FBD. An optimum intake of minerals and vitamins is also required. This can be accomplished with whole foods, juices, or high-dose multi-mineral and multivitamin supplements. Iodine is also helpful. On the negative side: coffee, cola, tea, chocolate, and other sources of methylxanthines should be avoided.

Fibroids and Endometriosis

Endometriosis involves series 2 prostaglandins. It should, therefore, be helpful to add w3 fatty acids from flax or fish to the diet to down-regulate excessive PG2 production. Often, candida is involved in endometriosis. This should be treated.

Soybean products and flax may also be helpful.

We should seek to support our healthy cells and tissues in doing their healthy work, by giving them the nutritional tools they need to organize the body along the lines dictated by our genes. Nutrient enrichment and better nutritional balance, improved life-style, and detoxification should improve endometriosis. More research is needed.

Fibroids may also respond to w3 fatty acids. They may also be helped by treatment with special forms of iodine, and may respond to some herbal combinations. Much is still unknown about fibroids.

Some researchers have suggested that like endometriosis, fibroids may involve allergies and/or candida yeast (or even viruses or other micro-organisms) in their cause. It is hard to imagine that the considerable disorganization of tissue growth presented by these two conditions can happen without some powerful disorganizing (reorganizing) influence similar to that which takes place in warts caused by viruses.

If allergies are involved, they must be treated. If organisms are involved, they must be treated. Underlying causes that allow infections to take root may include allergies, compromised immune function, nutritional deficiencies, and toxicity. All of these must be addressed.

As in *all* degenerative conditions, it is best to make use of a complete and balanced natural approach, rather than looking for 'magic bullets' to kill the symptoms.

Allergies, Arthritis, & Asthma 77

Allergies, arthritis, and asthma have environmental triggers and will, therefore, respond to environmental interventions. These three and several other conditions have a common denominator: they generally involve environmental triggers (antigens) from foods, water, or air. These antigens should not, but do, enter our body and blood, and stimulate our immune system to create neutralizing proteins (antibodies) which, when rechallenged by the antigen, produce biochemical reactions between antigen and antibody molecules, which can manifest as a wide variety of symptoms in any part of the body.

Allergies

Allergies are one of the most often missed, most often mis-diagnosed, most poorly addressed treatable conditions in the world. Allergies are estimated to affect between 20 and 40% of affluent populations (and an unmeasured percentage of people around the world); and probably *most* individuals have some kind of mild allergies and food incompatibilities.

Allergic reactions are our body's response to the repeated entrance of a foreign protein, or synthetic compound (an antigen) into our body. The most common route of their introduction is through our digestive system.[1]

Allergies can be due to genetic limitations that make some foods incompatible with our digestive system for life. Allergies may also result from poor maternal nutrition, resulting in a 'leaky gut' or poor digestive function in the mother, and a leaky mother-child barrier that allows some proteins from the mother to pass into the circulation of the fetus, triggering allergic response in the fetus. Allergies might also be due to nutritional stress (deficiency, toxicity, etc.) occurring at any time in life, or any kinds of stress (such as toxic chemicals like pesticides, PCBs, paint remover, tobacco smoke, alcohol, air pollutants, ozone and nitrogen dioxide, etc.) that take a further toll on an already compromised nutritional situation. Alcohol, for instance, affects our digestive tract in such a way as to make it more likely that undigested proteins (antigens) pass into our body through a 'leaky' intestinal wall.

Symptoms of allergies may appear immediately on contact or may be delayed, for minutes, hours, or up to about four days. If symptoms of allergy are immediate, their source is easy to identify and eliminate. Sources of delayed symptoms are more difficult to pinpoint and avoid, because we forget what we ate a few days ago. A systematic approach like keeping an ongoing diary of foods, environments, and symptoms can be used to identify delayed symptoms of allergies.

Allergies may be lifelong, or they may be temporary. They may get better with time, or worse. Each person has a unique set of genes interfacing with unique life situations that are changing all the time, and therefore has unique ways of reacting to internal assault by antigen molecules.

Usually, food or airborne proteins are the triggering antigens for allergies and the diseases that arise from them. Sometimes hydrocarbons, organochlorines, or other organic substances serve as triggers by aligning with proteins. In both cases, something that should have stayed out of our body enters it.

A Standing Army

Our immune system is alerted to an intruding substance, and after one or more exposures, builds a standing army against it. Each time the intruder makes its entrance, the army comes out, a battle ensues, and the intruder is destroyed.

The cost to health can be severe. We may experience the symptoms of allergic reactions in any part of our body: aching muscles, joints, or bones, back pain, stiff neck, headaches, heartbeat abnormalities, respiratory conditions, sensory dis-

---

[1] It has been estimated that over a normal lifespan, our body processes 10,000 kg (22,000 pounds) of antigens from foods, compared to 200 to 400 kg (440 to 880 pounds) from water, and 400 to 600 kg (880 to 1320 pounds) from air.

turbances, fuzzy thinking, foggy consciousness, mood swings, abnormal behavior, and other symptoms.

Allergies place an enormous burden on our immune system. Their load on this system makes us more susceptible to other environmental factors: toxic metals, toxic gases, physical and mental stress, and infections by virus, fungus, bacteria, and protozoa. Often, allergies are forerunners of cancer.

Untreated, allergies can become so severe that a person may tolerate so few foods that he or she requires intravenous nutrient support. A few sufferers are so sensitive to environmental triggers that they must live in a protected 'bubble' environment.

Treating Allergies

Some allergies can be helped with nutrient enrichment, adrenal support, or certain herbs. A supplement of digestive enzymes can be remarkably helpful, by improving digestion and minimizing the absorption of allergy-triggering, incompletely digested protein components of foods. For some allergy sufferers, these simpler treatments do not go far enough, and a more painstaking, meticulous approach must be followed.

Severe allergies can be treated with a clearing program of powdered nutrients for 10 days. Such a program provides all essential nutrients, but no allergens. During clearing, there may be symptoms of withdrawal from foods we are addicted to: weakness, tiredness, headaches, aches and pains in one or more parts of our body, or mood swings. After 10 days on this powdered program, most symptoms of allergic reactions have run their course and been cleared out (hence the term 'clearing program').

The clearing program is followed by a careful introduction of single foods, one every 4 days, and symptoms are recorded in a journal. Foods that produce no symptoms are incorporated into the program of allowable food choices. Foods or food combinations that produce symptoms are removed from the list of allowable foods. Each time allergic reactions occur, one can fall back on the powdered clearing program for a few days, then try new foods again. In this way, one deliberately develops one's own diet of foods compatible with one's unique digestive capabilities.

When a mother introduces her young child to solid foods, she follows a similar method. As foods are introduced, she notes symptoms, if any. Diarrhea, diaper rash, vomiting, colic, crying, and skin rashes are some of the symptoms that indicate that a new food should be stricken (for now or forever) from the baby's 'compatible foods' list.

As adults, each of us is in the best position to make these food assessments ourselves, on the basis of our own symptoms, because *we* experience them fully. We may have internal symptoms that our mother could not possibly have identified, because they showed no external signs. She could only guess what exactly her baby experienced when a new food was introduced.

Few people take the time necessary to systematically develop their own compatible food program unless severe symptoms force them to do so. Its development should be part of the rite of passage of each child into adulthood – the point at which we become responsible for our own choices.

A program of compatible foods must be both complete (contain all essential nutrients in optimum quantities) and allergy-free. One can use the powdered nutrient program to make up for nutritional gaps that result from food restrictions due to allergic responses. Such a food program heals, because it eliminates digestive, absorptive, and deficiency problems, and prevents the damaging immune and metabolic reactions that result from consuming incompatible foods.

'Unconscious' snacking and favorite bad food 'habits' are the greatest obstacles to success. Another obstacle is the fact that allergies can change over the course of our lifetime. We may lose some allergies. Others may start. The approach remains the same: identify and eliminate offending foods, improve nutrition to help heal tissues, and remove toxins from the body.

Arthritis

In arthritis, joints, muscles, tendons, and ligaments are involved in degenerative changes, causing swelling of joints and tendons, joint bone deterioration, dryness of joints, stiffness, and excruciating pain. Allergies are often involved.

Essential fatty acids (EFAs) are necessary to produce secretions that lubricate our joints. They are also required to build and deposit bone material, and used to transport minerals. EFAs are also required to build our cells' membranes; those that line our digestive tract help prevent the entrance of undigested foreign materials into our body. They also strengthen immune cells that inhabit all body surfaces.

Further, EFAs and fats and oils of any kind slow down stomach emptying time and thereby allow more time for the digestion of foods – especially proteins that could cause allergic reactions – to be completed. Digestive enzymes and ginger help arthritics, at least partly because they promote good digestion. Completely digested proteins turn into amino acids, which *cannot* cause allergic reactions. Our body uses amino acids to make body-own proteins.

EFAs are also required for immune system functions.

Other nutrients such as magnesium, calcium, and vitamins B_6 and D may be helpful. Vitamin C and zinc help immune functions, healing, and tissue construction. Optimum amounts of all nutrients are necessary for health.

Sometimes nutrient enrichment can help the digestive tract to rebuild itself so that it is no longer leaky. Such a process may take several months.[2]

---

[2] Biological healing with nutrients requires more time than symptom management with drugs. The latter is quick, but only masks or suppresses symptoms while allowing deterioration of cells and tissues to continue. Appropriate biological treatments allow our body to rebuild itself, molecule by molecule, which takes more time but constitutes a real cure.

'**Rheumatism**'. Johanna Budwig (see Chapter 63, Budwig, Flax Oil, and Protein) claims that fat droplets found in muscle cells are the only microscopic feature that distinguishes rheumatic (a term commonly used in the 1950s for rheumatoid arthritis) cells from normal ones. She says these fats distort cells, setting off nerve endings whose activity causes excruciating pain. According to her, the fat droplets contain saturated or altered 'unreactive' fats that are unable to take part in cells' metabolic activity. When we consume excessive fat from pork, beef, and especially from altered, unnatural fat derivatives in margarines and shortenings (says she), our body can't use them properly, and dumps them somewhere. In rheumatism, that place is the muscles.

It is now clear that allergic reactions play an important part in *most* arthritic and 'rheumatic' complaints. They therefore should be treated as allergies, with EFAs, AOs, other essential nutrients, enzymes, adrenal support, and/or a clearing program of powdered nutrients followed by the careful introduction of foods to develop a diet consisting of foods compatible with the individual's digestive and immune systems, as explained above.

Altered and hard fats, as well as nutrient deficiencies and the presence of other toxic molecules, can worsen an allergic situation and should therefore be eliminated.

Asthma

Asthma is almost always allergy-based. The offending allergen may come from food or water, affecting our respiratory system indirectly by absorption into our body through our digestive tract, or it may be airborne (pollen, bacteria, molds, dander, dust, mites, etc.), affecting our lungs and breathing passages directly.

As outlined above, an allergy treatment and/or clearing diet should be followed with careful introduction of foods free of allergy response for the individual. Water may need to be filtered to remove chlorine, other toxic materials, and allergens. Air may need to be filtered to remove airborne allergens and noxious fumes and odors. Some people with severe airborne allergies provide themselves with a 'safe' room outfitted with a high quality filter. They can retreat to this room to recover when their allergies get too intense to bear. For allergy treatment programs and sources of filters, see Services Provided, at the back of the book.

78 Addictions, Mental Illness, and Violence

These behavioral difficulties continue to puzzle the 'experts'. The fact that both our brain and our body are made from foods suggests that our thoughts and our actions should both respond to changes in nutrition.

Physical substances can affect perceptions, moods, and thoughts, and the behavior that flows from them. Drugs – both pharmaceutical and street – prove that. Food molecules however, have been given much less attention. They deserve a great deal more.

Addictions

Addictions have two components. One is *hunger,* our need for substances that our body uses for normal functions. We may remain hungry because we are not getting the nourishment our body requires. We keep eating until we get it. Those of us who listen to our body and understand its messages can identify a craving for specific foods that contain what our body needs. Others are not so sensitive, and may continue to eat foods that do not supply the missing ingredients. The hunger remains until the need is filled.

The second component of addictions is *withdrawal.* Withdrawal symptoms suggest that allergies may be present (see Chapter 77, Allergies). Often, withdrawal symptoms are so severe that it seems preferable to continue being addicted. Another drink 'cures' the hangover. At first, a fix brings a 'high'. Eventually, each fix only prevents the 'low' of withdrawal.

Fats and Addictions

Fats help with both components of addictions. Fats provide essential fatty acids (EFAs) that are necessary nutrients. Fats also slow down stomach emptying time, leading to better protein digestion, resulting in fewer potential allergens (antigens).

EFAs help build membranes better able to keep antigens from being absorbed into our body. They should be part of any nutritional treatment program used to help addicts.

Johanna Budwig, who researched fats in the 1950s, suggests that EFAs help treat addictive behaviors, including tobacco, alcohol, and drug addictions, as well as addictions to sex and violence that we consider voluntary, 'sick', 'criminal' behavior rather than molecularly based addictive behavior. EFAs increase the amount of tension that a person is able to bear. This is because electrical properties of EFAs heighten the capacity for electric tension across our membranes (membrane potentials). They keep brain and nerve function more stable under stress and tension. They help make it easier for people not to 'fly off the handle' at the small provocations, the day-to-day frustrations that lead to the use of alcohol, drugs, and addictive behaviors in the first place.

Other Nutrients

To treat addictions, a completely balanced, highly nutritious food supply is necessary. A high dose multi-mineral-multivitamin supplement is appropriate. In particular, large doses of vitamin C, other antioxidants, and niacin help to detoxify the body, and minimize withdrawal symptoms. Food allergies/addictions, yeast infections, and other addictive triggers must also be identified and treated.

Criminals. Alexander Schauss, a criminologist and researcher in biosocial research (how nutrition affects behavior) has shown that episodic and chronic violent criminals show distinct hair mineral patterns. These two types of criminals can be identified and separated by hair mineral analysis. Appropriate mineral supplements hold out promise to change criminal behavior by adjusting the mineral balance in their body.

This new work is particularly exciting because we know that incarceration and rehabilitation without nutritional changes have a low success rate (20%). Most criminals end up in jail again and again. In jail, cigarettes, coffee, sugared foods, and processed nutrient-poor foods are standard fare. These continue the biochemical problems from which at least some criminals suffer.

When criminals are taught to eat more nutritious foods, their behavior also improves. A large percentage of these nutritionally rehabilitated criminals change their life-style and stay out of jail. In one study, 80% of criminals who received nutrition counseling were completely rehabilitated, compared to only 20% who received no nutrition counseling and therefore did not improve their food habits.

Eighty to ninety percent of criminals measured in one study were shown to be suffering from hypoglycemia or food-, water-, or airborne allergies. It has been suggested that the majority of crimes are committed by people while hypoglycemic, a state in which our higher brain centers (critical thinking, socially acceptable behavior, conscience) fail to function because they are deprived of glucose, their fuel. Hypoglycemia activates our primitive 'lizard brain', which is responsible for fight (anger) or flight (fear) – survival behavior. In lizard brain mode, higher rational perceptive functions are distorted by the emotions involved in stress. The finer points of discriminatory capability are lost. We tend to lash out (fight) or tear through the shrubbery (flee). Criminal behavior is just one of the irrational possibilities. Crying spells, irrational fears, paranoia, violence, and wild mood swings are others.

Figures on the relationship of criminal behaviors and allergies are not widely available yet, but there are enough reports of individuals who changed their criminal behavior by avoiding specific trigger foods that thorough studies are warranted.

Mental illness. The relationship between mental illness and allergies has also received little attention, but individual clinical successes indicate that such relationships exist. One of the best known is an allergy to wheat. In certain individuals, the behavioral symptoms brought on by eating wheat-containing foods cannot be distinguished from the classical behavioral signs of schizophrenia. These schizophrenic behaviors completely subside within a few days of completely removing all traces of wheat from the diet of these 'patients'. Another, highly unusual case showed a reaction to very small amounts (drops) of red wine that elicited murderous behavior. This person does not belong in a jail, because he is completely normal as long as he *completely* avoids red wine.

When the underlying malnutrition, allergies, and toxicity are addressed, these conditions, the behaviors they generate, and the people who perform these out-of-control behaviors may settle down, at least in some cases. For these people, nutritional improvement is a cost-effective, humane, and life-transforming possibility well worth a little effort.

79 'Bugs': Candida Yeast, Fungi, Bacteria, and Chronic Fatigue

Our world is teeming with one-celled natural creatures: yeasts, fungi, bacteria, and protozoans. They are present in our soils, on our foods, in our water, and in the air we breathe. We find them on our skin and inside our intestinal tract. They are everywhere. Whether they harm us, help us, or simply leave us alone depends to a large extent on factors that are within our control.

'Bugs' are normal. Normally, most bugs mind their own business and live harmoniously inside or outside of us. A few are always disease-producing. Others attack us only when our body is run down and our immune system is not functioning properly, and it has been suggested that these bugs are scavengers that eat the molecular garbage in our body. Our body also has natural immune mechanisms at its disposal to protect us from being overtaken by these tiny organisms.[1]

In our intestines, yeasts, fungi, and bacteria fulfill normal, natural, even beneficial roles, and most of the time cause us no harm. Natural intestinal mechanisms control their growth and numbers. But bad things can happen when these natural creatures get out of control.

Good nutrition and life-style habits, a strong constitution built from whole, nutrient-rich foods, fresh water, clean air, and sunlight, and a strong, effectively functioning immune system (also made from food, water, air, and light) normally

---

[1] Most bacteria are a few hundred times smaller than cells, viruses a few hundred times smaller than bacteria, and molecules a few hundred times smaller than viruses.

controls internal one-celled organisms and effectively repels and resists external ones.

Thoughtless habits. When we replace health-building habits with convenient or thoughtless ones, we undermine our health, our physical constitution, and the capabilities of our body's natural defense system. We then become prone to infections, and may need to use toxic medicines (drugs) and methods to fight the invaders. Most of these methods and medicines do not strengthen, but further weaken us. They compromise our health and increase our dependence on these toxic substances in much the same way as killing birds and natural predators of insects with poisonous pesticides has made us even more dependent on these poisons for pest control. We have become addicted to them.

Addicts. As a society, we are as addicted to the use of medical drugs and pesticides as any alcohol, cigarette, or drug addict is to *their* poison. Drug-oriented, high-tech medicine seriously undermines the foundations of human health, adds to our toxic load, and produces unwanted side effects that are themselves full-blown diseases.

To break this dependence requires recognition of the danger, commitment to change, and deliberate effort. Withdrawal symptoms (healing reactions) can be expected. They may be worse for a time than the symptoms of the disease they were used to suppress. They can be minimized by high levels of essential nutrients. For people, these include essential fatty acids (EFAs), minerals, vitamins, good protein, and antioxidants (vitamins C and E, carotene, selenium, and sulphur) in larger quantities.

Antibiotics. The wonder drug 'magic bullet' antibiotics kill bacteria that can make us sick when they infect our weakened body, but antibiotics also kill friendly bacteria that keep our intestine healthy. When the friendly ones get killed, yeasts like candida flourish and grow out of control. When this happens, we can experience bloating, gas, intestinal pain, yeast toxin production and absorption, food allergies, deficient immune function, and may eventually succumb to cancer. Antibiotics are often prescribed to combat viral infections such as colds and flus but, while effective against bacteria, antibiotics are completely ineffective against viruses.

The routine use of antibiotics in cattle feeds to increase growth has resulted in another dangerous situation. Bacteria like *E. coli*, normal microorganisms in our intestine, have developed antibiotic-resistant strains that can cause life-threatening disease and has killed some children. Antibiotic-resistant, virulent bacteria have caused several outbreaks of sickness in people eating poorly-prepared hamburgers at some fast food outlets. The issue of resistance to antibiotics – and the failure of our magic bullets – was not clearly explained.

We need to restore the balance of friendly bacteria and yeast in our intestine, rebuild our immune system, and strengthen our body so that it can deal with bugs without outside help or interference. We do this with fresh vegetables, whole grains, wild fish, and organically grown meat (no pesticides, antibiotics, or steroids). Drugs should be used only in life-threatening emergencies.

Fats and bugs

By slowing down stomach emptying time, fats promote more complete digestion and help ensure that no undigested food enters our colon to feed yeasts, fungi, and strange bacteria. Fats and oils also inhibit the growth of fungi and yeasts.

Short-chain fatty acids such as butyric acid (4:0) found in butter serve as food for beneficial bacteria in our intestine. Others, like caprylic acid (8:0) slow down the growth of yeast cells. Researchers believe that yeasts incorporate this fatty acid into their membranes, which thereby weaken and rupture, spilling the yeast's insides, killing it.

EFAs and bugs. EFAs increase metabolic rate by increasing oxidation and metabolic rate. Candida, yeasts, fungi, and some (anaerobic) bacteria thrive in environments with decreased oxidation, lower body temperature, and lower metabolic rate.[2] They dislike oxygen. Increased oxidation inhibits their ability to proliferate out of control.

Besides increasing oxidation rate, metabolic rate, and body temperature, EFAs also:

- enhance immune functions by improving immune cells' ability to produce hydrogen peroxide (made by oxidizing essential fatty acids) that they use to kill bugs;
- speed up the rate of immune reactions;
- help reestablish population control over yeasts like candida that are normally present in our intestinal tract and over bugs that are not normally present; and
- make more energy available for cellular housecleaning;

More specifically, w3 fatty acids have been used in studies to kill both malaria and staph. Even better results can be expected if the treatment consists of a *complete* nutritional package that, besides w3 and w6 EFAs, includes zinc and vitamins A and C, which enhance immune functions, as well as antioxidants that snag free radicals produced by metabolism, bugs, and EFA oxidation.

Other Factors

Certain kinds of *fiber* provide food for beneficial bacteria in our intestines. The most effective kinds of fiber for this purpose include the fiber from okra, psyllium, and flax.

Strong hydrochloric acid in our stomach kills most of the bacteria that we take in with foods. *Zinc* and *protein* are required for its production. *Enzymes* ensure complete digestion of foods. A lack of stomach acid can allow bugs to sur-

---

[2] Fever increases oxidation rate and body temperature, and is one of our body's mechanisms for fighting infections.

vive our stomach and cause problems in our intestinal tract and colon. Lack of enzymes gives bugs more to feed on.

Vitamin C has been used effectively against all viruses and bacteria against which it has been tried. The dose necessary for effective therapy against some viruses may be 30 to 40 grams per day, while that against other viruses may be as high as 100 or even 200 grams per day. If the dose is too low, maximum therapeutic effect is not obtained. Effective dose is determined by 'bowel tolerance' limit, beyond which diarrhea occurs.

Sulphur-containing molecules such as N-acetyl cysteine and sulphur compounds from garlic also have antiviral, antifungal, and antibacterial effects.

A less well known group of substances known as *lignans,* which are most abundant in flax seeds, also have antiviral, antifungal, and antibacterial properties.

Garlic helps deal with infections in several ways: it contains substances that are bacteriocidal; it is rich in selenium and sulphur that act as antioxidants; and it keeps others who could transmit bugs from coming close enough to infect you.

Finally, it must be pointed out that defenses against bugs involve iron, zinc, copper, magnesium, potassium, phosphate, calcium, vitamin A, the B complex, C, D, amino acids, proteins, and essential fatty acids. All must come from foods, and only a nutrient-rich diet provides them in sufficient quantities.

Chronic Fatigue

Chronic fatigue has many possible causes: infection by viruses, fungi, yeasts, or bacteria, as well as allergies. All of these lower immune status. Besides improving nutrition overall, especially by improving digestion and immune support, there are foods to avoid.

Hard and altered fats interfere with oxidation and lower metabolic rate. Processed, nutrient-poor foods increase bug growth because they provide too many calories but too few essential nutrients. Processing also destroys enzymes that help digest the (raw) foods that contain them. Toxins that interfere with oxidation and immune function should be avoided. Foods that produce allergic responses must be better digested or avoided.

Sugars feed yeasts, fungi, and cancer cells. All simple sugars should be avoided for this and other reasons given in other chapters. Soluble fiber discussed above slows down sugar absorption and decreases the sugars available for yeast and fungal growth.

80 *Cancer*

On a nationwide radio talk show hosted by an announcer with strong conservative views, I made the bold statement that cancer could be reversed, and *only* by natural means. He disagreed and challenged me, so I tried to give him the kinds of considerations that are found throughout this book. During commercial breaks, we argued out those objections that we couldn't hash out on the airwaves due to lack of time.

I must confess that I felt overexposed and alone. But then the phones began to ring. During the two-hour show, several people who had cured themselves of cancer by natural means phoned in and briefly told their stories. By the time it was over, even my host was open to the possibility of healing by nature. It was one of my greatest successes in communication. After the second hour, he asked me to stay a third hour. The phones were ringing off the hook.

Thirty-three percent of the U.S. population is diagnosed with cancer at some time during their life. Twenty-three percent of all deaths each year (almost half a million individuals) result from cancer. The total cost for cancer treatments in the U.S. is about $72 billion each year.

Cancer as Fatty Degeneration

Cancer involves fatty degeneration in many different ways. It can be reversed by appropriately enriching our cells with nutrients, and detoxifying them.

Budwig on cancer. Johanna Budwig, a lipid researcher, claims that microscopic studies in the '50s revealed a common feature of all types of cancer cells, confirmed by electron microscopic examinations in France: the presence, within cell plasma and nucleus, of fatty materials that appear not to take part in cell functions, and are not found in healthy cells. Her information is probably incomplete and the picture of fats in cancer more complex. Remember that Budwig did her research in the early 1950s when techniques were rather primitive. Many experiments were carried out more recently, using more sensitive and accurate technical methods.

She also says that hard tumors have a hard, rubbery, sulphur-containing protein core surrounded by oils that cannot form associations with proteins. Belonging together, these two essential nutrients separate because oils are altered by chemical processes including light, oxygen, heat, and hydrogenation. Altered, they are unable to fulfill their protein-associated biological roles.

Budwig considered cancer not as rapid and uncontrolled cell growth, but as retarded cell growth. She claims that rapidly growing tissues always contain higher concentrations of essential fatty acids (EFAs) and sulphur, and always have increased oxygen consumption. In tumors, essential fatty acid concentration and oxygen consumption are always depressed, according to her. She considers tumors to be the result of debris that our cells cannot remove because they lack the energy needed to do so. This energy must be supplied by EFAs, sulphur-containing proteins, and oxygen (along with other essential nutrients).

Updated picture of cancer. Healers generally agree that cancer results from a combination of malnutrition and internal pollution of the cells throughout the entire body. Tumors are the last stage of poisoning that affects the entire organism, manifesting in various locations, before the poisoned body dies. To cure cancer, it is not enough to treat the localized tumorous manifestations. The entire body must be nutritionally enriched and detoxified if cancer is to be permanently reversed.

Healers also agree that cancer usually requires months or years to develop, gradually, through consistent, long-term mistakes in living. Mutations that produce cancerous cells are thought to occur routinely in healthy people, but are neutralized by an uncompromised immune system and therefore can't proliferate. The deterioration of immune function that eventually allows cancer cells to multiply may begin with allergens in foods or air. It may result from chemical toxins, heavy metals, viral or fungal agents, chlorine and other toxic chemicals, X-rays, radioactive elements, high-voltage power lines and other types of electromagnetic radiation, physical or mental stress, isolation, negative attitudes, overexertion, or any other influence that taxes our immune system beyond its capacity to respond. Increased chances of cancer also result from poor food choices that result in malnutrition, nutritional imbalances, or nutritional deficiencies that lower the functional capacities of the cells of our immune system and vital organs.

Most healers further agree that any influence that decreases the functional capacity of our liver increases our risk of cancer. This is because our liver, the main detoxifying organ in our body, must neutralize the toxic materials brought to it through our blood stream and lymphatics by our immune system. When our liver fails to process all that is brought to it, toxins back up in our immune system, which then loses its capacity to deal with more toxic influences. When all of our immune system's garbage trucks are full, so to speak, they cannot be further loaded.

Cancer represents the most extreme form of nutritional collapse. Metabolic rate is decreased. Oxygen uptake is inhibited. Cell division often remains incomplete. The polarity of cells is disrupted and all their functions are crippled. Membranes are defective. Red blood cells fall apart. Cell functions are disorganized.

Microbes and cancer. A number of pioneering researchers from several continents have independently observed that cancer involves the presence of microbes. Drs. Antoine Bechamp (Louis Pasteur's contemporary), Virginia Livingston-Wheeler, Johanna Budwig, Gaston Naessens, Guenther Enderlein, and others are among these researchers. They have had little support from orthodox medicine. Working independently, these researchers have given different names to the microbe involved. Observing them *alive,* these researchers report that like us, the microbes change form during their life cycle (are pleomorphic). They resemble a virus at one stage, a fungus at another, a bacterium at still another, and still other forms in further stages. Some of these changes in form follow changes in the food (medium) on which they grow. Some of the forms of these microbes are benign, while others are disease-producing (virulent). An asparagus medium will produce a benign form while a pork medium will transform the bug into its virulent form.

The virulent bug they observe in cancer, they say, is normally present in our body in its benign form when we are healthy, and probably serves functions that keep us healthy. Virulent bugs can be transformed back into benign bugs if we make our body into a different medium by dietary changes – away from meats and toward vegetables.

One way to maintain health is to adhere to food habits that make our body a medium that is *un*conducive to the development and growth of virulent forms of bugs. This is true not only for cancer, but also for other degenerative conditions involving bugs – including viruses, fungi, yeasts, bacteria, and protozoa. We change the medium of our body by changing our food habits, since our body – *their* food medium – is made from foods. These changes involve moving from meats toward increased use of fresh vegetables and whole grains, from altered fats toward fresh oils, from w9s and w6s toward w3s.

Part of the reason why the pleomorphic view has not been widely accepted is the way in which microbes are observed. In university, we observed dead microbes stained to identify different parts of their cells. We saw them in a static form, which led us to conclude that these 'bugs' *have* only one form (are monomorphic), which *is* true for dead, preserved bugs.[1]

Genes and cancer. Newly identified genetic markers for cancer genes (such as for colon cancer) make high-tech routes of intervention seem attractive,[2] but the nutritional environment is still the most important prevention and reversal factor that we can control. Genes that mediate some cancers, just like viruses that cause others,[3] act one way in a body made from junk food and another way in a body made from nutrient-rich foods. For instance, high levels of antioxidants, especially vitamin C, prevent viruses from being able grow, and vegetarian mediums prevent some cancer microbes from being able to express their virulent forms. This might also be true for cancer genes, but has not been researched

---

[1] Unidentified 'blips' on slides were explained away as 'artifacts' of no importance, without giving them further thought.

[2] Early detection obviously improves five-year survival, but it does not necessarily improve *actual* survival time or length of life. A real increase in survival time takes place only through more effective treatments. Early detection helps in either case. Prevention is even better.

[3] Viruses and genes are similar in that their central nature is genetic material that can replicate.

because it is not high-tech enough to be able to generate large profits.

Several questions need to be answered. What specific molecules turn cancer genes on? What specific molecules turn them off or prevent them from turning on in the first place? What intracellular (intranuclear) molecular conditions trigger their expression? Why don't cancer genes usually express themselves before birth or in infancy but must wait for years of unnatural food and life-style habits before they can come to expression? Why are cancer and food habits and general health associated? Why do some molecules (toxins) cause cancer to grow, while others (nutrients) inhibit its growth? Why, if cancer is genetic, can it sometimes be reversed by nutritional intervention?

Genes must always, and can only express themselves in an environment of molecules. The nature of these molecules determines whether or not they express themselves. We did not choose our genes, but we control their expression through choosing the nature of their molecular environment – our body. We build this molecular environment by choosing what we eat, drink, and breathe in, and by how we live.

Fats and Cancer

The association between fats – meaning saturated fats, refined w6s, rancid fats, processed oils, and altered fats – and cancer, (but excluding w3s and fresh, natural, unrefined oils) has long been documented. Long-chain saturated fatty acids interfere with oxygen use in our cells, as do altered fatty acids and fat products created by processing seed and marine animal oils. Heat, hydrogenation, light, and oxygen produce chemically altered fat products that are toxic to our cells (cytotoxic). Products altered by processing include margarines, shortenings, partially hydrogenated oils, deep-fried oils, refined and deodorized oils, oils exposed to light or oxygen during storage, oils fried in food preparation, and oils that have become rancid from exposure to air after opening. These fats kill people.

The healing fats in cancer include EFAs and the fresh, unrefined oils that contain them. EFAs, especially w3s, enhance oxygen use in cells, decrease tumor formation, slow tumor growth, decrease the spread of cancer cells (metastasis), and extend the patient's survival time. In clinical practice, they are used to help dissolve tumors. W3 EFAs are found in the fresh seeds of flax, hemp, soybean, and walnut, or their fresh oils. Flax is the richest w3 source and the only oil recommended for cancer patients. W3 derivatives are found in oils of fresh, high-fat, cold-water fish (see Chapter 55, Oils from Fish and Seafoods).

Minor natural components in fresh, unrefined, unheated oils may also play important roles in preventing cancer growth. These have not been systematically studied, but processing systematically removes them.

Fats and Mutations

Unsaturated fatty acids in fresh, natural, unheated oils are anti-mutagenic, which means that they protect our genetic material from being attacked by toxic chemicals that cause mutations. Oleic acid (w9), linoleic acid (w6), and alpha-linolenic acid (w3) are all effective. Saturated fatty acids do not have this protective ability.

Heating these oils above 150°C (302°F) makes them lose their protective power, and they become mutation-causing. *All* mass market oils except virgin olive oil have undergone heating during deodorization, which is carried out at above 200°C (392°F) that converts them from protective to destructive. When we use virgin olive or other unrefined oils for sautéeing, frying, or deep-frying, we overheat them, destroying their protective, anti-mutagenic properties.

All hydrogenated and partially hydrogenated products have also been overheated. Cancer patients should therefore avoid all margarines, shortenings, convenience foods containing partially hydrogenated vegetable oils, candies, pastries, fried and deep-fried foods, and bland-tasting, colorless, odorless, refined mass market oils in transparent bottles.

Essential Nutrients and Cancer

Deficiencies of the mineral and vitamin co-factors, which protect EFAs from damage and metabolize fatty acids and sugars, slow down oxygen use within cells. Several B-complex vitamins, and the minerals potassium, magnesium, and manganese are used in the production of energy by oxidation within our cells, and iodine (in thyroid hormone) increases metabolic rate by increasing oxidation rate. Vitamins E and A protect the integrity of EFAs and cell membranes. Vitamins C, B_3, and B_6, the antioxidant proteins using minerals zinc, manganese, and copper as co-factors, as well as selenium and sulphur-containing amino acids prevent oxidation of cholesterol and fatty acids and facilitate the production of prostaglandins. Iron allows hemoglobin to carry oxygen to all our cells, but an excess of free iron and copper increases the damage that oxygen can do to oils.

Our immune system, which is vital for destroying cancer cells, requires EFAs, vitamins C, B_6, and A, and zinc to function, and requires an exceptionally rich nutrient supply of *all* essential nutrients for its high level of complex cellular activities.

Deficiencies of EFAs and toxic, man-made synthetic drugs that interfere with essential fatty acid functions can create the conditions of fatty degeneration collectively known as cancer.

Animal studies carried out before 1965 had already shown that, besides deficiency of EFAs, low levels of any one of the following can cause, enhance, or be associated with the growth of cancer cells: vitamins A, B_2, B_6, D, and E, pantothenic acid, choline, copper, iodine, methionine, essential amino acids, and protein. Liver damage, refined w6s, hard fats, margarines and shortenings, and fried fats were also known to be associated with the growth of cancer before 1965. This is not new information.

Since 1965, carotene, the rest of the B-complex, bioflavonoids, vitamin C, glutathione, cysteine, fiber, fish and flax oils, magnesium, potassium, selenium, zinc, acidophilus bacteria, digestive enzymes and immune system- and liver function-enhancing herbs have been added to the list of nutrients that protect against, and help reverse, cancer. The newest member of the promising natural substances is shark cartilage extract, administered rectally.

Otto Warburg, a Nobel prize-winning researcher, discovered in the 1920s that by depriving tissues of oxygen (35% less than normal), he could induce cancer in tissues almost at will.

Poisons. Toxic influences work against our immune system and liver, and can lead to cancer. Examples of such influences include antibiotics, cortisone, many drugs, pesticides, heavy metals, smoke, alcohol, synthetic chemicals, and other toxins.

Allergies. Often overlooked, foods that produce allergic reactions are one of the greatest stresses on our immune system. When our immune system's load, from all sources of stress combined, becomes greater than its capacity to deal with these stresses, cancer cells can escape its control and then the manifestations of cancer become likely.

Cancer Can Be Reversed

There are now many natural protocols for reversing cancer. All include fresh vegetables and whole grains, and decreased consumption of animal products. All avoid altered and hard fats. All avoid processed foods containing white flour, white sugar, and 'white' oils. All forbid coffee, tobacco, and alcohol. All make liberal use of fresh carrot juice. Vitamins C and B_3, potassium, and iodine are particularly important in addition to w3 EFAs. Some herbal programs bring results in some cancers. Digestive enzymes are commonly used in natural and orthomolecular treatments of cancer.

Successful reversals of cancers, in which cancer totally disappeared and the person was still alive and cancer-free 10, 20, 30, and even 40 years after the diagnosis of 'terminal' cancer was made, have been documented.

Contrast this with the medical definition of 'cancer cure', which means: still alive five years after the initial diagnosis was made. According to one source, this has now been reduced to three years. When a person 'cured' of cancer (as documented in medical literature) dies of cancer in the sixth (or fourth) year, one cannot *realistically* call that a cure.

Documented cancer reversals with natural treatments include all types of cancers. Melanoma and lung cancer, which kill most quickly, have been cured. Brain tumors have been taken apart molecule by molecule, leaving no scars, by the body's own healing mechanisms when given the materials necessary to do this work. Pancreatic, colon, breast, ovarian, uterine, liver, and bone cancers have been completely reversed. Carcinomas, sarcomas, gliomas, and skin cancers have been reversed.

These results are accomplished by supporting healthy cells, liver, and immune system with nutrient-rich, non-toxic foods and practices that help the body rid itself of toxins that have built up in cells and tissues. Healthy cells know how to deal with cancer. Supply the body with its requirements as determined by nature, and you reestablish its natural state of functioning, which is health.

Point of No Return

Not all cancers can still be reversed by natural (or any other) means. If vital organs have been destroyed by cancer, they fail, and cancer kills. No one knows exactly when that point has come, so cancer patients should neither write themselves off, nor take recovery for granted, even though remarkable recoveries are possible. Cancer must be taken very seriously.

Some key points. If the liver has been destroyed by cancer, toxins, radiation, or drugs, it can no longer detoxify our body. In this case, remission may still take place, but reversal or cure of cancer is unlikely.

Don't expect to *cure* cancer with radioactivity (X-rays, gamma-rays, or rays from radioactive cobalt, cesium, iodine, radium, gold, or other element) that is known to *cause* cancer. While these rays *do* kill cancer cells, they also harm normal ones, making them new sources of toxicity and cancer. Their use constitutes dangerous practice.[4]

Don't expect chemotherapy drugs to cure cancers. These drugs are liver-toxic, work against the body's defenses, and make healing cancer even more difficult than it already is. While they can shrink tumors, they increase the total toxic burden of an already poisoned body. Their success rate is poor. People who get *no* treatment survive as long as those treated with chemo. Chemo drugs are not proven but experimental. You are the guinea pig. Drug companies profit. Toxic treatments should be avoided if at all possible, and used only as a last resort.

---

[4] Three anecdotes of carelessness in the use of these rays:
- When we emigrated from Europe to North America in 1952, we had to have a 'medical examination'. I remember my mother standing behind a screen, and us children wide-eyed with fascination. We could see her ribs, her skull, her teeth, and the bones in her arms, legs, and pelvis. Another view of mother! The doctor proudly declared that she had eaten cabbage that day, because radio-opaque cabbage showed up on his screen. The X-ray and his explanation took about 5 minutes (rather than present-day X-ray exposure of a fraction of a second). What damage was done in that time?
- I remember watching the bones in my feet move as I wiggled my toes inside new shoes. Instead of *asking* how they fit, X-rays were used – no need for the shoe salesman to communicate.
- The first woman I loved (after my mother) was born with a birthmark on the upper eyelid of her right eye. Doctors burned the birthmark off with a piece of (radioactive) radium taped to her eyelid. The birthmark is gone, but so is most of the vision in her right eye because the radioactive rays emitted by the radium also burned her retina.

Summary

Cancer, a serious condition that needs serious attention, is our body's way of letting us know that we have neglected ourselves too long and must start making life-affirming changes.

Natural treatments should be tried before toxic ones. At the first diagnosis of cancer, a serious program of natural therapy should be undertaken. Foods, water, air, and light should all be cleaned up. Toxic light, air, water, and foods must be avoided. Beliefs and life-style need to be examined and, where necessary for healing, changed. Many people with cancer have poor self-esteem, and put out more effort than they have energy for, to prove to others that they are worthy. They literally kill themselves for others. No 'other' is worth this kind of slow suicide. From nature's point of view, we are worthwhile because we are alive.

Finally, remember also that the human body *is* a terminal condition. We are all *terminally* alive. Because the body was born, it will one day die. We must come to terms with this fact.

If the diagnosis of 'terminally ill' has forced us to re-think our priorities for living, it has served a valuable purpose. Positive changes in how we appreciate that time, how we think, and eat, and act are likely to follow. Some of these changes may even bring us back to health and postpone our eventual termination.

AIDS **81**

AIDS or *acquired* immune deficiency syndrome – that kills about 50,000 individuals a year (in 1993) – results from a shutdown of the immune system. Note that the name indicates that the condition is not genetic but acquired – due to non-genetic (environmental) causes. Hence they should respond to environmental interventions that include changes in both nutrition and life-style. Causes of AIDS (besides the AIDS virus that gets so much attention, and unprotected sex, needle sharing, and tainted blood transfusions that spread it) include inadequate nutrition, use of immunosuppresive drugs and other toxins, opportunistic infections by other foreign organisms, stress, immune inhibition caused by sperm released during anal intercourse near lymphatics that circle the inside of the human anus,[1] and other life-style factors over which we can exercise control.

Regardless of whether AIDS is caused by a virus, or the virus is weak and kills only a body ravaged by other destructive influences, or whether the AIDS virus was

---

[1] The immuno-suppressiveness of sperm helps make pregnancy possible. Without it, the woman's immune system would attack and reject the 'foreign' tissue that constitutes sperm cells, and that would be the end of future generations.

spread through contaminated vaccines produced in a World Health Organization laboratory, or is part of a conspiracy to control the world (or gay) population, or came from African green monkeys, or is just syphilis unrecognized by a medical profession that thought it had conquered that disease with antibiotics and now is no longer trained to recognize its symptoms – all these suggestions have been advanced by various groups or individuals – or none of the above, AIDS shows what can happen when our immune system fails in its functions.

It is a clear reminder to keep our body strong, Like most other degenerative diseases, AIDS has no *medical* cure.

Oils and AIDS

Like cancer, AIDS responds to natural treatments and nutrient enrichment. In California, one clinic uses about 120 grams (8.5 tablespoons [4 ounces]) of flax oil per day in its treatments, along with a complete program of large doses of all other essential nutrients, many in supplement form. Although it is too early to say for sure, they appear to be successfully prolonging survival.

The exact mechanism for flax oil's action is not yet clear, but answers may be found in its ability to increase oxidation, increase peroxidation (which kills cancer cells and infectious microorganisms), develop cell membrane functions, and form prostaglandins.

One should expect w3 oils, sulphur (from garlic, N-acetyl cysteine, or reduced L-glutathione), and large amounts of vitamin C to be particularly effective in slowing down the deterioration of AIDS patients, since AIDS patients usually succumb to infectious organisms. Oil and sulphur are effective against yeasts, fungi, and bacteria. Vitamin C in large enough doses is effective against viruses and bacteria. Other antioxidants should also be helpful. Immune system-enhancing herbs should also be used.

Clinical Experience

Researchers in nutrition recommend keeping the body saturated with antioxidants (AOs), because AOs prevent viruses associated with immune deficiency from being able to replicate in our cells. Those at risk for or fearing infection with the AIDS virus should also keep their body saturated with AOs in whose presence the viruses cannot replicate.

Mainstream medicine is fooling around with high-tech methods for stopping the AIDS epidemic. So far, they have had little success. Perhaps the approach is wrong. Strengthening the body is easier – although less financially rewarding for doctors and drug companies – than finding yet another patentable magic bullet for a virus that, like flu and cold viruses, seems to be able to mutate almost at will, faster than we can develop new vaccines in our laboratories.

Joan Priestley, a clinician practicing in California, who has treated several dozen AIDS patients, claims that if the patients stay on her regime of complete, high-dose mineral, vitamin, and essential fatty acid enrichment, they can continue to live even though their immune system (specifically their T-cells) remains non-functional. The nutritional program does not rebuild their destroyed immune cells.

Defense and Healing Hierarchy?

Priestley's clinical observations suggest an interesting and important possibility: that our body's defenses are organized as a hierarchy of several levels.

At the bottom of the hierarchy is hygiene: clean food, clean water, clean air, 'clean' light, clean surroundings in which to live, and disposal of wastes and pollutants in ways that keep disease-producing microorganisms (viruses, fungi, bacteria, protozoa) from multiplying and then taking hold. With specific regard to AIDS, it means abstinence or safe sex.

The second level of the hierarchy is direct protection by nutrients from foods. This includes especially vitamin C, but also other antioxidants (AOs): carotene, vitamin E, sulphur, selenium, bioflavonoids, and other AOs naturally present in foods. These AOs protect our cells by neutralizing free radicals, oxidation products, and microorganisms (viruses, fungi, bacteria, protozoa) and making survival of foreign (pathogenic) microorganisms in our body impossible.

The third level includes several factors made by our body. On the one hand, our cells make AO proteins such as catalases and superoxide dismutase (SOD) from amino acids supplied by foods. These proteins use essential nutrients such as zinc, manganese, and copper (from foods) in their activity. Our cells use essential fatty acids (EFAs) from foods to make peroxides that kill foreign microorganisms. Chelating agents such as sulphur- and selenium-containing amino acids from foods grab toxic materials (they work like pliers or claws) and remove them from our body with wastes. There are many others.

A fourth level of protection is our cell membranes, barriers made from foods that can help keep toxins and organisms from entering our cells while allowing nutrients to enter and metabolic wastes to exit. These are made from EFAs, other fatty acids, cholesterol, proteins, vitamin E and carotene. Foods supply all the components of membranes.

A fifth level of complexity involves regulating substances – hormones – whose building blocks are nutritional. These are made by our cells (prostaglandins) or by special glands in response to triggering conditions in our body. Hormones speed up or slow down chemical reactions necessary for normalizing abnormal conditions in our body. For instance, infectious agents stimulate the production of pituitary and thyroid hormones that increase oxidation and metabolic rate, which speed up chemical reactions.[2] We experience this as the 'fever

---

[2] *Cold water*, properly used, also stimulates hypothalamus, pituitary, thyroid, and sex glands. It improves circulation, enhances immune function, helps alleviate PMS and menopausal flashes, increases vitality, rejuvenates, and improves general health.

that breaks the infection'. When modern medicines are used to bring down a fever, they interfere with our body's defense system. This is wise only if the fever is life-threatening.

A sixth level of complexity in our body's defenses is cellular, involving specialized cells made by our immune system. Immune cells are made from nutrients, and use nutrients in special ways as weapons to protect the integrity of our body. They engulf toxins and organisms, kill the latter with oxygen, peroxides, or enzymes, digest them, and transport the debris to lymph glands for filtering, further processing, and recycling. These cells can also make specific proteins that recognize, react with, and neutralize toxic materials and foreign organisms, and then digest or transport these materials for further processing.

A seventh level of complexity in defense organization is our liver (also made from food), a factory in which thousands of chemical reactions take place. These reactions include normal metabolic changes, but also involve filtering out and further processing toxic materials brought to it by our immune system. Once chemicals have been processed to neutralize or minimize their harmfulness, these materials are dumped into our intestine with bile, and leave our body with stool.

A Pyramid of Food

As complex as this healing pyramid is, every atom, molecule, and energy dynamic of its makeup comes from food, water, air, and light. Every part of this system completely depends on the presence of adequate amounts of the 50 essential factors in order to fulfill its health-protecting functions, and must be kept as free as possible of toxic interfering influences in order to function at optimum levels.

No matter what the offending substance in degenerative conditions – free radical, toxic molecule, virus, fungus, bacterium, protozoan, sliver, cut, or break – food, water, air, and light are the foundation of *all* our body's defenses and healing mechanisms. This is why AIDS can (and *must* ultimately) be stopped, prevented, and cured with nutrients, orthomolecular substances, and other natural means. The health of all cells and all levels of our body's defense capabilities depend on them.

82 *Auto-Immune Conditions*

Auto-immune conditions include multiple sclerosis, Hashimoto's disease, juvenile onset diabetes, glomerular nephritis, some forms of arthritis, and many rare and difficult conditions. These may be genetic in origin, or may begin with food allergies due to poor nutrition and/or stress at any time in life, from prenatal through adulthood. There may be some hope even for these difficult conditions.

It has now been suggested that juvenile diabetes starts with an allergy to whey protein in cow's milk. When undigested whey protein gets into a child's body, its immune system produces antibodies against this foreign protein; these antibodies neutralize whey protein every time it enters the child's body undigested. But the antibodies against whey protein also attack the body's own proteins in pancreatic cells that produce insulin (islets of Langerhans), because islet cells contain proteins that resemble the antibody-initiating stretch in whey protein. Niacinamide (a form of vitamin B₃) slows down the destruction of islet cells, but the damage would be better *prevented,* by nutrients that support the complete digestion of proteins, preventing the absorption of undigested whey protein in the first place. Avoidance of dairy products would be a second way to prevent the problem from being able to occur – three-quarters of the world's population is dairy-free without suffering malnutrition.

Similarly, antibodies that were originally made by our immune system against proteins that got into our system undigested and were recognized as foreign, may attack the body's own proteins with similar structures in the thyroid gland (Hashimoto's disease), nerve sheaths (multiple sclerosis), kidney tubules (glomerular nephritis), and other cells, tissues, and organs.

Permanent Destruction

Once a set of cells with specific functions has been completely destroyed, it cannot be repaired, and the function of that set of cells must then be taken over by externally injected materials or high-tech life support systems.

It is therefore important that auto-immune attack be prevented altogether, or detected and stopped before a set of cells is completely destroyed.

A high-tech solution after permanent destruction of islet cells makes use of transplants of encapsulated islet cells from animals. The capsules keep the human body from rejecting the transplanted tissue by preventing immune cells from being able to make contact with the islet cells but allowing the insulin made by these cells to leave the capsules to fulfill its functions in the body. In future, similar methods may replace tissue that has been surgically removed, destroyed by toxicity, or destroyed by our own immune system. While this is an intelligent high-tech development, *preventing* the problem by supporting health from the beginning is a cleaner and less costly route.

Role of Fats and EFAs

Fats may play a role by slowing stomach emptying, improving digestion, and leaving less undigested protein against which antibodies can be made.

EFAs may help by building better membranes and preventing undigested proteins from getting into our body. They may also protect certain proteins from auto-attack by physically associating with these proteins.

Allergy Prevention

The program described in Chapter 77 can help eliminate foods incompatible with our digestive system, foods against which our body may make antibodies because it cannot digest them properly.

It is wise to start such a program as early in a person's life as possible, to prevent the problem from arising in the first place. Even if this program was not started early, starting later may still help. If our body continues to be challenged by food antigens, it keeps the standing immune army on red alert. Many immune system soldiers are trained, and some of them may mistakenly attack the wrong side: tissue proteins in our own cells. In war, this is called 'friendly fire'. This is not meant to imply that it is a friendly kind of fire, but that one is being fired upon by friends. Auto-immune diseases are this kind of situation.

Auto-Immune Reversal?

Auto-immune diseases are considered irreversible. Once an organ, tissue, or cell type has been *completely* destroyed by auto-immune friendly fire, it is (obviously) beyond repair. But there may be some hope for people who are at the beginning of an auto-immune deterioration, because the process of auto-immune destruction takes time to be completed.

If the condition is triggered by food allergies, and one removes the offending foods from one's diet, eventually the standing army of antibodies may be taken down for lack of work. Antibody (missile) factories and immune cell (army) bases might be taken down when they are not needed. This would take time and persistence, but should be successful in at least some cases of auto-immune disorder.

Basic factors vital to any possible recovery include nutritional improvement, nutrient enrichment, supplementation with digestive enzymes, stress reduction, removal of allergens, detoxification, and changes in understanding and life-style.

Prevention?

When we live in line with nature, we attain the most positive possible results in *any* condition that faces us, up to the optimum that our genetic endowment allows. Most people will not require special high-tech help.

The time and care now given to those whose problems result from self-neglect could be given to those who, due to unfortunate genetic circumstances, require that help. If we refuse to look after our own biology and health, we deprive those who *need* that extra help.

This chapter gives helpful hints for multiple sclerosis, cystic fibrosis, fatty degeneration of liver, kidneys, and other organs, glandular atrophy, gall and kidney stones, and mineral metabolism. All can be helped with better nutrition.

For these and all degenerative conditions, a complete and balanced program of optimum nutrition will optimize our body's ability to function. In addition, there are specific hints for each of these conditions.

Rare Conditions of Fatty Degeneration

Multiple sclerosis (MS) is fatty degeneration. In one study, people who got MS were eating diets high in white bread, biscuits, cheese, pies, and prepared foods. None ate liver and only 2 out of 67 ate fish and fresh green vegetables more than once a month. In places where essential fatty acid (EFA) consumption is high, multiple sclerosis is rare. People with MS use essential fatty acids to arrest or slow the deterioration of nerve fibers that slowly destroys their nervous systems. After diagnosis, the sooner treatment with EFAs and diet begins, the better the outlook for the sufferer.

MS has been successfully treated with whole-foods diets (fresh vegetables and whole grains) with the addition of fresh, unrefined sunflower and/or flax oils. Evening primrose oil (refined) has also been used in MS treatment programs. Unrefined safflower and sesame oils should also work. The key criterion is that the oils are fresh and unrefined. Nutrient enrichment and supplementation are also helpful. Anecdotal evidence exists for the regeneration of nerves by octacosanol, a 28-carbon alcohol present in wheat germ oil.

Fresh juices, digestive enzymes, antioxidants, and balanced supplements will also help.

Cystic fibrosis (CF) is fatty degeneration, at least partly due to a genetic mutation. The body is unable to properly change the essential linoleic acid (LA, 18:2w6) into more highly unsaturated fatty acids, and there appears to be interference with the production of prostaglandins.

In CF, cells produce a thick mucus that clogs lungs and respiratory passages, and also interferes with digestion of foods and absorption of nutrients. EFAs can help make mucus more liquid. Nutrient enrichment is important. Increased intake of water may also be helpful, as well as mucilage fiber from flax and psyllium. But none of these are a cure for the genetic condition that produces the problems of CF.

Intravenous nutrient enrichment on a regular basis may also be helpful.

Glandular atrophy can result from deficiency of EFAs, which are necessary to produce the secretions of our glands, the mucus that lines the air passage to our lungs, and the lubrication for the lining of our joints. These conditions therefore belong to fatty degeneration. The mineral and vitamin co-factors of EFA metabolism should be part of a treatment program.

Other Conditions

The most common type of **gall** and **kidney stones** results from diets too high in the hard, sticky saturated fats and cholesterol. Fried fats and oxidized cholesterol can help gall and kidney stones. Processed, oxidized, and fried polyunsaturated oils can also enhance stone formation. Excess calcium, and/or deficiency of magnesium and vitamin B_6 may also be involved. A person with these problems needs to avoid saturated and altered fats: animal fats, butter, shortenings, and margarine. The stones are slowly dissolved by a reduction in hard and altered fats, an increase in the use of fresh, EFAs-containing oils, and lots of liquid.

Gall and kidney stones also respond to increased intake of magnesium and vitamin B_6, increased fiber and water, supplementation with taurine and glycine, and malic and other organic acids. Hydrangea herb is also used in some treatments. The best cure is prevention. Don't wait for stones – do it now!

Fatty degeneration of inner organs – liver (cirrhosis), kidneys, heart, and brain – can come from hard fats, *trans-* fatty acids, altered fats, fried oils, and many toxic substances. The solutions have been discussed in other places in this book.

Calcium metabolism is closely linked to EFA metabolism. This makes calcium problems at least a first cousin to diseases of fatty degeneration. Fatty acids are also involved with the metabolism of other minerals. This area needs a lot of further study.

Cellulite is another member of the family of fatty degeneration. Cellulite fat results from lack of exercise and poor diet. It is not different from other fats, except for the possibility of the presence of toxins in fat tissues.

Problems of **sense organ** function may result from lack of the high-energy w3 fatty acids our senses need for their very active metabolism. Use of good oils may improve vision, hearing, and mental clarity.

Every **organ** in our body is bathed in its own supply of liquid high-energy oils when it is healthy. Our *eyes* float in an oil bath. Our *kidneys* sit in their own 'oil can'. Our *heart* is surrounded by its oil supply of EFAs. Our *ears'* source of energy sits in close proximity to our inner ear. *Bone marrow* cells rely on a stored fat supply in our bones. Our *liver* requires a supply of EFAs in order to function. Lack of EFAs in the diet, wrong fats, altered fats, and lack of other essential nutrients all impair the functions of these and other organs.

Brown skin spots called **aging spots** or 'cemetery flowers' indicate fatty degeneration. These become especially pronounced on parts of our body that are exposed to direct sunlight frequently, like the back of our hands, our bald spot, and our face. These spots also indicate deficiency of the antioxidants vitamin E and/or selenium.

Depositions of fatty material on our eyelids or on the white of our **eyeballs** are signs of fatty degeneration. There are several different types of these deposits. Appropriate changes in oils, nutritional habits, and essential nutrient balance can help deal with these.

For most of these diseases, modern medicine has no cure. Affected parts can be surgically removed, burned by radiation, chemically treated, or 'zapped' with ultrasound. But without knowing their cause, these conditions cannot be reversed. All are largely due to malnutrition and/or internal poisoning. The best treatment is simply to return to living in balance with our nature and its nutritional requirements for health.

Aging and Longevity 84

The quality of diets and life-styles can shorten or lengthen the human life span. Diets high in fats speed up the rate at which children mature. The average age of first menstruation (menarche) in girls during the 17th century was 17 years old, on a diet containing about 20% fat. The present average age of first menstruation is 13 years old, on a diet containing 42% fat.

Faster Growth Rate
High-fat diets increase growth rate and adult body size. This is one reason why physical stature of human beings has increased over the last 100 years. It also explains why Japanese people who live in Japan are shorter on the average than Caucasians. Their diet contains about 15% fat, compared to ours at over 40%. When Japanese people and members of other racial groups come to North America and adopt Western food habits, the next generation becomes taller. In Japan, diets have increased in fat content, and Japanese in Japan are also growing taller now.

Shorter Life Span
Earlier maturity and taller stature are balanced by shorter life span. People on high-fat diets burn out quicker.

Aging. One theory to explain aging suggests that oxygen and free radicals (see Chapter 21, Light, Free Radicals, and Oils) produced from fats in our body cross-link genetic material, proteins, sugars with proteins, and connective tissues, and also produce toxic chemicals that hinder metabolism.

Aging also results from an accumulation of toxic breakdown products of normal metabolism, which slow down or clog up the wheels of our body chemistry, interfere with enzyme functions and slow down these wheels until they stop (and we die).

Still others talk about biological aging clocks, which run down like the spring in a watch. When our spring runs down, however, unlike the watch, we don't get rewound. We get recycled back to soil, water, and air.

Free radicals are involved in aging. Metabolites are also involved. The presence of each enhances the production of the other. Like chicken and egg, it's impossible to say which one came first, because both refer to the same total process. The production of metabolites involves biochemical reactions whose intermediates are free radicals.

Sugar. Refined sugars shorten life span, partly through their tendency to produce fats. They rob our body of minerals (especially chromium, potassium, magnesium, and zinc) and vitamins (especially Bs). They prevent mobilization of essential fatty acids from storage. They stress our pancreas and adrenal glands. They produce hard fats and cholesterol that interfere with insulin function, inhibit our immune system, interfere with the transport of vitamin C, feed yeasts (such as candida), feed bacteria that produce acid which dissolves the minerals in our teeth, and cross-link skin proteins, causing wrinkling. They also produce free radicals that may escape from confinement and cause random, degenerative reactions.

Exclusion of refined sugars from our diet slows aging and lengthens life span. Restriction of calories also slows aging. Rats on calorie-restricted diets without sugar live 50% longer.

Slow down aging. The presence of antioxidants (AOs) and other essential nutrients slow down the aging process. Vitamins C and B_3 have been shown to increase human life spans by six and two years, respectively, and chromium can extend animal life spans (not yet tested in humans) by 33%.

Other AOs can also be considered anti-aging nutrients. Selenium, vitamin E, carotene, sulphur, bioflavonoids, and several other minerals take part in antioxidant functions.

The use of flax grain (freshly ground, 1 tablespoon per day) is associated traditionally and anecdotally with long life, although no controlled studies have been done. Its fiber, lignans, and w3 fatty acids may all be involved in its effectiveness.

Diet Manipulation

If you want tall children who will live for a long time, feed them a high-fat diet while young, and teach them to eat a lower-fat, no-sugar diet as adults. In nature, infant mammals (including us) are fed breast milk containing about 4% fat, which constitutes just over 50% of human breast milk's calories. As young animals mature, they benefit from being switched to lower-fat (grass for cows, vegetables for humans) diets.

If you want children to mature more slowly, raise them on a lower-fat, no sugar diet from the time of weaning. But don't overdo it.

Caution: Infants *require* fat to grow. Parents who feed their babies low-fat

Pritikin-type diets – skim milk, vegetables, and no fats – find that these babies fail to thrive, and have dry skin. When overambitious adults impose no-fat diets on infants, these infants can also develop allergies.

Dietary manipulation is common in nature. Bee larvae that are fed one kind of food become sterile workers who die after six weeks. Bee larvae that are fed royal jelly become queens that live up to eight very productive years.

Dietary manipulation certainly works for humans. It can prevent and reverse degenerative diseases. It can build health. In so doing, it can extend both the quality *and* quantity of our life.

Longevity

A long life span is the cumulative result of doing a lot of little things right. It results from a balance of the following factors:

- fuels that build the fire of life necessary to keep cells active and clean;
- antioxidants that provide spark control;
- avoidance of external and internal toxic influences
- digestive efficiency;
- optimally functioning bowel flora;
- the right kinds of fiber that keep our colon clean;
- clean water to drink and bathe in;
- clean air;
- sunlight;
- physical activity that keeps our body fit;
- rest and relaxation;
- challenges worth meeting;
- good feeling about oneself;
- positive goals and constructive activities;
- mutually supportive relationships;
- a clean and natural environment;
- independence in thinking and livelihood;
- emotionally healthy beliefs;
- a sense of humor;
- faith in nature, life, and the human body;
- enjoyment of our own life;
- positive regard for life in general.

Obviously, nobody scores perfect on all of these factors. Each of us can identify for ourselves those factors on this list that need the most work. We can challenge ourselves to make the necessary improvements in all areas, beginning with those most likely to bring the greatest positive returns for our effort.

85 *Infants and Oils*

Low-fat diets for infants can seriously harm their health. There are healing fats and killing fats in infant nutrition. In our craze to lower the fat content of our diets for health reasons, overambitious parents sometimes do their children's health a (well-meant) disservice when, misinformed by media and medicine, they place them on low-fat or fat-free diets.

Seeds of Health – Good Foods Make Smart Babies

The 'seeds' of good adult health are sown before conception, during pregnancy, and during infancy. *All* of these 'seeds' of good health are nutritional, because our body is made from foods, water, and air. To begin life in good health, foods must be nutrient-rich and toxin-free, and water and air must be free of pollutants and poisons. Given these conditions, the genetic material of the fetus, infant, and child builds a body that is optimally normal and healthy.

Prenatal. Before birth, the unborn child is *completely* dependent for its health and normal development on its mother's habits. A mother attending to her own optimum health needs – nutrient-rich, toxin-free, allergen-free nutrition – is in the best position to give birth to a healthy child.

A mother who neglects her own health may thereby deform her baby for life. For instance, *dietary deficiency* of folic acid (a B vitamin) increases the chances of her baby being born with a neural tube defect (spina bifida). Deficiencies of w3 fatty acids can lead to permanent learning disabilities because of their importance in brain development and functions, as shown in animal studies. Lack of other vital nutrients can negatively affect fetal development in other ways, specific to the functions for which that nutrient is needed during the complex sequence of developmental processes and events.

Toxic substances can lead to congenital deformation and subnormal intelligence that will limit the child for life – and could have been avoided. The most common toxic influence is Fetal Alcohol Syndrome (FAS), where afflicted infants have widely spaced eyes and suffer mental deficiencies.[1] Mercury poisoning can also bring about physical deformation and permanent brain damage. Lead toxicity results in decreased intelligence. Pharmacological drugs can interfere in many ways with fetal development, and may result in miscarriage as well as deformation and mental deficiency. Even lack of arms has resulted from the interference of drugs with developmental events (thalidomide). Pregnant women should use no drugs at all, if possible.

---

[1] Alcohol is so toxic that, to protect their unborn child, mothers-to-be should *completely* abstain from alcohol.

380

If the mother eats foods to which she is allergic, these take a toll on her nutritional and immune status, and may also produce toxic substances. All of these can negatively affect the health of the child she carries.

Mother's milk. More than 50% of the calories contained in a mother's breast milk come from the fats her milk contains. Mother's milk is by no means a low-fat product. Babies need this fat in order to grow optimally.

The fatty acid composition of her milk reflects the fatty acids consumed by the mother. Measurements show that human breast milk can contain as little as 1% linoleic acid (African women on high carbohydrate, low-fat diets), and as much as 15% (Jordanian women on high-polyunsaturate diets). In studies, w3s in breast milk have been increased from 0.1% to 4.8% by feeding the mothers 47 grams of marine oils for 8 days, showing that milk fat content responds rapidly to dietary changes.

If the mother's diet contains both essential fatty acids (EFAs) in their natural form (from seeds or fresh, unrefined oils), their presence in her body will be accompanied by the natural 'minor' components that seeds and unrefined oils contain (see Chapter 54, Virgin Olive Oils). These substances play protective and health-promoting roles in the body.

Minerals and vitamins are also passed to the newborn child through her milk, to the extent that they are optimally present in her body through her food choices. Iron is an exception. Mother's milk is iron-poor. This protects the newborn from damaging pro-oxidant reactions that iron can have. Adequate iron in the mother's diet builds iron reserves in the fetus that will last for the first six months of the newborn's life, until its digestive system has developed the ability to digest solid foods.

Fats for Infants

Before birth, the fetus is fed through the umbilical cord, and nutrients from the mother's blood are passed into the infant's blood. The fetal digestive system is inactive until after birth. A newborn infant adapts to oral feeding within a few weeks. In those weeks, bile secretion from the liver and fat-digesting enzyme secretion from the pancreas develop. During this time, the fats provided should be easily digestible. Mother's milk is perfect for the infant's needs. It contains fat-splitting enzymes which, since it is an unheated product, remain active (pasteurization would destroy their activity). These enzymes, even though they are made of protein, resist digestion by the infant's stomach acid.

Unlike adults, who digest fats mainly in their small intestine with enzymes produced by their pancreas, infants also produce fat-digesting enzymes in their salivary glands (responsible for 20 to 30% of their total fat digestion) and in glands lining their stomach (responsible for 50 to 70% of their total fat digestion). These enzymes also resist stomach acidity.

Improved digestion. Fats and oils increase the time that foods spend in the stomach, resulting in better digestion of proteins. Dietary fats and oils thereby make the infant less likely to develop allergies in response to absorption of undigested or incompletely digested proteins. Both saturated and unsaturated fats help digestion in this regard, but unsaturated fats (oils) are better for health because of their content of essential fatty acids (EFAs).

EFAs influence the structure of the cells lining the intestinal tract, as well as the 'villi' through which absorption of nutrients takes place. They increase the thickness and surface area of the digestive-absorptive cells that line the inside of our intestine. This results in more effective digestion, better absorption of nutrients, less absorption of allergens, and better health.

The fats an infant needs *must* contain EFAs – linoleic (w6) and alpha-linolenic (w3) acids – as well as non-essential fatty acids. These are necessary to construct the cell membranes of all cells. They are also important for the functions of enzymes embedded in membranes, which transport substances in and out of cells, and in and out of subcellular organelles, affecting the efficiency of energy production (mitochondria), and the production of proteins (movement of ribonucleic acid [RNA] across the nuclear envelope). They are also necessary for the development of brain and nerve cells and for healthy liver function.

Deficiency. W6 EFA deficiency symptoms in a study of children included failure to thrive, diarrhea, skin problems, poor hair growth, and poor utilization of food energy. W3 deficiency symptoms included neurological and visual abnormalities. Besides preventing the effects of the deficiencies listed above, EFA-containing oils also appear to protect infants from developing food intolerances and allergies.

Oil Choices

Mothers-to-be and breast-feeding mothers should take particular care to choose fresh, EFA-rich, balanced, unrefined oils. Hemp oil is well-balanced, with w3 and w6 in a good ratio, and contains gamma-linolenic acid (GLA) as well. Flax can enrich a diet that has been lacking w3. Soybeans also contain both EFAs. A mixture of flax seeds with sunflower or sesame seeds can be used to balance w3 and w6 EFAs. Virgin olive oils are good for other reasons, but contain too little w3. They can be mixed 50:50 with flax or hemp seed oil to improve their EFA profile. Most other oils contain too much w6 and too little w3.

Margarines, shortenings, and partially hydrogenated oils (which contain *trans-* fatty acids), and fried and deep-fried oils and refined mass-market oils (which contain altered, toxic fatty acid derivatives) should all be avoided before conception, during pregnancy, while lactating, and forever. If the mother consumes them, they show up in her breast milk. *Trans-* fatty acids and altered fatty acid derivatives can have many deleterious influences on cell membranes, brain development, cardiovascular system, liver, and immune system of mother, fetus, infant, and child.

Baby Foods

Mother's milk ranges from 3 to 6% fat (averaging about 3.5%), but this fat makes up about half of its calories. The rest of the calories come from carbohydrates (mother's milk tastes sweeter than cow's milk) and proteins.

Infants absorb unsaturated (essential) fatty acids from oils almost completely (98%), and absorb short-chain saturated fatty acids (SaFAs) better than long-chain SaFAs. Stearic acid (18:0) is only 60% absorbed, and longer-chain saturated fatty acids are only 40% absorbed. If the minerals calcium and magnesium are added to infant formulas, fat absorption is decreased even further.

Expert committees have recently recommended that a minimum of 2.7% and a maximum of 6% of the calories in infant formulas should come from w6, and 0.5% should come from w3 fatty acids.

Medium-chain triglycerides from coconut oil, which contain 65% caprylic (8:0) and 30% capric (10:0) acids, improve fat absorption from the infant's intestine and are easy to digest. They can make up from 10 to 50% of the fat in the formula. Formula fats should contain less than 10% stearic (18:0) and less than 20% palmitic (16:0) acids. Less than 15% lauric (12:0) and myristic (14:0) acids are recommended.

Cholesterol is present in mother's milk, and is therefore also included in formulas, but in smaller concentrations than those found in breast milk.

Vitamin E is important in infant formulations to prevent the formation of peroxides that make red blood cells fragile. The recommended amount of vitamin E is 0.65 to 0.75 International Units (IU) per gram of polyunsaturated fatty acid.

Large doses of iron worsen the effects of vitamin E deficiency. By six months of age babies have low iron stores. Both iron and vitamin E must therefore be present in adequate quantities in baby foods. If the mother's prenatal diet was adequate in EFAs, vitamin E, and iron, the infant has stored these in its body and can draw on these stores during the first few months.

Trans- fatty acids are unacceptable ingredients in infant formula fat blends.

In tests comparing infant formulas with human milk, the latter comes out in front. Considering the complexities and genius of nature, it is not surprising to find that mother's breast milk is the world's best baby food.

Developing Habits

Early childhood is the time during which nutritional and taste habits that last a lifetime are learned. Because of the natural affinity of love that exists between mother and child, a conscientious mother imparts good food habits to her child with little effort. These habits, which last the child's lifetime, underscore both the power and the awesome responsibility of motherhood!

Good pre-conception, prenatal, and infant nutrition build the foundation of health for the adult. Problems created by poor nutrition and toxic influences during this time are much more difficult to fix later on.

Clean, whole, nutrient-rich, toxin-free foods, clean water and air, and full spectrum sunlight are more important during pregnancy and early childhood than at any other time in life, because more growth, development, tissue movement, differentiation, and structural organization takes place during these early years than at any other time in life. Optimum nutrition and freedom from toxic influences is the only assurance that these delicate and easily disrupted processes will occur in the normal, natural ways encoded in the developing body's genetic blueprint.

Maternal nutrition should be supported by both family and community, which must otherwise bear far higher costs for the results of its neglect. Time, energy, and money invested at this early time in life is the most cost-effective health care possible. An ounce (or penny's worth) of prevention is worth a pound (or dollar's worth) of cure.

The importance of each mother's choice of good oils and good nutrition during pre-conception, pregnancy, and early childhood cannot be overstated.

86 *Athletes and Oils*

Many athletes are junk food addicts who suffer more than necessary from bone, ligament, disc, joint, neck, shoulder, and spinal injuries. Those who practice nutrition at all believe in proteins because proteins build muscle and 'lean' body mass. They tend to avoid fats. But here, as in all aspects of fats and oils nutrition, a distinction must be made between the fats that heal and the fats that kill. The fats that heal are required for health, oxidation, energy production, regulation of cell functions, and healing of tissue injuries, sprains, and bruises. The fats that kill interfere with health and slow down athletic performance.

In this chapter, we delineate the difference, and give practical guidelines on what kinds of oils can enhance athletic performance, and how much might be appropriate for athletes.

Fats as Hormones Regulating Energy Production

It would be fair to say that *all* fats act like hormones. This is not a widely accepted view, so let me explain. Fats do not act like steroids, which build muscle mass (and have major negative side effects), but they regulate oxidation rate, metabolic rate, and energy production in all our cells. Whether they speed up or slow down these important cell functions depends on two aspects of their personality: how long they are, and how many double bonds they have.

Chain length. The chain length continuum is best illustrated by saturated fatty acids. The shorter the saturated fatty acid, the less it inhibits energy production. Our body easily metabolizes short-chain fatty acids (such as butyric in butter, and caprylic and capric in medium-chain triglycerides [MCTs]) to produce energy.

The longer a saturated fatty acid is, the more it inhibits energy production. Long-chain saturated fatty acids (such as palmitic and stearic acids in tropical fats, land animals, butter, and margarines, and arachidic acid in vegetable oils like peanut) slow down energy production.

Degree of unsaturation. The fewer double bonds there are in a fatty acid, the less it speeds up oxidation and metabolic rate, and the less it stimulates energy production. The more double bonds a fatty acid contains, the more it increases oxidation, metabolic rate, and energy production.

A saturated fatty acid of a particular chain length is 'slower' than an unsaturated fatty acid with the same number of carbons in its chain. Thus, among fatty acids with 18-carbon chains, stearic acid (18:0) is 'slower' than oleic acid (18:1), which in turn is 'slower' than linoleic acid (18:2), which in turn is 'slower' than alpha-linolenic acid (18:3).

Conversely, the more double bonds are present in a fatty acid, the more it increases oxidation rate, metabolic rate, and energy production. Obviously, this is important for athletes who want to increase their energy output in order to stay ahead of their competition. Alpha-linolenic acid is the best 18-carbon fatty acid for enhancing energy production, followed by linoleic acid, followed by oleic acid, followed by stearic acid.

As a ballpark estimate, monounsaturated oleic acid occupies a neutral position, neither speeding up nor slowing down oxidation, metabolic rate, or energy production.

Maximizing Energy Production

Athletes should make sure they get optimum amounts of both essential fatty acids (EFAs) in their foods. Generally speaking, diets contain enough w6s, although part of this is found in refined, rancid, or altered, toxic form. Most athletes get too little w3 EFA, because w3s have not yet been taken seriously by most coaches, are still quite new to nutritionists, and are still largely unknown to conservative 'old school' doctors and dieticians.

In order to maximize energy production, athletes should use short-chain saturated fatty acids, and increase their levels of w3s. At the same time, they should avoid the hard, saturated fats that slow them down. They should also avoid processed, altered, fried, deep-fried, hydrogenated, and rancid fats and oils, because these poison their cells and decrease cell (and athletic performance). Stated more precisely, they interfere with natural cell functions, and some inhibit cell oxidation (respiration) and energy levels. Some injure cell membranes, tissues, liver, and arteries. Others interfere with digestive processes, resulting in poorer absorption of nutrients, bowel irritation, 'leaky gut', and allergic reactions that require an enormous amount of energy to process, leaving less energy available for physical performance. They use up energy in immune defense reactions – energy that could otherwise be used for athletic activity.

Athletes who use w3s report increased stamina (longer performance before fatigue sets in), reach higher performance plateaus, and recover from fatigue after exercise more quickly than they did before taking w3s. These benefits are likely due to increased oxidation rate.

Because of their increase of oxidation and metabolic rate, w3s and other highly unsaturated fatty acids such as stearidonic (18:4w3), gamma-linolenic acid (GLA) (18:3w6), eicosapentaenoic acid (EPA) (20:5w3), and docosahexaenoic acid (DHA) (22:6w3) prevent fat deposition. These fatty acids help people lose excess fat as well as excess water held in tissues.

Fundamental assets. Optimum health, optimum cell, tissue, and organ function, optimum energy production, and optimum waste and toxin management are an athlete's fundamental assets.

Athletes who squander these assets break fewer records, win fewer matches, suffer more injuries, and take longer to heal at comparable levels of discipline, technique, and practice. Even if their spirit is willing, their flesh remains weak without good oils and good food habits. Optimizing the fundamental, natural assets of their 'athletic machine' leads to higher performance levels.

Whatever minimizes the energy needed to digest and absorb nutrients, process toxins, perform immune functions, and eliminate wastes gives an athlete an edge over the competition. Whatever maximizes energy production without creating toxic side effects widens the competitive edge. Whatever minimizes allergic reactions to foods supports higher peak athletic performance. Optimization of cell, tissue, and organ functions according to each athlete's unique genetic and physical makeup is key to peak performance.

Fatty Acids and Healing

Athletes report that bruises and sprains heal faster when they include w3s in their diet. According to these athletes, minor injuries take only one-quarter to one-third of the healing time previously required.

These reports should be followed up, both by athletes trying them and by serious controlled studies that either prove or disprove these reports. If they prove to be true, much can be gained in the world of sports and world records.

Although our knowledge of the biology and biochemistry of the w3s is incomplete, what we know about their effects on oxidation, membrane functions, and prostaglandin production predicts that they have a valuable role to play in extending the limits of human performance.

Quantities. One tablespoon of flax oil provides three times more than the *minimum* amount of w3 essential fatty acids, which in 1992 was set at 2 grams per day by an 'expert' government committee in Canada – the amount present in just under 1 teaspoon of this oil. Some people benefit from using up to 5 table-spoons of the oil daily. Whatever the initial amount may be, use the amount of oil necessary over the long term to keep skin soft and velvety feeling. When skin becomes dry, take as much oil as is needed to reattain velvety skin.

If hemp oil is used as the source of EFAs, 2 teaspoons contain the minimum recommended amount of w3s, and 2 tablespoons or more of hemp oil may provide optimum amounts of both EFAs.

Other Nutrients

The roles of w3s and other highly unsaturated fatty acids are fulfilled in the presence of other essential nutrients. Fats, oils, and EFAs require about 30 other essential nutrients to maximally perform their functions in our body. These have already been listed (see Chapter 35, Vitamin and Mineral Co-factors).

For athletes trying to maximize their performance, optimum amounts and balances of all essential nutrients are especially important. They need to find their individual optimum balance between pro-oxidant fuels that maximize energy production and antioxidants that prevent damaging free radical chain reactions (see Chapter 39, Antioxidants and the Fire that is Life). They need to find the levels of essential nutrients that optimize fuel and oxygen delivery to their cells and tissues for maximum energy production and, at the same time, efficiently detoxify waste products that build up during intense training and competition.

An optimum program must be individually designed for each athlete, because each athlete is a unique individual with unique biochemistry, and therefore needs a unique fuel mix for the highest possible performance short of burnout.

Product Quality

More than with any other nutrient group, oil quality and freshness is an important issue for athletes. This is because of the ease with which highly unsaturated fatty acids spoil and produce toxic substances when exposed to light, oxygen, heat, processing, and time. Like fresh vegetables, fruit, and meat, these oils are perishable, and should be treated like fresh produce.

The chemical reactivity of oils when exposed to light, oxygen, and heat, which makes them perishable, is also the quality that makes them useful for increasing energy production and physical performance.

Many oil products available on the market contain spoiled oil molecules. These are toxic because they interfere with energy-producing reactions, disrupt membranes, interfere with liver and immune functions, and can injure the cells lining the inside of arteries.

Conclusion

Fats and oils are vital to health and to athletic performance. Some enhance performance and some inhibit it. The field of athletics has barely begun to tap and exploit the potential of fats and oils. The right kinds of fresh oils, used in appropriate ratios as part of a complete program of super-nutrition for athletes, have much to offer.

87 *Pets and Oils*

The same degenerative conditions that plague humans also plague our pets. The same oils that are missing from our foods are missing from their foods. Similar nutrient deficiencies and similar kinds of toxins are present in the environments of our pets, and affect them in similar ways.

Between the fresh raw whole foods the ancestors of our pets ate in the wild, and the canned, kibbled, convenient foods we now feed them, there is a world of processing that creates an *enormous nutritional gap*. Neither pet foods nor pet food supplements bridge this gap completely. One veterinarian with whom I work believes that 80% or more of the animals he sees (he sees a lot of pets) are suffering from degenerative conditions. Most common are skin afflictions and allergic reactions. Obesity, infections, gastro-intestinal disorders, and geriatric conditions (mouth and teeth, immune, cardiovascular, kidney malfunctions) also respond well to improvements in nutrition that close the nutritional gap. Improved nutrition also speeds healing after injury, surgery, accidents, and broken bones. Food-related infertility is also common.

One area of neglect is our pets' need for raw, enzyme-rich, nutrient-rich foods. This topic deserved more attention that this book can devote to it.

Another area of neglect in pet foods involves essential fatty acids (EFAs). W6 EFAs are included in pet foods, but they are heated, refined, deodorized, cheap, easy to obtain, and mutagenic-carcinogenic. In addition, the fatty acids in pet foods are often rancid by the time our pet gets to eat them, because they are not protected from air.

W3 EFAs get less attention than w6s. They are five times more sensitive to destruction than w6s. They are not added into pet foods, and the w3 supplements on the market are overprocessed and rancid.

Pet food supplements that contain *fresh* w6 and w3 EFAs, and that bridge the nutritional gap that remains when our pets eat bagged and canned foods are now available. They are intended for use with bagged and canned foods. See Services Provided at the end of the book if you are looking for such products.

To protect the double bonds of EFAs in these products, one must understand the physics, chemistry, biochemistry, and biology of EFAs, and must also understand of machinery and custom design.

The Business and Politics of Health **88**

Learning how to keep healthy is about as difficult as learning to ride a bicycle. It is easier than learning how to do your job or learning a language. It is *certainly* easier than getting to the moon. It is natural to be healthy because health is a natural state.

But, you might ask, if health is a natural state that is quite easy to achieve, why aren't we healthy? Why does it cost so much to get treatments? Why do we remain sick after treatment? Furthermore, why are natural treatments so rarely used and so difficult to find? And why are those who attempt to provide natural treatments hounded by regulatory agencies? To attempt to answer these questions, this chapter takes a look at aspects of 'health care' that are not about science, knowledge, or care.

Deadly Humor

Business interests and the power politics of our so-called 'health care' system both complicate and interfere with the delivery of effective health care.

In one of its skits, the British comedy group Monty Python presents a dialog between a patient and his doctor. "What's wrong with me?" asks the patient. The doctor contemplates, then answers: "That depends on how much money you have. If you have a lot of money, your condition could get much worse." Later in the dialog, the doctor informs the patient that a radical 'cash-ectomy' will have to be performed. This skit, unfortunately, contains a kernel of truth, because what we call 'health care' today is more about profit and power than about health or care.

Drug companies, food processors, advertisers, insurance companies, governments, doctors, and citizens are *all* involved. Their most basic goals, preoccupations, and preconceptions keep truths about health from being sought, discovered, organized, widely disseminated, accepted, and applied. Our drug-oriented medical system continues to undermine our faith in nature, natural living, natural healing, and ourselves. It suffers from the inertia of ideas and habits we inherited from the past, and that we have not examined closely enough to discard and replace with better ones. Effective natural methods ('non-orthodox', as they are called by the medical establishment) of health care are difficult to obtain in affluent nations. For some natural treatments, patients must leave the country, creating further obstacles to achieving health.

History

History is filled with interesting stories about people and ambitions. Through inspired rhetoric, charismatic political individuals have changed the course of history by mobilizing people to accept and act on their views. Millions of people have enslaved and sacrificed themselves on altars of history erected to the gods of power, control, territory, ownership, 'national interests', freedom, status, and wealth. But so far, none of these ambitious, political individuals throughout history has given top priority to the health of the citizens who pay their way, support their power, and die for them.

Citizens *always* want health, but generally subvert their wishes to the political agenda of the day, even when that agenda results in chaos, war, poverty, and other factors that lead to disease. One must wonder why.

Past government involvement in so-called 'health care' focused on the important area of hygiene – water treatment, sewage disposal, food inspection – but beyond that, has been limited mainly to carrying out the wishes of those who market high-tech disease management and crisis intervention products and services for profit.

A more sensible approach to human health would be to clearly define the contexts, parameters, and components of health – based both on common sense and on research into human biology – and from this body of information to develop and make available to citizens, health care based on the biological roots of health. Much of the necessary biological research has already been done. It must now be properly organized.

Pioneers. Advances in our understanding of health have historically been pioneered and championed – often against strong resistance – by individuals who have unusual health problems, caring clinicians who take the suffering of their patients personally enough to search for real – even if 'unorthodox' – cures, and research investigators interested in the true nature of health, the body, disease, and healing.

Today, based on the failure of an enormously expensive crisis- and disease-management system that does not deliver health, the biological basis of human health is gradually being taken more seriously. For the first time in history, it is possible to define health and cure degenerative diseases by identifying and eliminating their root causes. Although we have far to go before real health care is instituted on a national and global scale, the signs of change are unmistakable.

Vested Interests

Vested interests reflect social values. Security, control, status, power, and wealth all rate higher than health in our society at the present time. This will change only when individuals and organizations put health higher on society's agenda.

Business interests, that work against a clean environment – and therefore against clean food, water, and air – include all industries that deplete, exploit, and pollute natural environments in order to make money. The bottom line in business tends to take a heavy toll on nature. When the economy improves, the environment gets polluted; when the environment is treated with respect, the economy suffers. Those who profit from the destruction of nature and of life put us all at peril. We must come to understand and embody the simple fact that, in the long term, life and nature are our only assets. Health results when we respect and align ourselves with both.

It is a mistake to measure our prosperity only by *economic* indicators. A country whose economy improves while its environment becomes more polluted, and its population less healthy is a *poor* country.

We need to learn to care more for nature and health than we do money, and to live with a view to maintaining the balance of the cycles of the natural system of which we are part and on which we depend.

Farmers. Decisions made a generation ago to use artificial fertilizers and intensive farming methods that take more from soils than they give back are coming home to roost as poor soils, poor foods, and poor health.

Pesticides, meant to decrease our losses to pests, are failing. Losses to pests ran at 6% of crops when we began to use them. Today, pests eat 13% of our crops. We eliminated no pests, but many of their natural predators by their use. We do not grow healthier foods, but poison ourselves and our children. A government study that measured pesticide levels in children, completed and scheduled to be released in 1989, is now 3 years overdue and still has not been made public.

We must now admit that the 'prophets of doom' who recognized the threat to our grandchildren were right. These 'prophets' of natural living, include the Kellogg brothers of the late 1800s (corn flakes are not what the Kellogg brothers recommended!), Sylvester Graham (graham crackers, named after him, are not what *he* used to eat!), Rachel Carson in the early 1960s with her book *Silent Spring*, and many others in both Europe and North America over the last two centuries.

Sustainable farming methods must fit natural cycles, make use of natural predators for pest control, and maintain fertile, mineral- and humus-rich soils teeming with soil bacteria and earthworms.

Nature is not an enemy but our friend, the source of our nurture and our nutriture.

Doctors. Special interests also mediate against health more directly. The economic interests of professional disease management (drug-, radiation-, surgery-, and high-tech-oriented medical practice) are strongly biased against instituting true health care. Disease is better business. Doctors get paid for treating – not for curing – diseases. If they were paid only for keeping people healthy, and lost their income when their patients got sick, medicine would completely change its approach without losing any of its self-interest.

Legally, the medical profession has exclusive ownership of a large part of the 'health care' territory. Others are not allowed to compete, even in areas where drug-oriented, 'orthodox' practices fail to bring health and even do harm.[1]

High-tech medicine as presently practiced is not viable for the society that uses it. Treatment costs have increased while levels of health have deteriorated. That's bad investment. For $900 billion each year in expenditures, we should expect, and are entitled to results. We should demand them.

The 'health care' (disease management) delivery system is not founded on understanding health. That was acceptable before we understood energy, electrons, atoms, chemical bonds, molecules, molecular interactions, essential nutrients and toxins, genetic material (DNA), its translation (RNA), proteins, enzymes, cell functions, glands and hormones, and the rest of biology and natural systems. But it is inexcusable now that we know enough to develop and then teach a systematically organized picture of human health appropriate for homes, schools, and colleges.

The use of unnatural methods for treating soils, foods, and illnesses has overdrawn our body's health account, mortgaged our soils, foods, water, air, and energy sources, spent our future for present convenience and now, like our governments, we are bankrupt.

We must turn again to nature as our doctor; to simpler, more natural, less stressful lives; to personal responsibility for learning to care for our health and practicing self-care; to live in line with nature and our own nature, rather than the demands of corporations and other vested interests that work against our health.

Drug manufacturers make synthetic, unnatural substances that they can patent to protect exclusivity and profits of 600% or more for 17 to 20 years. Since natural substances cannot be patented, competition pushes profits down – profit on vitamin and mineral supplements is about 100% before expenses – leaving less money to invest in research, advertising, and education.

In passing such laws, our governments have designed and built a profit system that mediates against the natural state of health. Synthetic drugs do not fit accurately into our molecular architecture. To the extent that they misfit, they produce 'side effects' – disease conditions caused by poisoning, from toxic properties in the molecular makeup of these unnatural substances.

Health is based on natural molecules. Drug profit is based on the sale of unnatural molecules. Respect for health, as a natural state, must take priority over drug patents and profits if health is to happen.

Giant food processors also have vested interests that mediate against health. Whole foods are relatively cheap. To increase profits, food processors change them into 'value added' products, because more can be charged for foods that have been changed by processing technology. Processing has little to do with health, but much to do with convenience and profit. From the point of view of health, processed products are 'value subtracted', since processing removes and/or

---

[1] The members of the medical profession, on whom we rely to lead us back to health when we fall ill, die from degenerative diseases at about the same frequency as the rest of us.

destroys nutrients, and/or adds toxins.

Food processing companies have played substantial political roles since the early 1900s in blocking efforts toward food laws that reflect the findings of science on the requirements for health. Such food laws would expose many processed products as nutritionally inferior and health-destroying.

Whole foods will always be our most important source of essential nutrients. The less processing they have been subjected to, the richer in health-building nutrients they are likely to be. Fresh local produce is preferable to imported produce in terms of freshness, nutritional value, control over pesticide levels, and minimization of toxic material released into our environment by transport vehicles.

Politicians elected by popular vote are subject to pressure by special interest groups. They must balance the often diverging interests of their wish to be re-elected with their job of protecting the public. Food companies, drug manufacturers, and the medical profession have three of the most powerful government lobbies.

The basis of our common wealth is found in the biology of soil, water, air, natural resources, and human resources. All ought to be passed on to our children in at least as good a state as that in which we inherited them from our parents. The last two or three generations have seen our resources neglected and squandered, and we must clean up a mess on all levels – from soil, to education, to government.

Laws that governments enact favor profits, monopolies, and economics, and give little attention to nature, the long term, and the natural basis of health.

The importance of harmonizing with nature should determine the direction of our lives. Health care, the environment, and other quality of life issues must be pioneered by individuals and groups who see the biological roots of human existence and push to have these roots reflected in our laws.

Educated consumers can bring about the necessary changes. Singly or in groups, working at grass roots levels, they are a powerful driving force for positive change in the system. When the people lead, the leaders *must* follow.

At present, *diseases* still get the lion's share of attention, while *health* is neglected. We study many diseases in great detail, but no university in the world educates us into the nature of health. As a result, consumers must rely on anecdotal and non-mainstream sources for their health education.

For health to become known, understood, and practiced requires deliberate effort. It does not automatically arise out of disease management. If even 5% of the money (over $3000 per person per year in the U.S.) currently spent on disease management were invested in discovering, and then learning, teaching, and practicing the principles of health, we would be a very healthy nation.

The scientific method is a relatively new way of trying to systematize our observations and findings. It is often applied dogmatically, like a religion – an unquestionable faith requiring no proof. We have successfully imposed this method to predict and control nature, but many scientists fail to acknowledge its limitations. Whatever falls outside its narrow range is not attended to – or worse – denied and decried.

In spite of studies in physics and psychology, which show that observers influence the outcomes of experiments, scientists still largely assume that *they* do not. Another fallacy is that one can do science without being aware of one's own biases. A third fallacy is the assumption, without proof, that one cannot be objective about oneself.

Probably the worst failing of the scientific method as presently practiced is that it is applied only to the external world while much of our life, including our health, is about inner experiences and feelings that *we* can clearly observe, but that may be difficult or impossible to verify. *External* situations and conditions (variables) can be manipulated, other investigators can verify observations, repeat experiments, and support or refute a theory with further experiments based on what a theory predicts.[2] In the world of health and human nature, which is internal, the scientific method cannot be carried out in the same way. One must learn to be still and to self-observe – thoughts, images, emotions, feelings – and to accurately report these (or at least acknowledge them to oneself). One can 'prove' to oneself the truth of one's own internal states, but not necessarily to anyone else.[3]

The stranglehold of the scientific method as presently practiced, over present research and research topics, slows down our discovery of health and human nature. To explore ourselves, we must become pioneers who break new ground outside of unquestioned assumptions, attitudes, and values held in common – the scientific method is one of these. These assumptions, attitudes, and values are failing us on a world-wide scale because, for all their apparent usefulness, they fail to solve our practical problems, and in fact often worsen them.

To be healthy, we must search, discover, feel, think, and act in new ways, different from those that kill two-thirds of us by degenerative conditions. We can do so only by looking deeper within ourselves, and discovering our own unknown. Health is one of the discoveries we'll make.

'Natural Laws'

We have studied nature for a few hundred years, and have discovered some of her laws. We have harnessed her powers in our technological inventions, by *obeying* these laws. We have never *conquered* nature, as some people claim.

We have taken what we learned by observing other organisms and applied it to ourselves. Sometimes this has worked. Sometimes it has led to mistakes (see

---

[2] In the end, one still ends up only with theory, never fact.

[3] One could also completely delude oneself, a capacity as uniquely human as our ability to be still, observe, and create. Hence it might be useful to be trained in objective self-observation by someone who knows their way around that elusive territory of human nature.

Chapter 20, Erucic Acid). We have yet to look at ourselves in the same thorough way in which we have looked at the organisms, objects, and forces around us.

There is a limit in the extent to which we can help our own health by relying on results from the study of other organisms. In some important ways, their biology, their needs, their food habits, their metabolism, their capacities, and their environments are different. Eventually, we must discover our own health at its source: in our own body, on its own terms. This can only be done by self-observation and self-discovery. In practical terms, it means becoming sensitive, observing what our body is telling us, learning what the signals mean, and responding appropriately – by adjusting how we eat, drink, breathe, and live.

This approach to health is new in the West, but has a long-standing history of success in older traditions and cultures. It holds exciting possibilities for the realization of optimum health. It goes far beyond what 'experts' or professionals can do, because each of us is the recipient of the messages from our own individual nature. 'Experts' and professionals can only guess. Science and technology can verify some of our self-observations by means of instruments, but cannot confirm others that may also be valid. Keep an open mind. The human body will continue to be the ultimate measuring instrument of its own state of health.

Individual Responsibility

Advancements in health result from work undertaken by individuals who take the time to examine the possibilities of attaining that natural state. Health belongs, to a large extent, in our own hands because it lives deep within us in places that only we can access. Our body expresses its needs as feelings. We can learn this language of feelings, learn what the feelings mean, and respond to our body's needs. As I said at the beginning, it's about as easy as learning to ride a bike, and much easier than learning a job or a language. Most of us have successfully done both by investing a bit of time and effort. With time and effort, we can also master health.

Health and environment are twins. When we poison our environment, we poison our bodies, because our bodies are this environment, taken in as foods, water, and air. Environmental pollution becomes internal pollution. This deceptively simple concept has enormously important consequences. Healers must also be environmentalists. Graffiti from the '60s sums up the health and environment issue: 'You can s... in your nest for only so long before you are nesting in your s...'

It is up to you – *'Tuum est'* – is the motto of the University of British Columbia where I studied Life Sciences. Nowhere is this motto more appropriate than in matters of health care.

To help us in our individual effort, we need a systematically organized, systematically learnable (and teachable) field of human health that accounts for and focuses on the effects of food, essential nutrients, water, air, light, and life-style, as well as pollutants and stress, on human biology.

Toward Total Health

Live Long and Feel Fat-astic!

This section gives general advice and recommendations to improve health, which follow from the topics that have occupied our attention throughout the book. It suggests what to do and what not to do to reverse degenerative conditions.

We explore the biological basis of the natural therapies that can cure most degenerative health problems, including many of the so-called 'incurable' diseases.

We conclude the book with a look at human nature, and the possibility of living a full life.

Recommendations for Health 89

My first piece of advice to the people I educate is not the usual, well-known, and overstated dictum to avoid hard fats, or even altered, toxic, killer fats. It is more important to identify and include those fats that affect health in a positive way – the fats that heal. It is more effective to find out what to do than what not to do.

By the time you have put the following positive recommendations into practice, you will have replaced many bad habits with good ones. You may not need to read the negative recommendations, but in case something has been missed, they are also given.

Positive Recommendations

1. Ensure adequate essential fatty acid (EFA) consumption. Our intake of EFAs should be at least one-third of total fat intake, no matter what our total level of fat consumption is. The best-balanced plant source of both EFAs is hemp seed oil. Flax is the richest source of the w3 EFA. Soybeans and walnuts contain both EFAs, but are richer in the w6 EFA. Safflower, sunflower, and sesame are sources of only the w6 EFA.

Fish like salmon, mackerel, rainbow trout, sardines, and eel contain large quantities of w3 EFA derivatives. Seaweed and shellfish supply both EFAs in small quantities. Dark-green vegetables such as spinach, parsley, and broccoli also contain small quantities of both EFAs. All whole, fresh, unprocessed foods contain some EFAs.

EFAs are extremely important for health and vitality. EFA deficiencies are correlated with degenerative diseases such as cardiovascular disease, cancer, diabetes, multiple sclerosis, skin afflictions, dry skin, premenstrual syndrome, behavioral problems, poor wound healing, arthritis, glandular atrophy, weakened immune functions, and sterility (especially in males).

Oils rich in both EFAs (hemp), mainly w3s (flax), and mainly w6s (safflower, sunflower, sesame) should be mechanically pressed (as opposed to chemically, solvent-extracted) from pesticide-free seeds at low temperature with light and oxygen excluded; should remain unrefined and unheated; and should be stored in opaque, inert metal, earthen, or glass containers, kept frozen in storage, and refrigerated or frozen in our home. For recommended quantities, see Chapter 64, Flax and Hemp Oil Recipes. When these conditions are not fulfilled, EFAs are unprotected and partially destroyed, losing much of their value to health through light-induced free radicals, oxygen-induced rancidity, or heat-induced molecular twisting and other changes. It is not conducive to health to consume such oils.

W3 oils such as flax are extremely sensitive to destruction. Some distribution systems keep these oils in transit too long. I recommend that flax and hemp seed oils be shipped by manufacturer directly to retail store. People with health problems should obtain fresh flax oil directly from a reputable manufacturer, air-shipped when appropriate to retain freshness.

Hemp seed oil, a balanced, natural EFA-rich oil, is somewhat more stable than flax, but should be treated with the same care demanded by flax oil. For highest quality sources of oils, see Services Provided, at the end of the book.

Fats and oils should make up about 15 to 20% of total calories consumed each day.

2. Ensure adequate intake of minerals, vitamins, protein, fiber, etc. A total of about 20 *minerals* and 13 *vitamins* are required for human health. Several of these help metabolize cholesterol and fats. Their presence in our body lowers cholesterol levels. Deficiency of these vitamins and minerals raises cholesterol. Vitamin C, niacin (B_3), chromium, and copper play key roles, but all minerals and vitamins are essential for health.

Minerals and vitamins protect EFAs from destruction by oxygen and free radicals. Vitamins A (or carotene), C, and E, the minerals zinc, manganese, copper, and selenium, and the element sulphur (contained in garlic and a few amino acids) are involved in this protection.

Vitamins and minerals are required to metabolize sugars and starches for the production of energy and help prevent them from turning into saturated fatty acids and hard fats. They include B complex vitamins and chromium. Potassium, magnesium, manganese, and iron are also necessary for energy production.

Adequate *proteins* containing all essential amino acids are required for health, but protein deficiency is rare in the diets of affluent people. Over-consumption of protein is more common than under-consumption.

All proteins are possible sources of allergy. Each person needs to find out which proteins are allergy-safe for them, because individuals differ in this regard.[1] Among meats, fish is preferable to chicken and turkey, which are preferable to lamb, beef, and pork. Eggs contain excellent protein. Yolk is nutritious and its

---

[1] The commonest food allergies are to dairy protein and wheat. Corn, egg, and pork allergies are also common. Vegetables and rice rarely produce allergic reactions, but some individuals *are* allergic to these. Therefore, allergies must be individually determined.

cholesterol poses no problems if our diet contains enough w3 and w6 EFAs, minerals, vitamins, and fiber. Among plant sources, seeds and nuts are rich in protein. Almonds and soybeans (tofu) contain especially good plant protein.

Increase the use of fresh vegetables and fruit, grains and beans, fish and seafoods.

Certain kinds of *fiber:* pectins, mucilages, and gums found in apples, potatoes, beets, carrots, okra, flax, beans, and oats tie up bile acids, cholesterol, and toxins, and carry them out of our body. They lower cholesterol levels and reduce our risk of cardiovascular disease. Other kinds of fiber help prevent constipation, weight gain, colon cancer, and gallstones. Some even increase glucose tolerance, which helps prevent hypoglycemia and diabetes (hyperglycemia).

Since much of the vitamins, minerals, EFAs, and fiber present in whole foods have been altered or removed during the processing of fats, oils, sugars, and starches we consume, we should nutrient-enrich our food supply with whole foods, fresh juices, super-foods, food concentrates, or supplements of vitamins, minerals, fiber, and EFAs. It is easy to get them back, by eating fiber-rich foods, taking a high-potency multi-vitamin, multi-mineral supplement, and using one of the fresh, balanced oils rich in both EFAs. Additional vitamins C, E, and carotene may be advisable, since even high-potency supplements contain less of these than most people find optimal for health.

Fiber supplements are also available. Fiber should be taken with lots of fluid, as some types of fiber absorb 20 to 60 times their volume of water. Lack of fluid can lead to abdominal pain, and may even be dangerous. If you are looking for sources, see Services Provided at the back of the book.

Friendly bacteria (acidophilus) help keep our colon healthy. They are easily destroyed by antibiotics and can be replaced by taking an acidophilus supplement, in dry or liquid, refrigerated form.

Hydrochloric acid, bile, and *enzymes* may help us digest our foods more completely. These take on increasing importance as we age.

Herbs contain natural factors that can help our liver (e.g., silybum), digestive (e.g., bitters), respiratory (e.g., mullein, angelica), circulatory (e.g., hawthorn), and immune (e.g., echinacea) and other systems function more efficiently.

3. Fresh water, fresh air, sunshine. Living in an ideal natural setting, we would eat natural, fresh, whole, sun-ripened, unprocessed, seasonal, locally grown, raw, toxin-free foods. We would drink clean, flowing water, and breathe clean, oxygen-rich air. We would be natural beings living a natural life-style in harmony with nature and our own nature. For every step we take away from this ideal natural setting, we pay a price in health. Each step we take back in the direction of the ideal natural setting has positive effects on health.

Our *water* should be clean and free of toxins. If it is chlorinated and contains other impurities, these impurities should be removed. Several technologies are available, but no one technology works well alone; they should therefore be combined to best protect health.

The *air* we breathe should be clean. Although outdoor industrial pollution gets much attention, our indoor air is often more contaminated than that outside. That's why we still go outside for a breath of fresh air. Indoor filters that remove particles, dust, bacteria, molds, gases, synthetic vapors, and odors can be installed. If you need help with technologies, see Services Provided, at the back of the book.

We are creatures of *light*. Human health requires full-spectrum sunlight including UV rays in moderation. It benefits our health to spend at least some time (one hour or more) each day outside in direct or indirect, unfiltered sunlight. Sunglasses that block UV should not be worn during this light-for-health time.

4. Exercise. Our body is made for activity. If there were nothing to do, we wouldn't need a body – we could just be disembodied spirits floating about. If our exercise consists only of the grinding movement of our jaws, the movement of our arms from plate to mouth, and the push away from the table, that's not enough. Lack of exercise results in poorer digestion, absorption, and metabolism of fats, carbohydrates, and proteins. Regular activity is extremely important for maintaining health. If our nutrition is optimal, being active is natural and comes easily. If we remain inactive, even good nutrition will not keep us healthy.

Exercise comes in three forms: squeak *(stretching),* which includes yoga, pre-workout limbering, and post-workout cool-down, where muscles are gently moved and stretched out; sweat *(aerobics),* which consists of workouts for lungs and cardiovascular system through sustained (20 minutes or more) rapid movement training; and grunt *(strength),* which includes muscle and body building by moving increasingly heavy loads increasingly often (reps).

All three forms of exercise are part of all-round physical fitness.

5. Relax, rest, pray, enjoy, and party with the gang. To balance a life of activity and busy-ness, we need to also make time for relaxation and rest. To unwind. To discover ourselves as nature made us rather than as society expects us to be. To come to terms with our smallness in relation to a vast universe. To find that which loves us unconditionally from within the core of our being. To enjoy being alive for no reason other than that life is inherently enjoyable. These too are important to health.

Harmonious social relations and the company of people with whom we have mutual acceptance, nurture, love, and trust is important for human health. Serving and contributing to others is also important.

Good old days? Some people long for the good old days, imagining that in less 'modern', less hectic times, people enjoyed more time with members of their family, tribe, or community; could trust most strangers; enjoyed more time with themselves; balanced solitary and social time better; were closer to themselves, to others, and to nature; had more faith in what they didn't know; expressed more gratitude and counted their blessings; and in the silence of the longing of their souls, were closer to what sustains us all.

Today, this seems a tall order. But in reality it is no taller an order today than it was in the past or will be in the future. In fact, every generation of the past, present, and future has had, has, and will have their share of problems to deal with, and their escapist images of better pasts and futures. And in every era, there have been, are, and will be individuals who manage to live full and content lives in spite of the circumstances of the time. They do it (and we can do it) by living consciously.

Living consciously means being aware of our feelings, emotions, and thoughts; being aware of the actions that flow from emotions and thoughts; being aware of the consequences of our actions, and learning from these consequences. Living consciously is necessary for realizing today, in *our* life, what we imagine were the 'good old days' or what we hope will be the 'better future'. Living consciously has always required the effort of being aware, present, alert, and deliberate. While the circumstances in which we face the challenge of living consciously change, conscious living is simply a question of values, priorities, and commitments. Conscious living has always been, is, and always will be possible for any person, under any set of circumstances – a matter of deciding and choosing how we live.

Negative Recommendations

6. Lower fat (and cholesterol) consumption. A large body of research indicates that if we want to remain healthier longer, we need to reduce our total fat consumption from over 40% down to between 15 and 20% of total calories. At this level, our chances of dying from cardiovascular disease, cancer, or other diseases of fatty degeneration become smaller, especially if our fats contain both EFAs in proper balance.

The easiest way to reduce fat consumption is to decrease our consumption of fatty foods (if a food is 20% fats by weight, it means that 45% or more of its calories come from fats), and increase our consumption of low-fat, high-fiber foods. Avoid obvious sources of poor-quality fat such as margarines and shortenings. Reduce butter (80% fat) to 1 tablespoon per day (14 grams; 101 calories).[2] Limit refined vegetable oils (100% fat) to 1 tablespoon per day (126 calories). Discard visible fats on beef, lamb, and pork, and the skin on chicken and turkey.

Avoid processed foods containing hidden fats, such as sausage. Reduce reliance on greasy burgers, cheese (except low-fat cheese containing less than 10% butter fat) and oily salad dressings. Avoid potato chips and fried foods.

For 30% of the population, dietary cholesterol intake increases blood cholesterol levels. For the other 70%, increased dietary cholesterol leads to decreased cholesterol production by their liver, keeping their blood cholesterol levels constant regardless of dietary intake.

---

[2] Butter and margarines contain about 20% water.

7. Avoid oxidized fats, oils, and cholesterol, and sticky hard fats. When our foods are processed and aged while exposed to air, and also lack antioxidant minerals and vitamins, we consume more oxidized cholesterol, oils, and fats than our body can handle.

Oxidized fats and cholesterol occur in cured, processed, and aged foods. Include meats, sausages, cheese, scrambled (as opposed to boiled) eggs, fried convenience foods, and stored foods on the list of oxidized foods that mediate arterial damage leading to the plethora of cardiovascular problems that have been wrongly blamed on cholesterol. Avoid them, and stick to fresh, whole foods that have not had air pushed into them, and that still contain their natural minerals and vitamins.

Over several years or decades, the consumption of oxidized cholesterol, oils, fats, and fatty acids together with deficiencies of essential nutrients result in arterial damage. Thickened arteries brought about by repair proteins narrow these blood vessels, impair circulation, and increase our risk of cardiovascular disease: stroke, heart attack, blindness, high blood pressure, kidney and heart failure. Hard fats and saturated fatty acids make platelets more sticky. In arteries damaged by oxidized fats and thickened and narrowed by plaque (atherosclerosis) formed largely due to lack of vitamin C and other essential nutrients, sticky fats increase the probability of a clot blocking an artery completely and resulting in heart attack, stroke, or embolism. Magnesium deficiency may help trigger a spasm in a coronary artery that begins the blocking event.

A strict vegetarian diet (no meat, eggs, or dairy products, but plenty of fresh vegetables and grains, as well as smaller amounts of seeds, nuts, and fruit) can lower a cholesterol level of 260 mg/dl to 160 mg/dl within a month, and also supplies an abundance of antioxidants, minerals, and vitamins. The death rate from cardiovascular disease of strict vegetarians is only one-quarter that of meat eaters. The average blood cholesterol level of a heart attack patient is 244 mg/dl. A level of 160 mg/dl or less is associated with virtually complete absence of cardiovascular disease.

8. Avoid altered fats. Altered fats do not fit into the precise molecular architecture of our bodies. This architecture is the framework on which life energy flows, keeping us alive and healthy. Altered fats are linked to mutations, cancers, atherosclerosis, and degeneration of cells, tissues, and organs. Some take part in uncontrolled free radical chain reactions within our body, resulting in toxic metabolic byproducts.

The main sources of altered fats are hydrogenated oil products. Avoid them. Shortenings, margarines (both hard and soft), shortening oils and partially hydrogenated vegetable oils (used in convenience, processed, and junk foods) make up the bulk of altered fats in our food supply. We also find them in bakery products, candies, french fries, fried and deep-fried foods, and processed convenience foods and snacks such as potato and corn chips and other bagged snacks. Avoid them all. Refined oils also contain some altered fats. Humans consume nearly 10 pounds of altered fats per person per year (10 to 12 grams per day), more than twice their consumption of all other food additives combined.

Fresh raw seeds and nuts – the raw materials from which come the oils that we ruin in order to make shortenings, margarines, and other altered fat products – contain no altered fats. Choose them for health-giving fats and oils.

Fresh oils containing EFAs and other natural factors are available. High on the list are flax and hemp oils. EFAs in these oils are destroyed if they are exposed to light and air during processing, storage, and display, by heat during processing; and by frying and deep-frying in home and restaurant. If you want them fresh and in their natural state, see Services Provided, at the end of the book.

9. Avoid refined sugars; reduce refined starches and calorie-rich foods. Our body transforms refined sugars into, hard, sticky fats and cholesterol. These interfere with the functions of EFAs and make our platelets more sticky. Sugars increase our blood fat (triglyceride) levels, which increase atherosclerosis, make platelets sticky, and increase risk of heart attack, stroke, embolism, high blood pressure, kidney failure, and heart failure. Sugars inhibit immune function, feed cancer, feed candida, yeast, and bacteria, prevent vitamin C transport (glucose and vitamin C use the same transport mechanism), rob our body of minerals, cause hypoglycemia and diabetes, burn out our adrenal glands and pancreas, increase internal stress which increases cholesterol production, can also cause tooth decay and unruly behavior. All refined and concentrated sources of sugars do this and should be avoided as much as possible. Even sweet fruit eaten in excess can have this effect in some people. Fruit should be eaten in moderation.

In 1815, sugar consumption was 15 pounds per person per year. In 1865, human beings consumed about 40 pounds of sugar per year. By 1900, sugar consumption had risen to 85 pounds per person per year. In 1970, sugar consumption was about 120 pounds per person per year, and today it stands at 135 pounds per person per year. Sugars are added to most processed foods including ketchup (which contains more sugar than ice cream), processed meats (which are extended with starch or sweetened with sugar), canned vegetables, and 'non-sweet' bakery products (which contain added sugar). Avoid these less obvious sources of sugar.

White flour, refined cornstarch, macaroni, noodles, and pasta also lack vitamins, minerals, and essential fatty acids necessary for health. They, and other concentrated, fiber-poor foods help produce chronic constipation suffered by 30% of the population. In the 1800s, white bread was used as a folk remedy to stop diarrhea, because it was known to constipate. Reduce or avoid refined starches.

Calorie-rich foods include eggs, meats, and cheese. Fiberless, they contain more calories than our body is made to handle, and also constipate. Reduce your consumption of these, and balance them with fiber-rich vegetables.

Cardiovascular disease, diabetes, and obesity result from increased use of refined sugars, refined starches, and calorie-rich foods. In the 1800s, cardiovascular deaths were extremely rare. They rose to 1 in 7 deaths by 1900, and today account for more than 1 death in every 3. Diabetes rose at a similar rate and, if one includes its cardiovascular complications, now accounts for 1 death in 20. About 30% of adults in Western society are obese, risking cancer, cardiovascular disease, diabetes, allergies, and a host of other degenerative ailments.

Human societies consuming traditional diets consisting of vegetables (including raw sugarcane) and whole grains rarely suffer from these afflictions. Returning to the use of natural foods – fresh vegetables and fruits, whole grains, and unprocessed seeds, nuts, and fish – eliminates many of the problems that refined sugars, starches, and calorie-rich foods bring on.

10. Avoid toxins including drugs, pesticides, and food additives. Some healers claim that *all* drugs, pesticides, and additives are liver-toxic and therefore increase our chances of cancer. This is because our liver is the main organ that must detoxify the toxic materials in our body.

The use of pharmaceutical drugs is so widespread that it has become a major problem. Most have *not* been adequately tested for safety. Being unnatural substances, we should *assume* that they are unsafe. The toxicity of many drugs produces side effects that are full-blown diseases themselves. Many drugs and synthetic molecules were sold for profit and used by human guinea pigs for years before their side effects became sufficiently well documented to force them off the market. Arsenic, mercury, thalidomide, and the cancer-causing food dyes (butter yellow and sudan red) are examples. Antibiotics and cortisone inhibit immune function. About 18% of all illnesses today are *caused* by medical treatments – these are called iatrogenic illnesses.

To reduce our need for synthetic drugs and poisons, we must strengthen our body's ability to resist disease by increasing the quality of our food intake, and by ensuring that we get all essential nutrients in sufficient quantities. In this way, we can meet our needs for growth and activity, for maintaining physical health, healing illnesses, and resisting stress, pollution, and toxic influences from the environment.

Pesticides are poisons developed to kill organisms that are part of the same natural system that is also our mother. They poison us too. To decrease our reliance on pesticides, we must strengthen soils, diversify our crop base, develop hardy plants, encourage natural predators of pests and, if all else fails, harvest insects as food.

To reduce our intake of pesticides and other food additives, we must avoid sprayed, highly processed, artificially colored and flavored foods, and return to pesticide-free foods – organically-grown, fresh vegetables and fruit, organically-grown whole grains, nuts and seeds, and wild meats (especially fish). These foods kept our ancestors free of fat-related degenerative diseases. They keep the so-called 'primitive' people and citizens of less developed nations healthy. They keep wild animals healthy. They will also keep us healthy.

The Biological Basis
of Natural Therapies 90

A few simple but fundamental concepts form the foundation for healing degenerative diseases by natural means. Effective natural, self-responsible treatments to prevent, reverse, and cure degenerative conditions must be based on principles similar to those set out here.

Incurable?

I remember overhearing as a teenager that cancer is incurable. I was outraged. "That's impossible," I remember protesting. "If you know what it is, and you examine what you did to get it, and you know what health is, then you should be able to reverse it by changing what you do!" It was obvious to me that the body is self-healing. Self-healing is not a difficult concept! Our body heals bruises, scratches, cuts, wounds, burns, and broken bones quite masterfully.

Sources of Disease

Degenerative diseases can have only three possible sources. The first is genetic, where an error (mutation) in our genes determines that a normal biochemical reaction takes place more slowly than normal, too quickly, or not at all. The total frequency of genetic conditions with serious health consequences has been estimated at about 5 per 1000 people in the population. Natural methods can help these people, but may not be able to cure them completely.

The rest of the people affected by degenerative conditions (995 per 1000 people in our population) are negatively affected by either malnutrition or internal pollution. Those suffering degenerative conditions due to malnutrition and internal pollution can be helped by natural means.

Malnutrition

Malnutrition includes deficiencies, imbalances, and/or excesses of essential nutrients or other natural substances.

Nutrient deficiencies are the most common form of malnutrition by which we depart from health – a lack in our foods of one or more of the nearly 50 essential factors. Reasons for nutrient deficiency are easy to identify. They include:

- *poor diet* due to market unavailability; poor soil management and growing practices; harvesting products unripe; transport and storage losses; removal of essential nutrients by processing; poor food choices based on inadequate or wrong information, poverty, infirmity, or physical and/or mental illness; or destructive food preparation;
- *poor digestion* due to genetic or acquired digestive imperfections, bad food

combinations, or allergic reactions;

- *poor absorption* that may be inherited, or nutrition-, age-, or toxin-related;
- *inordinately high nutrient requirements* that may be temporary or permanent; based on genetic limitations, disease, toxicity, allergy, environment, or related to stress or high performance.

Deficiencies are widespread in our society, because food growing, manufacturing, and preparation revolve around convenience rather than health requirements. Nutrient quality reflects these priorities. A poor diet will eventually result in poor digestion and absorption. Symptoms of degeneration alert us to the need to change our priorities.

Deficiency has been documented. It is widespread in affluent populations (see Chapter 13, Essential Nutrients). Young and old suffer most, but all age groups are affected. The scientific research literature is now filled with reports of deficiencies of essential nutrients in degenerative conditions. Diets of hospital dieticians themselves – the 'experts' in nutrition – have been shown to be nutritionally deficient. Hospital diets have been analyzed and shown to worsen nutritional deficiency in patients at a time when due to illness, their nutrition should be optimized. Patients on an intravenous before and after surgery usually get only a saline (fluid and electrolyte replacement) or a glucose drip, but not the minerals and vitamins required for glucose metabolism, health, and healing. Both saline and glucose drips are forms of fasting (nutrient deprivation), imposed on those who can least afford to be deprived of nutrients. Recovering patients need the complete range of essential nutrients in their drip. Such formulas are readily available.

Nutrient imbalances are a second type of malnutrition. They include imbalances in:

- the ratio of w3 to w6 essential fatty acids (EFAs);
- the ratio between non-essential and essential fatty acids;
- the ratios between different B vitamins;
- the ratios between different minerals;
- the ratio of concentrated, calorie-rich foods to fiber; and
- the relative amounts of fat, carbohydrates, and protein.

Nutrient excesses are the third type of malnutrition, with toxic effects. These include excesses of:

- vitamins A or D, which can be toxic;
- fats or proteins which have toxic effects on liver and kidneys;
- sugar, which has many toxic effects in all cells and tissues;
- oxygen and water; and
- in theory, we can get too much of any nutrient substance.

Government surveys. Two U.S. government-sponsored surveys, known as the Health and Nutrition Examination Surveys (HANES I & II) and National Food Consumption Survey (NFCS), as well as the Ten State Nutritional Survey, and a large Canadian survey measured intake of 13 of the nearly 50 known essentials in thousands of people, and found over 60% of the population getting less than the government-set Recommended Daily Allowance (RDA). Estimates for deficiency of other essential nutrients have been made by clinicians. This information was presented in Chapter 13.

Improved nutrition. We can prevent and reverse degeneration due to nutrient deficiency by means of improved, enriched nutrition. This can be accomplished by:

- a change from refined and processed foods to *fresh whole foods;*
- the use of *enzymes* that ensure complete digestion of our foods;
- the use of *fresh juices*, which are mineral-, vitamin-, and enzyme-rich, and require little energy to digest; our cells can use energy not needed for digestive functions – which normally consume a great deal of it – for healing and house-cleaning our body;
- the use of nutrient-rich *super-foods* such as kelp, brewer's yeast, flax, sardines, green and blue-green algae, barley and wheat grass, bee pollen, and others;
- the use of *food concentrates* that are rich in essential nutrients; and
- the use of *supplements* of key essential nutrients.

Whole foods, super-foods, food concentrates, and juices should exclude those that produce allergies, which place a great burden on our immune system. Essential nutrients in powder form are allergy-free.

An imbalance or excess of nutrients is balanced by adjusting the amounts of nutrients with respect to one another. This fine-tuning aspect of building health is important because an excess of one essential mineral may decrease the absorption of another, and an excess of one B vitamin may cause a relative shortage of others. Excess fats and sugar can interfere with the functions of EFAs, vitamin C, and other essential nutrients.

Internal Pollution (Poisoning, Toxicity)

By definition, internal pollution is due to poisonous, toxic molecules that interfere with biochemical reactions. These can come from many sources. They subvert our body's normal functions on the biological, biochemical, molecular levels. They interfere with the biochemistry of life by slowing down, rerouting, or blocking biochemical reactions.

Environmental. Some poisons exist naturally in nature. They include bee stings, ant, spider, and snake bites; poison oak, poison ivy, and poison mushrooms; and poisons from other wild plants, animals, microorganisms, and spoiled foods.

We have synthetically made other poisons that now pollute our soil, food, water, and air, and enter our body with what we eat, drink, and breathe – pesticides, synthetics, industrial chemicals, heavy metals, chlorine, smog, etc.

Still other poisons pollute our indoor home environment. They include 'outgassing' from synthetic fibers in clothing, drapes, and carpets; fumes from paints, varnishes, household cleaners, cosmetics, etc.; as well as radiation from TV, computers, electrical wiring and motors, cellular telephones, and other modern gadgets.

Alcohol and tobacco are poisons. Street drugs are poisons that affect thoughts, moods, and consciousness. Pharmaceutical drugs are poisons – their 'side effects' are the obvious signs of their poisonous properties.

Metabolic. Toxins are also produced within our body. Some are normal metabolic waste products that our body usually discards with ease through breath, sweat, urine, and stool. If they remain within our body, they can exert toxic effects. Others are absorbed from our colon due to poor digestion or fermentation activity of microorganisms in our intestines.

Infectious. Still other poisons may be produced within our body by infectious organisms: protozoa, bacteria, fungi, yeasts, and viruses. They result from normal activities of these pathogenic organisms.

Allergic. Further poisons may be produced by our body's defenses against foreign proteins, and other substances to which we have developed allergic responses. These create biochemical disorganization, and constitute an enormous burden for the molecular and cellular police force and army of our immune system which, when overloaded, can lead to immune collapse and cancer.

Stress. Our biochemical reactions to chronic physical and mental stress can also produce toxic substances within our body.

Pollution control (detoxification). For health, we need to practice pollution control. Many methods of detoxification are available, but they all try to perform one of the following functions:

1. Prevent poisons in our environment (soil, food, water, air) from entering our body. In the short term, this means choosing cleaner (organic) foods from the range of foods that is available to us. In the long term, it means learning to care for life and our planet enough to choose not to use processes that leave radioactive and chemical pollutants in our planet's soil, water, and air.

    Foods for healing degenerative diseases must be grown in fertile soils free of toxic chemicals, and foods should be free of pesticide and other toxic residues (organically grown). Water for both drinking and bathing/showering should be filtered if necessary. Bath and shower water are a greater threat to health than drinking water, because volatile toxins and chlorine enter and damage our unprotected lungs. Air can also be filtered if necessary, especially for those who suffer from airborne allergies.

    Avoidance of foods to which one is allergic is a method of preventing toxic reactions from taking place.

2. Remove poisons from our body at a faster rate than we take them in. Water carries toxic materials from our body. Saunas, increased fluid intake, and sweating from exercise help remove toxic materials from our body. Mucilage fibers help keep our intestines clean and carry toxins out of our body into the

toilet. Friendly bacteria help prevent pathogenic organisms from being able to grow. Charcoal may be helpful to absorb toxic materials from our intestine. It also lowers cholesterol.

Our colon can be kept clean by means of appropriate kinds of fiber, or by the judicious use of enemas. Properly supervised castor oil purges may also be helpful.

3. Neutralize poisons by changing them chemically into less poisonous or non-poisonous substances. Fevers increase the rate at which detoxifying chemical reactions take place.

Our liver, our most important detoxifying organ, which must neutralize the poisons in our cells and blood, needs to be encouraged in this function. A substance called silymarin from the herb milk thistle, specifically improves its ability to detoxify, and protects it from damage.

Vitamin C, niacin, vitamin E, carotene, and other antioxidants disarm toxic free radicals and poisons. Nutrients like iodine, w3 fatty acids, and niacin increase oxidation and metabolic rate, increasing energy available for all life functions, including detoxification.

A complete program. For natural therapy, a complete program is necessary. It requires more than the specific points listed above. A complete and balanced nutritional program, exercise, relaxation, social harmony, contentment – in short, a life-style in line with natural living – are necessary for complete healing by natural means. The essence of natural healing is to realign ourselves with the requirements of our own nature.

If health means wholeness, then we must eat clean, nutrient-rich foods, drink clean water, and breathe clean air, be active, develop harmonious relationships, live in harmony with the natural environment, and feel content with life (see Chapter 91, Health as Wholeness).

Time Required for Cure

A natural program that reverses degenerative conditions by addressing the underlying nutritional and toxicity factors involved in the development of these conditions takes about two years to complete if we do everything right, because the entire human body is completely rebuilt in that time (in university the more conservative estimate of seven years was given). Rapidly-growing and chemically active tissues like liver, intestinal lining, and skin replace themselves every 2 to 6 weeks. Slower tissues turn over more slowly.

Within 24 months, every atom within our body has been replaced by new atoms derived from foods, water, and air, without us losing body structure or personality. This means that if we eat optimally nutrient-rich, easily digested, toxin-free foods compatible with the capacities and limitations of our own digestive system for two years, our inherent rebuilding mechanisms can rebuild us a completely new body according to (within the limits set by) our genetic endowment, which built it in the first place.

A treatment program of this kind, with minor variations in helpful supplements, can reverse most major degenerative conditions, including cancer, cardiovascular disease, diabetes, arthritis, and even multiple sclerosis. Cured terminal cancer patients have been presented before the U.S. Senate since 1946 with full documentation. But the politics of the drug-oriented disease management business continue to keep natural treatments from being adopted by the medical profession or widely disseminated to the public (see Chapter 88, The Business and Politics of Health).

Thorough. A thorough program is time-consuming and painstaking. It it is built on the premise that degenerative diseases must be treated and reversed by nutrient enrichment and detoxification. This requires changes from food habits that led to the degenerative condition. Patients are advised to eat *organically-grown* whole, fresh foods, fresh juices from organic foods, superfoods and food concentrates, and specific nutrient supplements. Certain herbs can also be useful, and homeopathic remedies may also help.

For curing cancer, such a program adds supplements of digestive enzymes, hydrochloric acid, w3s, potassium, iodine, vitamin B_3, and other effective substances to the organic foods and fresh juices from organically-grown vegetables and fruit. For detoxification, it uses vitamin C, fiber, clean (filtered) water for drinking and bathing, and careful food selection to avoid foods that produce digestive and allergic reactions. For diabetes, chromium and zinc are critical to the success of the program.

A natural therapy program holds *all* drugs to be liver-toxic. Chemotherapy drugs are especially counterproductive to natural healing because of their toxicity to our liver, whose function of detoxification should be supported, not inhibited. Drugs are also toxic to our other organs, our rebuilding mechanisms, and our body's healing capacity.

Natural therapy is not a magic bullet approach or a quick-fix of symptom suppression, but addresses deficiency and toxicity in a thorough and deliberate way, based on understanding the nutritional causes of physical degeneration. Natural therapy directs itself to removing these causes.

Natural therapy is not complete as soon as tumors recede, because cancer is usually the end symptom of long-standing deficiency and toxification of the entire system. The body must receive the nutrients necessary for healing, and must be protected from the toxins that interfere with normal, natural cell functions. If these two needs are effectively met, cancer cannot grow and can often be reversed.

Cured terminal cancer patients whose tumors completely disappeared under such a treatment program, whose cancer and body toxicity were completely reversed, remain alive and completely cancer-free 10, 20, 30, and even 40 years after being diagnosed 'terminal' (which means: go home and die) by orthodox physicians.[1]

Cardiovascular disease and some types of diabetes are easy to cure. Arthritis, allergies, asthma, migraines, and many other conditions respond well to nutrient enrichment, improved digestion, selection of compatible foods, and detoxification.

Natural therapy works because it is in line with the body's nature and its requirements for optimum biological function, which *define* health.

It seems remarkable that as individuals or as nations, we only rarely practice healing and prevention based on clear understanding of the natural foundation of human health. We cannot attend a university anywhere in the world that grants degrees in a course of studies upon whose completion we can articulate the nature of human health in an organized and coherent fashion.

The Argument for Natural Therapies

Let me list, in point form, some of the main points to consider about the biological basis of natural therapies.

1. **Background observations from science.**
   a. The energy that keeps us alive never gets sick.
   b. The electrons and atoms that make up our body never get sick.
   c. Individual molecules never get sick.
   d. Since energy, atoms, and molecules do not get sick, sickness must originate on a more complex level – the level of molecular interactions and processes that form complex organizations characteristic of living organisms. Disease, then, is a result of intermolecular disorganization.
   e. Molecular interactions can follow the normal course of nature for an organism (health), or they can deviate from that course (disease).
   f. We can interfere with these interactions by withholding substances essential to their occurrence (minerals, co-factors, substances being acted upon during metabolism, etc.) or by 'poisoning' these molecular interactions (with heavy metals, natural 'poisons', special synthetic molecular poisons, etc.).

2. **Background observations from nature.**
   a. Wild animals living in their natural state rarely suffer degenerative diseases.
   b. Wild animals eat foods that are fresh, raw, live, organically-grown, sun-ripened, and in season. Nothing is processed.
   c. When we feed animals food processed by the methods we use for our own foods, they get degenerative disease similar to those that affect humans.
   d. Like the bodies of animals, the human body evolved, developed, and lives within nature. It is a part of nature.

---

[1] Orthodox medicine considers a cure to be 5 years' survival with no *clinical* evidence of the disease after initial diagnosis of cancer. This means that a 'cured' cancer patient can die of cancer the year after being cured. Earlier diagnosis would improve survival time even if ineffective treatments continue to be used.

3. **Health is a natural state.**

  a. Internally, its optimum possibility is determined by our genetic makeup, which includes complex and sophisticated digestive, absorptive, constructive, maintaining, dismantling, metabolic, protective, and healing mechanisms. Because individuals differ genetically, optimum health is also somewhat different for different individuals.

  b. Externally, health is determined by the natural environment, which provides:
  • the surroundings (setting);
  • the building blocks from which our body is constructed and continuously reconstructed; and
  • toxic substances that can interfere with processes that underlie health and healing.

4. **Our body is made from foods, water, air, and light energy.**

  a. The key to effective primary health care and disease prevention is found in living as we would live if we were in an ideal natural setting, where foods are fresh, alive, raw, sun-ripened, locally grown, in season, and pesticide-free. Water is clean. Air is clean. Light is full-spectrum sunlight.

  b. From foods, water, and air our body must derive nearly 50 essential factors that it must obtain to function in a healthy way, but that it cannot make from other substances. These include 20 or 21 minerals; 13 vitamins; 8 to 11 essential amino acids; 2 essential fatty acids; water; air; light; and a source of energy (usually carbohydrates). Processing removes essential nutrients from foods and may also destroy nutrients or change them into toxic substances. Deficiencies of essential nutrients and toxicity in foods have both been documented.

  c. For each essential factor, a minimum, maximum, and optimum level can be determined. Below minimum levels, there is deficiency resulting in physical deterioration. Beyond maximum levels, there may be toxicity leading to physical deterioration.

  d. Optimum levels of nutrients can vary by tenfold or more between different individuals. Each individual must therefore determine for him or herself their personal minimum, maximum, and optimum amounts for each essential substance.

5. **Disease is a departure from health.**

  a. A departure from health is a departure from the natural state – internally, externally, or both.

  b. All diseases have causes that can be discovered.

  c. Diseases that result from injury on organ, tissue, and cell levels must ultimately be expressions of change(s) on the molecular level.

  d. The most common causes of degenerative diseases include *malnutrition* (deficiency of essential substances, nutrient imbalances, nutrient excesses) and *internal pollution* (interfering substances: pollutants, heavy metals,

414

organic and inorganic poisons, drugs, metabolic waste products, toxins produced by organisms, toxins made in our body as a result of allergic reactions).

    e. Even when we are sick, most of the cellular processes throughout our body remain normal and function normally.

6. **Degenerative diseases can be reversed.**

    a. Reversal of degenerative diseases caused by malnutrition and internal pollution requires *improved nutrition* and *pollution cleanup* (detoxification).

    b. Nutrition can be improved by the use of whole foods, fresh juices, superfoods, food concentrates, and supplements in pill, powder, or liquid form.

    c. Detoxification requires clean sources of food, water, and air, and enhancement of our body's toxin-neutralizing and eliminating functions. Detoxification may include avoiding incompatible (allergy-activating) foods, increasing oxidation rate, increasing intake of detoxifying nutrients (vitamin C, antioxidants, etc.), using digestives (HCl, enzymes, bile), sweating and increasing activity (to improve circulation and oxidation), improving bowel hygiene (soluble fiber, enemas), using herbs that enhance liver and immune functions (silymarin, echinacea, etc.), and others.

7. **Our body is self-healing.**

    a. We have all experienced healing of cuts, bruises, injuries, and broken bones. Fascinating to watch. Marvellous to contemplate. Our body knows how to heal itself. When healing fails, we must ask: Why?

    b. In order for our body to reverse and cure degenerative conditions, we must supply it with the tools of nature which it needs for healing. We do not heal it, but we can support its inherent self-healing by providing appropriate molecules from nature.

    c. Clean food, water, and air – and the 50 essential factors they contain – are the natural sources of healing molecules.

    d. It takes about 2 years for the body to rebuild itself completely. Done properly, this is also the time it takes to completely reverse a malnutrition- and/or internal pollution-induced degenerative condition, and to remove accumulated toxins from the body.

8. **There is a point of no return.**

    a. Recovery by natural (or other) means is no longer possible when healing mechanisms or organs have become damaged beyond repair. We don't know where that point is for any disease.

    b. The point of no return can be reached through inappropriate treatments or, in the end, from natural aging mechanisms taking their inevitable course.

    Challenge. Think about these points. Question them. Understand their meaning. Pick them apart. Discuss them with others. You don't need a PhD to understand the biological basis of health and healing. Once you have understood that health is inherent (within limits determined by each person's unique genetic makeup) and that disease is a departure from health, the rest of the natural healing approach follows logically. It is then just a matter of gathering the details and putting a natural healing program into practice.

91 *Health as Wholeness*

In this closing chapter, I want to take a look at health as wholeness within the context of human nature.

The bulk of this book concentrated on a limited (though extremely important) part of only one of three components of human beings, the physical-nutritional component. Of about 50 known essential factors that make up this component of health, we focused mainly on two – the essential fatty acids – and to a lesser extent on the other 48. A simple-minded, search for a 'magic bullet' molecule, whether natural or synthetic, that can bring us health and cure our ills is unrealistic and leads to disappointment.

My journey to understand health and human nature began early. As long as I can remember, I've always hated illness and suffering. I didn't think it was necessary. I didn't want to see others suffer, and I didn't like being sick myself. When I was still a young boy, I started wondering what health might be. I thought that if I knew health, I would know both how to avoid and how to cure illness.

Health

Let's look at the word 'health'. The word 'health' is derived from the Old High German root word for 'whole', which implies that all parts are present, properly arranged, and properly functioning in harmonious balance. Other root word meanings of the word health include 'hale' (also meaning whole), and 'holy', which may also be related to the word 'health' in its original meaning.

Common usage does not reflect these original meanings of the word 'health'. We use the word more in the sense of 'freedom from disease, pain, or defect'. We are healthy when we are not sick. But if you examine it, this way of using the word misleads us. Health has to be the *presence* of something – all parts in proper arrangement, working in harmonious balance – that makes us whole, hale, holy, and healthy. When we lose that presence, those parts, that arrangement, that harmonious and balanced function, disease results. We need to search for, find, and embrace that presence.

Medical Students

By and large, medical students are not independent, brilliant thinkers. Rather, they tend to be conservative and hard-working, doing what they are told to do, learning what they are told to learn, questioning not very much. They enter the

416

profession that delivers 'health care' – a misleading term for both students and the public, that should be replaced by the more accurate term 'disease management' – as young adults, assuming that they will learn to deliver health care. After training, they tend to be skeptical about the connection between nutrition and health.

"If nutrition were important to health, we would have learned about it in medical school," one doctor told me. This is the medical profession's catch-22. Ignorance overlaid by professional arrogance is a deluding combination.

Medicine

When I enrolled in medical school, I knew my goal very clearly: I wanted to learn what health is. I had not yet discovered that medicine has more to do with 'sick-experts', business, careers, making money, image-making, politicking, vested interests, entrenched ways of thinking, turf protection, and powerful lobby groups than it does with health.

During my first year, I discovered to my dismay that medicine is not about health. Not a single course was offered on the nature of human health. Medicine teaches diagnosis of disease, and the use of drugs to fight or suppress the signs and symptoms of disease. With no definition of health that we might aim for, and with no notion of how to establish or reestablish health, we would not recognize health even if we stumbled and became impaled upon it.

We neglect our health (whatever that may be) until it fails. Then we consult doctors, in the stated or unstated expectation and hope that they can make our illness go away, and thus bring back our health. Doctors diagnose our illness(es) and, without knowing what health is, treat us – cure is *not guaranteed* – mainly by prescribing the 'medicines' of surgery, radiation, and drugs. Those who prefer more natural treatments of disease disparagingly call medicine the 'cut, burn, poison approach'.

More recently, modern medicine has also begun to concern itself with disease prevention, but disease prevention is not health, either. I wanted to learn about the nature of health.

Dialog

I took my dismay to the Dean of my medical school and a conversation, which went roughly like the following, ensued.

"What is health?" I asked him.

"We don't know," he answered. "We're working on it."

"Health must be more than just not being sick!" I suggested. He agreed, adding that the World Health Organization (WHO) had been saying that for years. WHO defines health as "a state of complete physical, mental, and social well-being and not merely an absence of disease or infirmity." This definition does not provide much help, because it fails to give *practical* guidelines for bringing someone who lacks physical, mental, and social well-being back to physical, mental, and social well-being – health. However, I felt encouraged by the Dean's remark, and went on.

"It's really important to know what health is! If we *know* health, curing illness becomes relatively easy. We know that illness is a departure, in some direction, from health. If we know what health is, we can just turn a sick person who wants to get well back in the direction of health."

"Yes, but we don't know what health is," the Dean reminded me.

At that point, I missed my cue to stop, because the Dean appeared open and friendly, and I was naive. "How about life itself?" I suggested, carried away by my enthusiasm. "Life energy creates, maintains, and repairs our cells, tissues and organs, using the nutrients present in our foods according to our inherited genetic program. It knows (though we don't know) exactly where to take each molecule and how to use it. Therefore it must also be the ultimate standard of health." His eyebrows rose but, on a roll, I went on. "Whatever brings us closer in harmony with life will bring us closer to health. All we need to do is discover it, get to know it, and live according to its nature." The conversation ended very quickly then. The feeling in the room had grown distinctly darker.

Later, reflecting on the conversation, I realized that the moment I used the term 'life energy', I lost the Dean completely. My notion was too ephemeral for him. Not hard enough for 'hard' science. For me, that conversation was the beginning of a long, independent search to discover the nature of health and of human nature, a search that led me through the fields of many sciences, especially biology, biochemistry, psychology, and consciousness.

Life and life's energy are facts. They are less controversial than new drugs and organ transplants; they have been around far longer than both of these high-tech inventions, and will still be around when both have been abandoned for something not yet imagined by medical scientists. Life's energy[1] is within everything that lives. While it is present, so much is possible. We walk, talk, eat, work, heal, digest, think, reproduce, feel, laugh, and play. Without it, nothing! We might as well have a look at it, get to know it, maybe even make friends with it. We might as well look at the other components of human nature as well. Our refusal to do so reminds me of a story.

Galileo's Apple Cart

Until Galileo's time, our planet was considered the center of the universe. The

---

[1] Life energy uses our inherited genetic DNA master plan, translates this into an RNA blueprint, and uses the RNA blueprint to manage the production of proteins, both structural and enzymatic. These proteins catalyze the building and assembly of molecules into the superstructure that we call the human body. Life's energy is the power that activates and drives translation processes. Without this energy, the genetic program is untranslatable, and *nothing* happens.

stars, moon, and sun were thought to revolve around the earth.

Along comes Galileo who, by using a telescope, charts the movements of the celestial bodies. He discovers that the earth revolves around the sun.

The scientists and theologians of his time were outraged at his proposition. It contradicted what they'd learned, believed, and taught. Galileo had upset their conceptual apple cart, and the apples were rolling everywhere. Instead of changing their mind, they threw him in jail. Today, we laugh at these 'learned' men, because though Galileo had telescope and mathematical proofs, and put everything at their disposal when he invited them to see for themselves, they wouldn't even look. Their minds were closed on the subject, because they thought they knew the truth.

We too are like the learned minds of Galileo's time, though not about the earth and sun anymore. That issue was settled in Galileo's favor. We *all* believe him now. Our preoccupation with disease and crisis intervention, and our refusal to take the time necessary to look for and find the nature of health is a modern version of Galileo's apple cart.

We believe in disease, but not in health. Countless sincere men and women have dedicated their lives to study and describe diseases in greater and greater detail. Huge institutions have been built around disease, including medical schools, research centers, and hospitals. Huge organizations have grown around the focus of diseases, including many 'professional' associations, government agencies, and support groups.

Enormous amounts of time, attention, money, and effort have fostered the growth of the monster of disease, while health has been left to grow without nurture.

A turnaround in our way of thinking is necessary if health is what we are *really* after. Health is not the absence of disease. Disease is the absence of health. Health is the presence of something.

Health, Wholeness, and Human Nature

Health as wholeness means living in alignment with human nature. If we want to know what health in the sense of wholeness is, we need to know more about the parameters of human nature, which consists of several components that synergize and synchronize to establish and maintain wholeness.

Wholeness is something within us that we feel and radiate when we live aligned with all aspects of our nature. I'd like to share with you a model for understanding health-wholeness, that I derived from observation, experience, study, and common sense. My view and my way of articulating this model are biased by my background in science and psychology, and my interest in consciousness, in life.

Three components. Human nature can be said to consist of three distinct components: what keeps us alive, what our bodies are made of, and what we've learned. In healthy people, all three components of human nature are integrated. They work together in harmony.

Each of these three components differs from the others in its makeup, its function, its properties, and its relationship to health. Each must be studied by a different method in order to be known; each requires a different kind of attention; each requires attention on a regular basis; each responds to a different kind of intervention. To establish and maintain health, we must work with each component in accordance with its distinctive nature.

Energy

According to physicists, the essence of energy is energy itself: it is stable, constant, unchangeable, indestructible, and indivisible. It cannot be burned, drowned, broken, or dried. Energy pervades our entire body, enlivens every cell, and powers us. It catalyzes the chemical changes that make life possible but it remains unchanged. It is beyond our narrow view of health and illnesses, beyond our beliefs and concepts, beyond learning.

Besides these more obvious and scientifically verifiable attributes of energy, there is a more subtle experiential attribute to life's energy. It can be felt. In the direct experience of life energy, one discovers a *feeling of contentment, completion, fulfillment – a feeling of well-being* deep within the core of one's being. This is the private, solitary, always existing, still, undisturbable part of our nature. Within the heart of our being, we are alone in our enjoyment of life. An individual can know this life energy and feel content regardless of circumstances.

The experience of life energy does not guarantee social change, improved moral character, more ethical behavior, greater physical and/or mental health, or money in the bank. Such changes are brought about through decisions and actions, all of which belong to the other two components of human nature. In other words, it is possible to feel content while the body is ravaged by terminal cancer, and in the midst of mental and social turmoil.

If we are unable to connect ourselves to the life energy within us, we may feel incomplete, discontent, or frustrated, even in situations which (we think) are ideal and *should* make us feel content, or we vaguely long – for what, we know not. If our own attempts to reach contentment are unsuccessful, someone may be able to provide guidance. If you don't succeed in being your own teacher of contentment, find a master of this aspect of human nature who is willing to teach, and become that master's student.

Body

Our body, the subject of *physical health*, is made from food, water, and air. It is made for *activity*. Physical health depends on two factors, within limits set by a third.

First, it depends on the quality of food, water, air, and light, from which we

420

must obtain ample (or optimum) quantities of about 50 different essential factors, including 20 minerals, 13 vitamins, 8 to 11 essential amino acids, 2 essential fatty acids, water, oxygen, a source of fuel, and light. Complete absence of any one of these 50 must eventually kill the body. Deficiency of any one of more of them results in less than optional functioning, in gradual deterioration, increasing degeneration, degenerative disease, and finally, death.

Second, physical health also depends on the absence of toxic substances – defined as those that interfere with normal biochemical and metabolic functions – from our food, water, air, and light.

Third, physical health is possible only within limits set by each individual's unique genetic makeup, inherited from parents made by nature created by life.

To the extent that they are not genetic (only about 5 in 1000 people have inherited genetic 'defects'), all degenerative conditions are caused by malnutrition (deficiency or imbalance of essential substances and excess of certain non-essential substances) and/or poisoning (toxicity, internal pollution) due to the presence of interfering substances – toxins. The reversal of non-genetic degenerative conditions therefore requires improved nutrition, through nutrient enrichment, balance, and moderation; and/or poison control, through detoxification and the avoidance of toxins.

Optimum food, water, and air, plus avoidance of toxic influences constitutes *self-responsible primary health care* or *self-care* – the basis of physical health – that each individual must attend to him or herself. For tools to help practice primary health care, look to nature.

A good primary health care program includes optimum quantities of all essential food substances from fresh foods grown in the most natural way possible, augmented where necessary by concentrates of these substances in pill, powder, or liquid form. Clean food, water, air, and light also require a clean environment – the major worldwide issue facing us in the future.

For life-threatening crises, broken bones, serious injury and infection, high-tech life support systems, and disease management, look to high-tech medical intervention, surgery and drugs. This is not health care but *crisis management by experts*. Our failure in health care is that we have applied disease and crisis management techniques to conditions begging for treatments in line with the nature of the human body, and have almost completely ignored the arsenal of nature and natural primary health care.

Made *from* food, our body is made *for* activity. If it is inactive, our body serves no purpose and degenerates. Besides food, water, air, and a non-toxic environment, activity is also necessary for physical health.

The body is created out of smaller units: atoms, molecules, cells, organs, and tissues. It will one day be destroyed, dismantled into these smaller units again. Physical health can therefore be described as a worthwhile but losing proposition!

Within this restriction, physical health based on fulfilling our body's requirements for food, water, air, light, absence of toxins, and exercise enables us to live fully functional, active lives.

Nutrition, health, and fitness are key disciplines that will eventually address this component of human nature more fully.

Mind

Mind, the subject of *mental health*, is complex, beginning with simple feelings of comfort and discomfort, which are elaborated into our emotions. To these, we anchor first sensory inputs from both environment and our own body; later, increasingly complex abstractions that we interpret and organize into belief systems – our 'cognitive blueprints for living'; our individually created 'style of life' (according to psychologist Alfred Adler) that determines the direction for our actions and thereby our destiny. Mind consists of emotional, mental, social, and environmental impressions mostly learned after birth.

According to Adler and his student Rudolf Dreikurs, the essence of mental health is a sense of belonging and constructive contribution to the well-being of the whole of which we are a part (self, family, humanity, nature, life). In addition to being private individuals, we are also social creatures living our lives in social settings with others. Through learning we choose, acquire, and embrace conceptual frameworks, or belief systems meant to adapt us to live harmoniously in complex, constantly changing social and natural environments.

This view is practical and optimistic. We *chose* the views and beliefs we hold, and when they fail to serve us because the situation has changed from the one in which we developed these views and beliefs, we can choose to learn others that work better in present contexts. Improving mental health is a matter of educating and reeducating ourselves toward better social integration, cooperation, and contribution.

People who lose their sense of belonging lose their feeling of kinship and equality with others. This is mental illness. They become discouraged, develop inferiority feelings, become preoccupied with having power over others rather than within themselves, and behave in socially useless and destructive ways. Helping discouraged people toward better mental health requires acceptance of their equality, encouragement, and acknowledgment of socially useful contributions.

Mind is located in the surface of our brain, that part known as the 'associative cortex'. It connects us outward, through our senses and perception, to the social and natural world within which we live, and inward to all parts of our body.

Key disciplines that must deal with learning and mind include parenting, education and, when these fail, counseling. When parents, teachers, and counselors all fail, lawyers, judges, mental hospitals, and jails take over.

Integration

In order to be fully human, we need to feel content, be physically healthy and active for as long as possible, and live in social and environmental harmony. Every day, we need to feel; need to eat, drink, breathe, and act; and need to learn and understand.

Our problems must be correctly identified within the component of human nature in which they originated. They can then be solved by moving to a deeper level in that component than that at which they originated, and operating from that deeper level.[2] Solutions are found behind (or beneath,) problems, not in their projections. Physical problems have physical solutions. Mental problems have mental solutions. Energy problems have energy solutions. When we embrace the essence of each component of our nature, we maximize our possibilities for complete well-being, health, and harmony.

We have to be open to learn, because there is a lot to learn, a lot to experience, a lot to enjoy. We can learn to be quiet and observe our habits and our ways of thinking – to become sensitive to ourselves.

We learn best, not by blindly following rules or opinions, but by relaxed attention; by watching with an open heart and a calm mind the ways of nature and of life. In this calm state of being, we can see clearly, and learning becomes discovery – easy and natural. It is a state to nurture. Life is a flow with its own texture, melody, and beauty.

To a lover, the whole world vibrates with love. It can be seen everywhere. Love is not an opinion or concept projected on the world, as cynics out of touch with love claim. A lover has discovered the depth of life's nature, sees that depth in everything, and feels grateful for the wonder and the gift of life.

If we expect to succeed in our quest for wholeness, we need to get to know, to respect, to trust, to love, and to merge in our own nature. And this is really the basis of health in its wider sense of wholeness – trust in life, in nature, and in human nature. In our 'transformation' to wholeness, we do not change ourselves. We simply discover more and more of the wonder that is always present within us, the wonder that is our life. Wholeness is achieved by discovering our own human nature and harmonizing with it, to all the way deep inside.

---

[2] Albert Einstein observed that we cannot solve our problems at the same level at which we were operating when we created them, but must operate from a deeper level in order to solve them.

Abbreviations

AA - arachidonic acid
AIDS - Acquired Immune Deficiency
    Syndrome
ALA - alpha-linolenic acid
ALD - adrenoleukodystrophy
ALENA - alpha-linolenic acid
AO(s) - antioxidant(s)
Apo(a) - Apoprotein(a)
BA - butyric acid
BHA - butylated hydroxyanisole
BHT - butylated hydroxytoluene
C - Celsius
CF - cystic fibrosis
CH_3 - methyl
COOH - carboxyl
CVD - cardiovascular disease
D6D - delta-6-desaturase
DGLA - dihomogamma-linolenic acid
DHA - docosahexaenoic acid
DNA - deoxyribonucleic acid
DPA - docosapentaenoic acid
EDTA - ethylene diamine tetraacetic acid
EFA(s) - essential fatty acid(s)
EPA - eicosapentaenoic acid
EPO - evening primrose oil
ETA - ecosatetraenoic acid
F - Fahrenheit
FAO - Food and Agricultural Organization
FAS - fetal alcohol syndrome
FBD - fibrocystic breast disease
FDA - Food and Drug Administration
FR - fractionation
GAS - General Adaptation Syndrome
GLA - gamma-linolenic acid
GRAS - Generally Recognized As Safe
GTF - glucose tolerance factor
H_2O - water
HANES - Health & Nutrition Examination
    Survey
HDL - high-density lipoprotein(s)
HEAR - high erucic acid rapeseed
IU - International Unit(s)
IUD(s) - intrauterine device(s)
kg - kilogram
LA - linoleic acid

LDL - low density lipoprotein(s)
LEAR - low erucic acid rapeseed
LNA - alpha-linolenic acid
Lp(a) - lipoprotein(a)
mcg - microgram
MCT(s) - medium-chain triglyceride(s)
MD - medical doctor
MDR - minimum daily requirement
meq/kg - milli-equivalents per kilogram
mg - milligram
mg/dl - milligrams per deciliter
mL - milliliter
mmol/L - millimoles per liter
MS - multiple sclerosis
MUFA(s) - monounsaturated fatty acid(s)
Na_2CO_3 - sodium carbonate
NAC - N-acetyl cysteine
NAG - N-acetyl glucosamine
NaOH - sodium hydroxide
NFCS - Nationwide Food Consumption
    Survey
OA - oleic acid
OH - hydroxyl
P5P - pyridoxine-5-phosphate
PA - palmitic acid
PABA - para aminobenzoic acid
PCB(s) - polychlorinated biphenyl(s)
PE - polyethylene
PG(s) - prostaglandin(s)
PG1 - prostaglandin 1
PG2 - prostaglandin 2
PG3 - prostaglandin 3
PhD - Doctor of Philosophy degree
Phe - phenylalanine
PKU - phenylketonuria
PL(s) - phospholipid(s)
PMS - premenstrual syndrome
POA - palmitoleic acid
PUFA(s) - polyunsaturated fatty acid(s)
PV - peroxide value
RDA(s) - Recommended Daily Allowance(s)
RNA - ribonucleic acid
SA - stearic acid
SaFA(s) - saturated fatty acid(s)
SDA - stearidonic acid

SH - sulphydryl
SOD - superoxide dismutase
SUFA(s) - superunsaturated fatty acid(s)
TBHQ - tertiary butyhydroquinone
TCP - thrombocytopenia
TE - transesterification
TG(s) - triglyceride(s)
THC - tetrahydrocannabinol
TPP - thiamin pyrophosphate
UV - ultra-violet
UFA(s) - unsaturated fatty acid(s)
vitamin A - retinol, retinal, and retinoic acid
vitamin B_1 - thiamin
vitamin B_2 - riboflavin
vitamin B_3 - niacin
vitamin B_5 - pantothenic acid
vitamin B_6 - pyridoxine
vitamin B_{12} - cyanocobalamin
vitamin C - ascorbic acid
vitamin D - cholecalciferol and ergocalciferol
vitamin E - tocopherols
vitamin K - phylloquinones and menaquinones
VLDL - very low density lipoprotein(s)
W - omega
W3 - omega 3
W6 - omega 6
W9 - omega 9
WHO - World Health Organization
4:0 - butyric acid; four-carbon saturated fatty
  acid
6:0 - caproic acid; six-carbon saturated fatty
  acid
8:0 - caprylic acid; eight-carbon saturated fatty
  acid
10:0 - capric acid; ten-carbon saturated fatty
  acid
12:0 - lauric acid; twelve-carbon saturated fatty
  acid
14:0 - myrisitc acid; fourteen-carbon saturated
  fatty acid
16:0 - palmitic acid; sixteen-carbon saturated
  fatty acid
16:1w7 - palmitoleic acid; 16-carbon
  monounsaturated fatty acid; double
  bond between carbons 7 and 8
18:0 - stearic acid; eighteen-carbon saturated
  fatty acid
18:1w9 - oleic acid; 18-carbon
  monounsaturated fatty acid; double

bond between carbons 9 and 10
18:2w6 - linoleic acid; 18-carbon
  polyunsaturated fatty acid; double
  bonds between carbons 6 and 7, and 9
  and 10
18:3w3 - alpha-linolenic acid; 18-carbon
  superunsaturated fatty acid; double
  bonds between carbons 3 and 4, 6 and
  7, and 9 and 10
18:3w6 - gamma-linolenic acid; 18-carbon
  polyunsaturated fatty acid; double
  bonds between carbons 6 and 7, 9 and
  10, and 12 and 13
18:4w3 - stearidonic acid; 18-carbon
  superunsaturated fatty acid; double
  bonds between carbons 3 and 4, 6 and
  7, 9 and 10, and 12 and 13
20:0 - arachidic acid; twenty-carbon saturated
  fatty acid
20:3w6 - dihomogamma-linolenic acid; 20-
  carbon polyunsaturated fatty acid;
  double bonds between carbons 6 and 7,
  9 and 10, and 12 and 13
20:4w6 - arachidonic acid; 20-carbon
  polyunsaturated fatty acid; double
  bonds between carbons 6 and 7, 9 and
  10, 12 and 13, and 15 and 16
20:5w3 - eicosapentanoic acid; 20-carbon
  superunsaturated fatty acid; double
  bonds between carbons 3 and 4, 6 and
  7, 9 and 10, 12 and 13, and 15 and 16
22:0 - behenic acid; 22-carbon saturated fatty
  acid
22:1w9 - erucic acid; 22-carbon
  monounsaturated fatty acid; double
  bond between carbons 9 and 10
22:1w11 - cetoleic acid; 22-carbon
  monounsaturated fatty acid; double
  bond between carbons 11 and 12
22:6w3 - docosahaxenioc acid; 22-carbon
  superunsaturated fatty acid; double
  bonds between carbons 3 and 4, 6 and
  7, 9 and 10, 12 and 13, 15 and 16, and
  18 and 19
24:0 - lignoceric acid; 24-carbon saturated
  fatty acid

Glossary

acetate: 2-carbon molecular fragments containing an organic (carboxylic) acid group; the basis of acetic acid, which is vinegar; the building block for fatty acids and cholesterol; an intermediate product when sugars and fatty acids are 'burned' to produce energy in our body.

adipose: the scientist's name for fat tissue or body fat.

adrenoleukodystrophy (ALD): a genetic, X-linked condition in which the body over-produces very long-chain saturated fatty acids (20- to 28-carbon chains) that destroy the myelin which is the insulation of nerves in the central nervous system. The disease is usually fatal in childhood, but its effects can be slowed down with a mixture of 20% erucic acid and 80% oleic acid (Lorenzo's oil).

AIDS – Acquired Immune Deficiency Syndrome: a failure of immune function thought to be caused be a virus that can be transmitted by sex, shared needles, and transfusions of tainted blood products. Patients often die of opportunistic infections against which the immune-deficient body cannot defend itself.

all cis- : in a fatty acid, the arrangement where the single hydrogens on both carbons involved in a double bond are found on the same side of the molecule, producing a bend or kink in its shape.

alpha-linolenic acid (LNA, ALA, 18:3w3): an 18-carbon fatty acid with 3 double bonds, positioned between w carbons 3 and 4, 6 and 7, and 9 and 10. It is the second of the 2 essential fatty acids. Our body cannot make it, requires it for life, and must therefore obtain it from food. It is vital to optimum health. LNA is extremely sensitive to destruction by light, oxygen, and high temperature. Deficiency is linked to degenerative disease. Modern diets contain only 1/6 as much LNA as traditional Western diets in 1850. LNA inhibits tumor formation. LNA sources include flax and hemp seeds and their oils.

amino acid: the building block of proteins; there are over 20 different amino acids present in nature.

antioxidant: any of a large group of natural or synthetic substances whose presence slows down oxygen- and free radical-induced deterioration of fatty acids and other substances.

apo(a): a sticky repair protein, made by the liver, that regulates thickening (repair) of arteries in vitamin C deficiency. Apo(a) is a strong risk factor for cardiovascular disease. Increased dietary vitamin C decreases apo(a) concentration.

arachidic acid (20:10): a 20-carbon saturated fatty acid found in peanuts.

arachidonic acid (AA, 20:4w6): a 20-carbon, 4 times unsaturated fatty acid made from the essential linoleic acid by enzymes in our body, and also found in animal foods (meat, eggs, dairy). It is the parent compound from which series 2 prostaglandins are made.

beta carotene: an orange plant pigment; 2 vitamin A molecules hooked tail to tail. While too much vitamin A can be toxic, beta carotene is non-toxic. The body stores carotene, and makes vitamin A from it only as it needs vitamin A.

bile acids: made from cholesterol in the liver and stored in the gallbladder, bile acids help to break fats into smaller droplets. This exposes a larger surface area of fats to the action of fat-digesting enzymes, speeding up fat digestion.

blood cholesterol: all cholesterol in transit from bowel to liver and body cells, and all cholesterol returning from cells to liver to be turned into bile acids and discarded into our intestine.

bond: see chemical bond.

butylated hydroxyanisole (BHA): an artificial preservative added to oils to slow down their deterioration; it replaces vitamin E, which is removed during oil processing.

butylated hydroxytoluene (BHT): an artificial preservative added to oils to slow down their deterioration; it replaces vitamin E, which is removed during oil processing.

butyric acid (BA, 4:0): a short-chain (4-carbon) saturated fatty acid found in butter. BA is beneficial to normal intestinal bacteria.

caproic acid (6:0): a short-chain (6-carbon) saturated fatty acid found in tropical oils and to a small extent in medium-chains triglycerides (MCTs).

caprylic acid (8:0): a medium-chain (8-carbon) saturated fatty acid found in tropical oils and in medium-chain triclycerides (MCTs).

carbon chain: carbon atoms linked to one another in a chain by bonds formed when atoms share electrons.

carboxyl (–COOH): a weak acid group found at one end of fatty acids (and many other molecules found in nature).

cardiovascular disease (CVD): collective term for diseases of the heart and arteries. CVD includes atherosclerosis, ischemic heart disease, strokes, heart attacks, high blood pressure, peripheral arterial disease, emboli, heart failure, heart enlargement, elevated cholesterol and triglycerides, abnormal blood clotting, and other conditions.

catalyst: a molecule that facilitates a specific chemical reaction that would not otherwise take place. Most catalysts in our body are protein enzymes.

cell membrane: a double layer of fatty material (phospholipids) and proteins that surrounds each living cell of all organisms.

chemical bond: atoms held together by sharing electrons with one another to form molecules. Two shared electrons, one each from two atoms, constitute a chemical bond between those atoms.

cholesterol: a complex fatty substance with many important functions in our body. It can be made in our body or supplied through foods of animal origin. Oxidized cholesterol may damage and be deposited in artery linings.

choline: a pseudo-vitamin involved in the metabolism of fats and in nerve function, and found in lecithin (phosphatidyl choline).

chylomicron: fat and cholesterol carrying vehicle, made in our intestinal cells and transported by our lymphatic system into our bloodstream. It is our body's way of getting digested food fats into the bloodstream for distribution to the trillions of cells that need these fats.

cis- configuration: see all *cis-* .

cold-pressed: a meaningless advertising term used to imply quality in edible oils.

complex carbohydrate: sugar molecules linked together in various ways to make digestible molecules such as starch and glycogen or indigestible molecules of fiber, which include cellulose, bran, pectin, mucilage and gum.

cross-link: bonds that form across molecules and result in complex molecular structures. Also, bonds that make tissues more rigid, leading to aging.

cystic fibrosis (CF): a genetic condition usually fatal in early adulthood, in which the secretion of thick mucus in respiratory and digestive systems (due to an error in chloride metabolism) inhibits oxygen and nutrient absorption.

deficiency disease: the negative effect on health of shortage or absence of any one or more of the 50 substances essential for normal functioning of human cells, tissues, and organs.

degenerative disease: loss of the capacity of cells, tissues and organs to function normally. Causes include deficiency of essential nutrients, presence of interfering substances, excess of substances or imbalance in the relative concentrations of substances.

Delta-6-desaturase (D6D): the enzyme that converts w6 linoleic acid (LA) to gammalinolenic acid (GLA), and w3 alpha-linolenic acid (LNA) to stearidonic acid (SDA).

deoxyribonucleic acid (DNA): the genetic material that carries the instructions for most living organisms.

desaturation: the enzymatic process by which 2 hydrogen atoms are removed from neighboring carbon atoms in a fatty acid chain and at the same time, an additional bond is created between these 2 atoms.

dihomogamma-linolenic acid (DGLA, 20:3w6): a fatty acid, the second w6 derivative; made from GLA; DGLA is the parent of hormone-like series 1 prostaglandins which have many beneficial effects on health.

docosahexaenoic acid (DHA, 22:6w3): a 22-carbon fatty acid with 6 double bonds in its chain. It is found in large concentrations in cold-water fish and marine animals, and also in retina, brain, adrenals, and testes. It can be manufactured in healthy human tissue from the essential alpha-linolenic acid (18:3w3).

docosapentaenoic acid (DPA, 22:5w6): the last member of the w6 family. It may pinch-hit for w3 deficiency.

double bond: a linking of adjacent atoms in the carbon chain by sharing 2 pairs of electrons between the carbons instead of the usual 1 shared pair of a single bond.

ethylene diamine tetraacetic acid (EDTA): a chelating (claw-like) molecule used to remove heavy metals and calcium from the human body. It is one way of treating heavy metal toxicity and atherosclerotic deposits in arteries.

eicosapentaenoic acid (EPA, 20:5w3): a 20-carbon fatty acid with 5 double bonds in its chain. It is found in large quantities in cold-water fish and marine animals. The oil of Chinese water snake is the richest known source of EPA. EPA is the parent substance from which the body makes series 3 prostaglandins that decrease inflammation, water retention, and blood pressure by inhibiting the production of pro-inflammatory, water-retaining, artery-constricting series 2 prostaglandins.

eicosatetraenoic acid (ETA, 20:4w3): an intermediate in the conversion of the w3 essential fatty acid to EPA.

elongation: the enzymatic process by which a fatty acid is lengthened by 2 carbon atoms.

emulsify: to break fats into smaller droplets by the action of detergents such as lecithin.

enzyme: a protein produced by the body to catalyze (facilitate) particular chemical reactions. The enzyme that catalyzes the reaction is not itself changed thereby.

essential amino acid: any one of 8 amino acids that the body requires but cannot manufacture and must therefore obtain from foods. For children, 10 amino acids are essential. Premature infants require 11.

essential fatty acid (EFA): either of 2 fatty acids that the body requires, cannot make from other substances and must therefore get from foods. The names of these 2 EFAs are linoleic acid (LA; 18:2w6) and alpha-linolenic acid (LNA: 18:3w3).

essential fatty acid deficiency: shortage of one or both of the essential fatty acids and the attendant effects on health.

essential nutrient: any of about 45 nutrients that are known to be necessary for body structure and physical health. 20 or 21 minerals, 13 vitamins, 8 to 11 amino acids and 2 essential fatty acids must come from foods we eat, since the body cannot manufacture them out of other factors.

essential factor: any of about 50 principles known to be necessary for health. In addition to 45 essential nutrients, a source of calorie energy, water, oxygen, and light are included. Sometimes fiber and intestinal bacteria are also included in the list of essential factor.

esterify: to chemically link an alcohol or acid with another substance in a particular way called an ester linkage.

evening primrose oil (EPO): a w6 plant seed oil containing 9% GLA, which is used in the treatment of Sjogren's syndrome, PMS, arthritis, and type II diabetes.

fat: three free-swinging fatty acid molecules hooked to a glycerol molecule in ester linkages. In common usage, it refers to those substances that fit the above description and are hard at room temperature because they contain mostly saturated fatty acids.

fatty acid: a carbon chain with an organic acid group at one end, and hydrogens attached to the rest of the carbon atoms. The chain length can vary from 4 to 26 or more.

fatty degeneration: fat-related interference with normal biological functions, commonly found in arteries, around tumors, and in liver and other internal organs.

fetal alcohol syndrome (FAS): the developmental effect of maternal alcohol consumption on children: wide spaced eyes, mental retardation, motor problems, emotional lability.

fiber: any of several undigestible complex carbohydrates that make up the 'roughage' of plant material. They promote bowel regularity, help stabilize blood sugar, and help eliminate bile acids and cholesterol from the body.

flax: an ancient plant whose seed oil is the richest source of alpha-linolenic acid (LNA; 18:3w3), which is rare in our foods. It also contains protein, minerals, and vitamins. It is a rich source of mucilage and fiber, which help the body eliminate cholesterol, and help prevent reabsorption of toxic wastes from the large intestine. Flax is also the richest known source of lignans, which have anti-viral, anti-fungal, anti-bacterial and anti-cancer properties. Its oil is used in natural programs for the reversal of cardiovascular disease, cancer, diabetes, premenstrual syndrome, inflammatory conditions, arthritis, etc.

Food and Drug Administration (FDA): government agency charged with controlling the safety of foods and drugs. Has come under fire for biased enforcement favoring drugs over nutrients.

fractionation (FR): a process used to separate fatty acids or triglycerides on the basis of their distinct physical and chemical properties.

free radical: a molecular fragment with a single unpaired electron which, wanting to be paired, steals electrons from other pairs. Free radical reactions occur normally in biological processes.

free radical chain reaction: uncontrolled free radical reaction that is damaging to biological processes.

gamma-linolenic acid (GLA, 18:3w6): a substance made from the essential linoleic acid (18:2w6) by healthy cells, also found in hemp, borage, and evening primrose oils. GLA may help in conditions in which the body's ability to make it from linoleic acid may be impaired. Its best successes are in arthritis and premenstrual syndrome.

General Adaptation Syndrome (GAS): the body's mechanism for responding to stress of all different kinds.

generally recognized as safe (GRAS): the classification used by the FDA to denote a food substance that is considered to be safe for human consumption.

glucose tolerance factor (GTF): a combination of chromium, niacin (vitamin B_3), and amino acids. Found in brewer's yeast, GTF improves the body's ability to metabolize glucose.

glycerol: a molecule that consists of 3 carbon atoms, hydrogen and oxygen. It is the backbone of the fat or oil molecule and of the membranes' fatty components. Two glycerol molecules can be hooked together to make a sugar molecule.

glycogen: glucose molecules hooked together in long-chains and stored in the liver and muscle of animals as energy reserves. It is also called 'animal starch.'

Health and Nutrition Examination Surveys (HANES): government-sponsored surveys that measured nutrient intakes of Americans during the 1970s. These surveys turned up widespread nutrient deficiencies in all age groups and socioeconomic levels of the population.

hemp: an ancient plant also known as marijuana; one of the first fiber plants cultivated by humanity for making cloth and rope; also cultivated for seeds, which provide both proteins and essential fatty acid-rich oil. Hemp seed oil is a reasonably well-balanced natural oil. It contains both essential fatty acids in a ratio conducive to continuing essential fatty acid balance over the long term. Hemp oil also contains up to 2% GLA. The oil is green and tastes like sunflower oil.

high-density lipoprotein (HDL): one of the vehicles found in the bloodstream, which carries fats and cholesterol. It returns excess cholesterol from cells to liver. Our liver changes cholesterol into bile acids, and pours them into the intestine to aid in fat digestion on their way out of the body.

high erucic acid rape seed (HEAR): rape and mustard seeds as found in nature and used for food in India and China for several thousand years. They contain 20 to 45% erucic acid.

hydrogenation: a commercial process by which liquid oils are turned into plastic or hard fats, by breaking double bonds in fatty acids and and forming bonds with hydrogen instead, thereby 'saturating' carbon atoms with hydrogen.

hydrolysis: breakdown of molecules by (enzyme-controlled) addition of a water molecule.

International Unit (IU): the internationally agreed upon unit of measurement for vitamins A, D, and E.

intrauterine device (IUD): a device made of copper, plastic, or other material that, inserted into the uterus, prevents conception (in most cases).

Inuit: Eskimo name for Eskimos. 'Inuit' means 'the people.'

isomer: a chemical substance that is identical to another in composition, but differs in its 3-dimensional spatial arrangement, and that therefore has different properties.

ketone: a type of chemical substance; ketones are involved in acidosis, a toxic condition of the blood and fluids of poorly managed cases of diabetes.

Krebs cycle: the body's main way of releasing the energy stored in chemical bonds, making that energy available for the body's energy needs. Carbohydrates are its main fuel, but fats and proteins may also be used. Also called tricarboxylic acid cycle or citric acid cycle.

lecithin: a nutritional substance containing fatty acids, glycerol, a phosphate group and choline. Its health value depends on its content of essential fatty acids and choline. Soybeans are the usual source of lecithin containing both essential fatty acids. Lecithin is part of the structure of membranes of cells and organelles.

life energy (or life force): sunlight energy stored in the chemical bonds between atoms in molecules, released in the process of metabolism, and stored in special molecules called CP, ATP, and others, which make this energy available to 'drive' the chemical reactions that build, maintain and repair the body and make activity possible.

linoleic acid (LA): an 18-carbon fatty acid with 2 double bonds, positioned between w carbon atoms 6 and 7, and 9 and 10. It is one of the 2 essential fatty acids. The body cannot make it, requires it for life, and must therefore obtain from food. It is sensitive to destruction by light, oxygen and high temperatures, and extremely important to health. Its absence is fatal. Deficiency causes severe problems in every cell, tissue, and organ. The body makes several other important substances from LA. LA-rich foods include the seeds and oils of safflower, sunflower, hemp, and soybeans.

linolenic acid: see alpha-linolenic acid.

lipid: the chemist's collective name for fats, oils, cholesterol, and other fatty substances.

lipoprotein: fatty substances (fats, oils, cholesterol, carotene, vitamin E) carried in an envelope made of protein and phospholipid (lecithin-like) materials. Specifically, it refers to transport vehicles for fats and cholesterol in our blood and lymph fluids. Lipoproteins carry lipids between our intestine, liver, and body cells.

lipoprotein(a): an LDL-like carrier vehicle of fats and cholesterol, which contains a sticky repair protein known as apo(a), a strong risk factor for cardiovascular disease.

long-chain fatty acid: a fatty acid containing more than 14 carbon atoms in its chain.

low-density lipoprotein (LDL): vehicles that transport fats and cholesterol via the bloodstream to the cells. An excess of these vehicles is said by medical dogma to be associated with cardiovascular disease; hence it is also called the 'bad' cholesterol. When measured separately from apo(a), LDL is only a mild risk factor. See also: lipoprotein(a).

low erucic acid rape seed (LEAR): newly bred rape seed varieties that contain less than 5% erucic acid. Also called canola.

medium-chain fatty acid: a saturated fatty acid that has between 6- and 12- carbons in its chain.

medium-chain triglyceride (MCT): artificial fat molecules made from a fraction of tropical oils that contain mostly 8- and 10-carbon saturated fatty acids as well as some 6- and 12- carbon chains.

metabolism: all chemical changes in the body that make physical life possible.

methyl (– CH$_3$): the free end of a fatty acid. Methyl is a carbon singly bonded to three hydrogen atoms.

methylene interrupted: in fatty acid chemistry, the situation where double bonds start 3 carbons apart. This is usual in fatty acids in their natural state.

milliequivalents per kilogram (meq/kg): a measure of rancidity in a product containing fats and oils. The units used to measure peroxide value (PV). A PV of 100 means about 2 to 3% rancid molecules.

milligrams per deciliter (mg/dL): old measure used by doctors for determining serum cholesterol.

milliliters (mL): thousandths of a liter; same as cubic centimeters.

millimoles per liter (mmol/L): new measure used by doctors for determining serum cholesterol.

mineral: any of several of the basic elements, including metals. In the body, about 20 minerals are required for biochemical life functions.

minimum daily requirement (MDR): also called the 'Recommended Daily Allowance' (RDA); for those essential nutrients for which an RDA has been set by government committees, it is the amount of each of these essential nutrients required daily to prevent the symptoms of deficiency in a normal, healthy person.

molecule: 2 or more atoms held together by means of a pair of electrons shared between them.

monounsaturated fatty acid (MUFA): a fatty acid containing one double bond between carbon atoms somewhere in its fatty chain.

Multiple Sclerosis (MS): an auto-immune condition that leads to neural damage, motor paralysis, respiratory paralysis, and death. MS responds relatively well to nutrition and detoxification if treatment is started early.

National Food Consumption Survey (NFCS): a survey that measured nutrient levels and found deficiencies in the U.S. during the 1970s.

oil: a liquid fat. The shorter the fatty acid chains or the more Omega 3 or Omega 6 double bonds present in them, the more liquid the oil.

oleic acid (OA, 18:1w9): an 18-carbon fatty acid with one double bond between carbons 9 and 10. OA is a monounsaturated fatty acid found in olive, peanut, canola, pecan, macadamia, and other oils.

omega: symbolized by w, it refers to the methyl end of a fatty acid.

omega 6 (w6): a family of related fatty acids essential for human health. These are amply supplied by Western diets. In fact, their consumption has doubled in the last 50 years. From w6 fatty acids, the body makes series 1 and series 2 prostaglandins. Excess of the latter can cause inflammation, water retention, increased blood pressure, sticky platelets, and decreased immune response.

omega 3 (w3): a second family of related fatty acids essential to human health but lacking from most Western diets. Our intake of these has decreased to 1/6 of their level in 1850. From w3 fatty acids, our body makes series 3 prostaglandins, which prevent the negative effects of series 2 prostaglandins by preventing their production.

omega 6:3 balance: the balance of w6 to w3 fatty acids that leads to optimum health. Researchers consider four or five omega 6 to each omega 3 a good balance. Most Western diets are between 10 and 20 to 1 in favor of omega 6, far too high in omega 6, which encourages overproduction of series 2 prostaglandins with negative effects on health. Therapeutic w6:w3 balance for Western diets is about 1 to 2.

optimum: most effective. In nutrition, it is the daily dose of a nutrient or nutrient combination that results in the most effective biochemical and metabolic functioning of the organism. Optimum nutrition results in the best possible physical health.

organelle: literally, a little organ. In the cell, various kinds of biochemical 'machinery' that carry out different specialized cell functions. Mitochondria, lysosomes, vesicles, Golgi, nucleus and nucleolus are organelles.

orthomolecular: of the right molecules. In nutrition, it is the maintenance of health and the treatment of disease by varying the concentrations of substances normally present in the body (vitamins, minerals, fatty acids, amino acids, enzymes, hormones).

oxidize: the addition of oxygen, subtraction of hydrogen, or addition of electrons to a substance, often accompanied by a release of energy.

palmitic acid (PA, 16:0): a 16-carbon saturated fatty acid found abundantly in tropical oils. PA increases cholesterol levels.

palmitoleic acid (POA, 16:1w7): a 16-carbon fatty acid with a double bond between carbons 7 and 8.

partially hydrogenated: an oil in which some but not all double bonds have been destroyed by adding hydrogen to the fatty acid molecules under pressure and high temperature in the presence of a nickel-aluminum catalyst. A semi-solid plastic fat results. Many chemical changes take place in the fatty acid molecules during this process.

peroxide value (PV): a measure of rancidity in oils.

phenylalanine (Phe): an essential amino acid.

phenylketonuria (PKU): a genetic mutation that makes carriers unable to metabolize the amino acid phenylalanine (Phe). Unless dietary Phe is carefully restricted, babies with PKU become mentally disabled during early development.

phosphatide: see phospholipid.

phospholipid: a class of fatty compounds found in membranes, consisting of 2 fatty acid molecules, a glycerol molecule, a phosphate group, and some other groups hooked to the phosphate. Lecithin is the best-known example.

plastic: synthetic materials used for packaging; those used for oils may cause contact derivatives in sensitive individuals; contrary to marketing hype, they are neither biodegradable nor truly recyclable. As a result, dark glass is preferable for oil packaging.

platelet: small, colorless disks in circulating blood, which aid in blood clotting. Platelets become more sticky (form clots easier) when we consume hard or hydrogenated fats, and less sticky (form clots less readily) when we consume w3 essential fatty acids. Less sticky platelets protect against heart attacks and strokes.

433

polychlorinated biphenyl (PCB): organic (aromatic) molecules that have been reacted with chlorine. Such molecules are extremely toxic, and also cause cancer.

polyethylene (PE): a type of plastic used as packaging material for dry foods. Amber glass is preferable packaging material for oils because of environmental concerns and unanswered health questions. Many plastics are toxic.

polymerize: the process of forming complex or giant molecules by linking together many smaller units. Fatty acids containing many double bonds may polymerize under certain conditions of processing. Our body lacks the capacity to metabolize such molecules easily.

polyunsaturated fatty acid (PUFA): a fatty acid that contains more than one double bond between carbon atoms in its chain. The term includes both natural, health-enhancing as well as unnatural, health-destroying kinds.

precursor: parent substance; a substance out of which another substance is made by chemical modification.

premenstrual syndrome (PMS): a nutrition-related degenerative condition affecting women before the onset of the monthly period. Water retention, bloating, mood swings, and behavioral difficulties are often involved.

preservative: any of a large number of possible compounds that slow down chemical deterioration.

prostaglandin (PG): a fatty acid partially oxidized in a very specific and controlled way by enzymes made in the body for just this purpose. Prostaglandins have hormone-like functions in the regulation of cell activity. Over 30 different prostaglandins are known.

protein: a group of complex molecules with specific and precise structural and chemical functions. They are made by linking together amino acids (over 20 different kinds of amino acids are known) in a specific linear sequence and then folding these chains in particular 3-dimensional ways. Enzymes, muscle, and egg white are examples of protein.

Recommended Daily Allowance (RDA): the daily dosage of essential nutrients required by an average healthy person in order to prevent the occurrence of deficiency symptoms. It is a minimum requirement rather than an optimum for good health. It does not take into account increased requirement during pregnancy, breast-feeding, infancy, growth, adolescence, athletic activity, hard physical labor, healing, convalescence, aging, disease, stress, or individual biochemical differences.

refined: refers to processed sugars, starches and fats and oils. Essential substances are removed from foods, and thus refined substances rob the body of its stores of these essential nutrients, leading to deficiency diseases and degeneration. In terms of health, refined means 'deficient' and 'nutrient-impoverished'.

ribonucleic acid (RNA): messages translated from genetic material (DNA), that are used by our cells to synthesize proteins.

saturated fatty acid (SaFA): a fatty acid with no double bonds in the carbon chain, and with every possible position on the carbon atoms taken up by hydrogen atoms.

short-chain fatty acid: a fatty acid with 6 or less carbon atoms in its chain.

simple carbohydrate: a simple sugar. Glucose, fructose and lactose are examples, as well as sucrose (table sugar). Simple carbohydrates are absorbed into the bloodstream rapidly; consumption may lead to hypoglycemia, diabetes and cardiovascular problems, as well as obesity. They also inhibit immune function.

starch: glucose molecules hooked together into branching chains by plant cells. Digested and absorbed slowly, starches supply energy at the rate at which the body uses it.

stearic acid (SA, 18:0): an 18-carbon saturated fatty acid abundant in hard fats.

stearidonic acid (SDA, 18:4w3): an w3 fatty acid derivative. SDA is the first step in the production of EPA, the parent of hormone-like series 3 prostaglandins.

superoxide dismutase (SOD): an enzyme made in our body that neutralizes free radicals that could otherwise cause damage to cells.

superunsaturated fatty acid (SUFA): another name for w3 fatty acids, that distinguishes them from w6 fatty acids.

tertiary butyhydroquinone (TBHQ): an artificial preservative for oils, which replaces natural vitamin E and carotene, which are removed during oil processing.

tetrahydrocannabinol (THC): the molecule in hemp (marijuana) that produces the 'high' when a person smokes or eats marijuana leaves or flowers.

thrombocytopenia (TCP): a low number of platelets in the blood.

toximolecular: of toxic molecules. The use of substances foreign to the body in the treatment of disease. This commonly accepted approach of drug-oriented medical practice does not make sense for long-term health care, because it goes against human biology.

toximolecular medical practice: rests on the fact that synthetic, toxic (drug) molecules can be patented, protecting large monopoly profits for 17 to 20 years. Toximolecular practice is based on business decisions. Health-based decisions would force a more biological approach.

trans- configuration: the spatial arrangement in which hydrogen atoms on the carbons involved in a double bond are found on opposite sides of the molecule.

transesterification (TE): an industrial way of randomizing fatty acid positions in a triglyceride (fat or oil). It can be used to make a hybrid oil from two different kinds of oil.

trans- fatty acid: a fatty acid in which the hydrogen atoms on the carbon atoms involved in a double bond are situated on opposite sides of the fatty chain.

triglyceride (TG): a molecule of fat or oil. It consists of 3 free-swinging fatty acid molecules hooked to a glycerol backbone. This is the form in which fatty acids are stored in the body's fat tissues and in the seeds of plants.

ultraviolet (UV): the skin-burning part of the sun's spectrum.

unrefined ('crude'): in its natural state; not altered, nutrient-rich.

unsaturated fatty acid (UFA): a fatty acid with one or more double bonds between carbons in its chain.

vegan: a person who eats no animal products whatsoever. No meat, no fish, no eggs, no dairy products.

very low-density lipoprotein (VLDL): vehicles made in the liver for transporting fats and cholesterol.

vitamin E: a natural antioxidant and essential vitamin found in seed oils. It is required by the body to prevent the destruction of membrane fatty acids by oxidation.

vitamin: any of 13 essential nutrients that the body cannot make from other substances, requires for health and life, and must therefore obtain from external sources. Food processing removes much of the content of these essential nutrients and therefore causes deficiency, deterioration, and degeneration of cells, tissues, organs, and human health.

Bibliography

Introduction

Two different approaches are used in published material on fats and oils. One approach serves the industry. It emphasizes the technical, complex nature of fats and oils, and stresses the processes by which raw materials can be changed into marketable products. This approach also concerns itself with customer appeal of products through taste, smell, color, texture, convenience, shelf-life, etc. This material is generally written for other experts in the field, and is often boring to read. It downplays the health, nutrition, and safety aspects of fats and oils products.

The other approach serves the 'lay' public, and emphasizes the effects on health of fats and oils products. It also concerns itself with the nature of the chemical changes to which industry subjects natural raw foodstuffs and the effect of these changes on nutritional qualities and health. Both kinds of published material contain valuable information, and both can contribute to our understanding. References to both are given.

References marked with an asterisk (*) are, in the author's opinion, outstanding works.

Fats, oils, essential fatty acids

Bates, C. *Essential Fatty Acids and Immunity in Mental Health.* Tacoma, WA. Life Sciences Press. 1987.

*BeareRogers, J. (ed) *Dietary Fat Requirements in Health and Development.* Champaign, IL. AOCS. 1988.

*Brisson, G.J. *Lipids in Human Nutrition.* Inglewood, NJ. Burgess. 1981.

*Budwig, J. *Das Fettsyndrom,* Freiburg, Germany. Hyperion Verlag. 1959. (The Fat Syndrome).

*Budwig, J. *Die elementare Funktion der Atmung in ihrer Beziehung zu autoxydablen Nahrungstoffen.* Freiburg, Germany. Hyperion Verlag. 1953. (The basic function of cell respiration in its relationship to autoxidizable nutrients).

Cambie, R. *Fats for the Future.* New York, NY. Avi London, Van Nostrand-Reinhold. 1989.

Eastman, W. *The History of Linseed Oil Industry in the U.S.* Dennison & Co. Publishers, Minneapolis, MN. 1968.

Enig, M.G. *Trans- Fatty Acids in the Food Supply: a comprehensive report covering 60 years of research.* Silver Springs, MD, Enig Associates. 1993.

*Gunstone, F. et al. *The Lipid Handbook.* London, England. Chapman & Hall. 1986.

Hamilton, E. et al *Nutrition Concepts and Controversies.* St. Paul, MN. West Publishing. 1988.

Horrobin, D.F. *Essential Fatty Acids: A Review.* In: Horrobin, D.F. (ed) Clinical Uses of Essential Fatty Acids. London, England. Eden Press. 1982.

Kabara, J. *Pharmacological Effects of Lipids.* Champaign, IL. AOCS. 1978.

Kabara, J. *Pharmacological Effects of Lipids II.* Champaign, IL. AOCS. 1985.

Kabara, J. *Pharmacological Effects of Lipids III.* Champaign, IL. AOCS. 1989.

Kiritsakis, A. *Olive Oil.* Champaign, IL. AOCS. 1990.

Kunau, W. & Holman, R. *Polyunsaturated Fatty Acids.* Champaign, IL. AOCS. 1977.

Lands, W.E.M. (ed) *Polyunsaturated Fatty Acids and Eicosanoids.* Champaign, IL. AOCS. 1987.

Lees, R. & Karel, M. *Omega 3 Fatty Acids in Health and Disease.* Basel, Switzerland. Dekker. 1990.

Lusas, E. *Food Uses of Whole Oil and Protein Seeds.* Champaign, IL. AOCS. 1989.

*Mead, J.F. and Fulco, A.J. *The Unsaturated and Polyunsaturated Fatty Acids in Health and Disease.* Springfield IL. Charles C. Thomas. 1976.

Minor, L. *Standards for Fats and Oils.* Westport, CT. Avi Publishing. 1985.

Nettleton, J.A. *Seafood Nutrition.* Huntington, NY. Osprey Books. 1985.

Page, L. *Healthy Healing: an alternative healing reference,* 8th Ed. San Francisco, CA. Author-published. 1990.

*Perkins, E. C. and Visek, W. J. (eds) *Dietary Fats and Health. Champaign,* IL. American Oil Chemists' Society. 1983.

Pique, G.G. *Omega -3 - The Fish Oil Factors.* San Diego, CA. The Omega 3 Project. 1986.

Pryde, E. et al. *New Sources of Fats and Oils.* Champaign, IL. AOCS. 1981.

Rudin, D.O. & Felix, C. *The Omega-3 Phenomenon.* New York, NY. Rawson Associates. 1987.

Ruzicka, T. *Eicosanoids and the Skin.* Boca Raton, FL. CRC Press. 1990.

Salunkhe, D. et al. *World Oil Seeds: chemistry, technology, & utilization.* New York, NY. Avi Books. 1992.

Sevanian, A. *Lipid Peroxidation in Biological Systems.* Champaign, IL. AOCS. 1988.

Shahaidi, F. *Canola and Rapeseed: production, chemistry, nutrition & processing technology.* New York, NY. Avi Books. 1990.

Sinclair, H.M. *Essential Fatty Acids.* London, England. Butterworths. 1958.

Snyder, H. & Kwon, T. *Soybean Utilization.* New York, NY. Avi Books. 1987.

Somogyi, J.C. and Francis, A. *Nutritional Aspects of Fats.* New York, NY. Karger. 1977.

Stier, B. *Secrets des Huiles de Premiere Pression a Froid.* Quebec City, QU. Rodet Presse. 1990.

WHO/FAO. *Dietary Fats and Oils in Human Nutrition.* Report of an expert consultation. UN Food and Agricultural Organization. Rome, Italy. 1977.

Willis, A. *Handbook of Eicosanoids: prostaglandins and related lipids* (Vol. I – Chemical and biochemical aspects). Boca Raton, FL. CRC Press. 1987.

Willis, A. *Handbook of Eicosanoids: prostaglandins and related lipids* (Vol. II - Drugs acting via the eicosanoids). Boca Raton, FL. CRC Press. 1989.

Nutrition & related topics

Arasaki, T. & Arasaki, S. *Vegetables From the Sea.* Tokyo, Japan. Japan Publications. 1983.

*Ballentine, R. *Diet and Nutrition: a holistic approach.* Honesdale, PA. Himalayan International Institute. 1978.

*Beasley, J.D. *The Betrayal of Health.* New York, NY. Times Books. 1991.

Bieler, H.G. *Food is Your Best Medicine.* New York, NY. Vintage Books. 1973.

Bland, J. (ed) *Yearbook of Nutritional Medicine,* New Canaan, CT. Keats Publishing. 1985.

Braly, J. *Dr. Braly's Food Allergy & Nutrition Revolution.* New Canaan, CT. Keats Publishing. 1992.

*Braverman, E.R. and Pfeiffer, C.C. *The Healing Nutrients Within: facts, findings and new research on amino acids.* New Canaan, CT. Keats Publishing. 1987.

*Cleave, T. L. *The Saccharine Disease.* New Canaan, CT. Keats Publishers. 1975.

*Colgan, M. *Your Personal Vitamin Profile.* New York, NY. Quill Books. 1982.

Crook, W.G. *The Yeast Connection.* Jackson, TN. Professional Books. 1989.

Davis, A. *Let's Get Well.* New York, NY. Harcourt Brace Jovanovich. 1965.

Dunne, L. *Nutrition Almanac,* 3rd Ed. New York, NY. McGraw-Hill. 1990.

Fredericks, C. *Carlton Fredericks' High Fiber Way to Total Health.* New York, NY. Pocket Books. 1976.

*Gislason, S. *Nutritional Therapy.* Vancouver, B.C. PerSona Publications. 1991.

Guthrie, H.A. *Introductory Nutrition.* 6th Ed. St. Louis, MO. Mosby, 1986.

*Hendler, S.S. *The Doctors' Vitamin and Mineral Encyclopedia.* New York, NY. Simon and Schuster. 1990.

*Hoffer, A. *Orthomolecular Medicine for Physicians.* New Canaan, CT. Keats Publishing. 1989.

*Howell, E. *Enzyme Nutrition.* Wayne, NJ. Avery Publishing Group. 1985.

Hunt, S.M. & Groff, J.L. *Advanced Nutrition and Human Metabolism.* St. Paul, MN. West Publishing Group. 1990.

*Kollath, W. *Die Ordnung unserer Nahrung (The organization of our nutrition).* Heidelberg, W. Germany. Haug Verlag. 1977.

*Koop, E. *The Surgeon General's Report.* Washington, DC. U.S. Department of Health and Human Services, Publication No. 88-50210. 1988.

*Kunin, R.A. *Meganutrition.* New York, NY. McGraw-Hill. 1980.

Mindell, E. *Earl Mindell's Vitamin Bible.* New York, NY. Warner Books. 1979.

Nutrition Reviews. *Present Knowledge in Nutrition.* 5th Ed. Washington, DC. Nutrition Foundation. 1984.

*Ott, J. Health and Light. New York, NY. Pocket Books. 1976.

*Passwater, R. & Cranton, E. *Trace Elements, Hair Analysis & Nutrition.* New Canaan, CT. Keats Publishing. 1983.

*Passwater, R.A. *The New Supernutrition.* New York, NY. Pocket Books, 1991.

*Pauling, L. *Vitamin C, The Common Cold, and The Flu.* San Francisco, CA. Freeman Book Co. 1976.

*Pauling, L. *How to Live Longer & Feel Better.* New York, NY. Avon Books. 1987.

*Pfeiffer, C.C. et al. *The Schizophrenias: ours to conquer.* Wichita, KS. Biocommunications Press. 1988.

*Pfeiffer, C.C. *Mental and Elemental Nutrients.* New Canaan, CT. Keats Publishers. 1975.

*Philpott, W.H. and Kalita, D.K. *Brain Allergies.* New Canaan, CT. Keats Publishers. 1980.

Pickarski, R. *Friendly Foods: gourmet vegetarian cuisine.* Berkeley, CA. Ten Speed Press. 1991.

Pottenger, F. *Pottenger's Cats.* La Mesa, CA. The Price - Pottenger Foundation. 1983.

*Price, W. *Nutrition and Physical Degeneration.* La Mesa, CA. Price - Pottenger Foundation. 1945.

*Reading, C.M. and Meillon, R.S. *Your Family Tree Connection.* New Canaan, CT. Keats Publishing. 1988.

Rousseau, D. *Your Home, Your Health, and Well-Being.* Vancouver, BC. Hartley & Marks. 1989.

Scharffenberg, J.A. *Problems with Meat.* Santa Barbara, CA. Woodbridge Publishers. 1979.

Schmid, R.F. *Traditional Foods are your Best Medicine.* Stratford, CT. Ocean View Publications. 1987.

*Schroeder, H.A. *The Poisons around Us.* New Canaan, CT. Keats Publishers. 1978.

*Shils, M.E. & Young, V.R. *Modern Nutrition in Health and Disease,* 7th Ed. Philadelphia, PA. Lea & Febiger. 1988.

Smith, L. *Feed Your Kids Right.* New York, NY. Delta Books. 1979.

*Werbach, M. *Nutritional Influences on Illness.* Tarzana, CA. Third Line Press. 1988.

*Werbach, M. *Nutritional Influences on Mental Illness.* Tarzana, CA. Third Line Press. 1991.

*Williams, R.J. *Nutrition against Disease.* New York, NY. Bantam Books. 1971.

Williams, R.J. and Kalita, D.K. *A Physician's Handbook of Orthomolecular Medicine.* New York, NY. Pergamon Press. 1977.

Wynn, M. & Wynn, A. *The Case for Preconception Care of Men and Women.* Bicester, Oxon, U.K. AB Academic Publishers. 1991.

Cardiovascular disease, cholesterol, serum lipids

American Health Foundation. *Plasma Lipids: optimum levels for health.* New York, NY. Academic Press. 1980.

*BeareRogers, J. (ed) *Dietary Fat Requirements in Health and Development.* Champaign, IL. AOCS. 1988.

Cooper, K.H. *Controlling Cholesterol.* New York, NY. Bantam Books. 1988.

Cranton, E. & Brecher, A. *Bypassing Bypass: the new technique of chelation therapy.* Herndon, VA. MEDEX Publishers. 1984.

Day, C.E. and Levy, R.S. (eds) *Low-Density Lipoproteins.* New York, NY. Plenum Press. 1976.

Despopoulos A. and Silbernagl, S. *Color Atlas of Physiology.* Chicago, IL. Year Book Medical Publisher, Inc. 1981.

Fox, E.L. et al. *The Physiological Basis of Physical Education and Athletics,* 4th Ed. Philadelphia, PA. Saunders College Publishing. 1988.

Hietanen, E. *Regulation of Serum Lipids by Physical Exercise.* Boca Raton, FL. CRC Press. 1982.

Kowalski, R.E. *The 8-Week Cholesterol Cure.* New York, NY. Harper & Row. 1987.

life-style Counterattack. Symposium on diet, exercise, and health. Simon Fraser University, Burnaby, BC, Canada. April 13-15, 1984.

*Ornish, D. *Dr. Dean Ornish's Program for Reversing Heart Disease.* New York, NY. Random House. 1990.

*Passwater, B.A. *Supernutrition for Healthy Hearts.* New York, NY. Jove Books. 1977.

**Rath, M. &Pauling, L. *Solution to the Puzzle of Human Cardiovascular Disease: its primary cause is ascorbate deficiency leading to the deposition of lipoprotein(a) and fibrinogen/fibrin in the vascular wall.* Journal of Orthomolecular Medicine, Vol. 6, p. 125 - 134, 1991.

Smith, L.L. *Cholesterol Autoxidation.* New York, NY. Plenum Press. 1981.

Stare, F. et al *Balanced Nutrition: beyond the cholesterol scare.* Holbrook, MA. Bob Adams Publishers. 1989.

Cancer, immunity, aging, AIDS

Bodanski, O. *Biochemistry of Cancer.* New York, NY. Academic Press. 1975.

Booth, G. *The Cancer Epidemic: shadow of the conquest of nature.* Lewiston, NY. Edwin Mellen. 1979.

*Cameron, E. and Pauling, L. *Cancer and Vitamin C.* New York, NY. Warner Books. 1979.

Deutsch, E. (ed) *Molecular Base of Malignancy.* Stuttgart, W. Germany. Georg Thieme Verlag. 1976.

Galeotti, T. et al. *Membranes in Tumor Growth.* New York, NY. Elsevier Books. 1982.

Galland, L. *Superimmunity for Kids.* New York, NY. Delta Books. 1988.

Jochems, R. *Dr. Moerman's Anti-Cancer Diet: Holland's revolutionary nutritional program for combatting cancer.* Garden City Park, NY. Avery. 1990.

Kidd, P.M. & Huber, W. *Living with the AIDS Virus.* Berkeley, CA. HK Biomedical - Education. 1991.

Kimball, J.W. *Introduction to Immunology,* 2nd Ed. New York, NY. McMillan Publishers. 1986.

Masoro, E.J. (ed) *Handbook of Physiology in Aging.* Boca Raton, FL. CRC Press. 1981.

McCabe, E. *Oxygen Therapies.* Morrisville, NY. Energy Publications. 1988.

Moss, R.W. *The Cancer Syndrome.* New York, NY. Grove Press. 1980.

National Research Council. *Diet, Nutrition, and Cancer.* Washington, DC, National Academy of Science. 1982.

Newbold, H. L. *Vitamin C against Cancer.* New York, NY. Stein and Day. 1979.

Bibliography

Pearson, D. and Shaw, S. *Life Extension.* New York, NY. Warner Books. 1983.

Peter, F. M. (ed) *Diet, Nutrition & Cancer.* False Church, Virginia. American Institute for Cancer Research, Committee on Diet, Nutrition and Cancer, Assembly of Life Sciences, National Academy of Sciences. 1982.

Reingold, C.B. *The Lifelong Anti-Cancer Diet.* New York, NY. Signet Books. 1982.

Shaw, C.R. *Prevention of Occupational Cancer.* Boca Raton, FL. CRC Press. 1981 .

*Szent-Gyorgyi, A. *The Living State and Cancer.* New York, NY. Dekker. 1978.

Tache, J., Selye, H., and Day, S.B. *Cancer, Stress, and Death.* New York, NY. Plenum Press. 1979.

Tizard, I. *Veterinary Immunology.* Philadelphia, PA. W.B. Saunders Co. 1992.

Walters, R. *Options.* Garden City Park, NY. Avery Publishing Group. 1993.

*Weiner, M.A. *Maximum Immunity.* Boston, MA. Houghton Mifflin Co. 1986.

Wolstenholme, G. E. W., Fitzsimmons, D. W., and Whelan, J. (eds) *Submolecular Biology and Cancer.* New York NY. Ciba Foundation. Excerpta Medica. 1979.

Wood, R. *Tumor Lipids: biochemistry and metabolism.* Champaign, IL. American Oil Chemists' Society. 1973.

Body composition, fat tissue, membranes

Alberts, B. et al. *Molecular Biology of the Cell.* New York, NY. Garland Publishing. 1983.

Beck, J.S. *Biomembranes: fundamentals in relation to human biology.* New York, NY. McGraw-Hill. 1980.

Behuke, A.R. and Williams, J.H. *Evaluation of Body Build and Composition.* Englewood Cliffs, NJ. Prentice-Hall. 1974.

Bloch, K., Bolis, L., and Tosteson, DC. (eds) *Membranes, Molecules. Toxins, and Cells.* Littleton, MA. PSG Publishers. 1981.

Brozek, J. M. (ed) *Human Body Composition: approaches and applications.* New York, NY. Symposium Publications Division, Pergamon Press. 1965.

Lundberg, O. *Brown Adipose Tissue.* New York, NY. Elsevier Books. 1970.

National Research Council. *Body Composition in Animals and Man.* Washington, D.C. National Academy of Science. 1968.

Parizkova, J. *Body Fat and Physical Fitness.* The Hague, Netherlands. Martinus Nijhoff BV/Medical Division. 1977.

Peeters, H. (ed) *Phosphatidylcholine.* New York, NY. Springer Verlag. 1976.

*Robertson, R.N. *The Lively Membranes.* Cambridge, England. Cambridge U. Press. 1983.

Diets, eating disorders, obesity, weight loss

Angel, A. (ed) *The Adipocyte and Obesity: cellular and molecular mechanisms.* New York, NY. Raven Press. 1983.

Atkins, R.C. *Dr. Atkins' Diet Revolution.* New York, NY. Bantam Books. 1972.

Darling, K. *Weight No More.* Mill Valley, CA. Whatever Publishing. 1984.

Gittleman, A.L. *Beyond Pritikin.* New York, NY. Bantam Books. 1988.

Jablow, M. *A Parent's Guide to Eating Disorders and Obesity.* New York, NY. Bantam-Delta-Dell. 1992.

Kunin, R.C. *Meganutrition for Women.* New York, NY. McGraw-Hill. 1983.

Pritikin, N. *The Pritikin Program of Diet and Exercise.* New York, NY. Bantam Books, 1979.

Remington, D. et al *How to Lower Your Fat Thermostat.* Provo, UT. Vitality Hours. 1983.

Riebel, L. & Kaplan, J. *Someone You Love is Obsessed With Food: what you need to know about eating disorders.* New York, NY. Hazeldine Ed. Press. 1989.

Riebel, L. *Understanding Eating Disorders: a guide for health care professionals.* Sacramento, CA. Robert J. Anderson Publishing. 1988.

*Schwartz, R. *Diets Don't Work.* Houston, TX. Breakthru Publishing. 1982.

Tannenhaus, N. *What You Can Do About Eating Disorders.* New York, NY. Dell Medical Library. 1992.

Psychological aspects, behavior, crime

Cheraskin, E. and Ringsdorf, W.M. *Psychodietetics.* New York, NY. Bantam Books. 1974.

Cousins, N. *Anatomy of an Illness.* New York, NY. Bantam Books. 1979.

Fredericks, C. *Psychonutrition.* New York, NY. Grosset & Dunlap, 1976.

Gardner, H. *Frames of Mind.* New York, NY. Basic Books. 1983.

Kanarek, R.B. & Marks-Kaufman, R. *Nutrition and Behavior: new perspectives.* New York, NY. Avi Books. 1991.

*Padus, E. *Emotions and Your Health.* Emmaus, PA. Rodale Press. 1986.

*Rapp, D. *The Impossible Child.* Tacoma, WA. Life Sciences Press. 1986.

Rapp, D. *Is This Your Child?* New York, NY. Quill Books. 1991.

Reed, B. *Food, Teens & Behavior.* Manitowoc, WI. Natural Press. 1983.

*Schauss, A. *Diet, Crime, and Delinquency.* Berkeley, CA. Parker House. 1980.

*Selye, H. *The Stress of Life.* New York, NY. McGraw-Hill. 1956.

Selye, H. *Stress Without Distress.* New York, NY. Harper & Row. 1974.

*Simonton, O.C., Matthews-Simonton, S. and Creighton, J.L. *Getting Well Again.* New York, NY. Bantam Books. 1978.

*Smith, L.H. *Improving Your Child's Behavior Chemistry.* Englewood Cliffs, NJ. Prentice-Hall. 1984.

Wilson, E.O. *The Diversity of Life.* Cambrige, MA. Harvard U Press. 1992.

Politics of nutrition, medicine, and environment

Armstrong, D. & Metzger-Armstong, E. *The Great American Medicine Show: illustrated history of hucksters, healers, health evangelists and heroes from Plymouth Rock to the present.* New York, NY. Prentice-Hall. 1991.

*Beasley, J.D. and Swift J.J. *The Kellogg Report: the impact of nutrition, environment & life-style on the health of Americans.* Annandale-on-Hudson, NY. The Institute of Health Policy and Practice, The Bard College Center. 1989.

Carson, R. *Silent Spring.* New York NY. Fawcett Crest Books. 1962.

*Epstein, S. *The Politics of Cancer.* San Francisco, CA. Sierra Club Books. 1978.

Griffin, G.E. *World Without Cancer.* Westlake Village, CA. American Media. 1974.

*Hall, R.H. *Food for Nought: the decline in nutrition.* New York, NY. Random House. 1974.

*Jensen, B. & Anderson, M. *Empty Harvest.* Garden City Park, NY. Avery Publishing. 1990.

Mendelsohn, R.S. *Confessions of a Medical Heretic.* New York, NY. Warner Books. 1979.

Sobel, D. *Ways of Health: holistic approaches to ancient and contemporary medicine.* New York, NY. Harcourt Brace Jovanovich. 1979.

Journal & magazine articles

Adams, C. *The Nutritive Value of American Foods in Common Units.* Washington, DC. U.S. Dept. of Agriculture (US Printing Office). 1975.

American Oil Chemists' Society. *The Journal.* Champaign, IL. 1924-present.

Aquaculture, Vol. 25,1981. pp. 161-172. Fatty acid composition of salmon oils. Amsterdam, Holland. Elsevier Scientific.

Bibliography

Blix, G. (ed) *Polyunsaturated Fatty Acids as Nutrients*. Symposium of the Swedish Nutrition Foundation. Vol. IV. Stockholm, Sweden. Almquist Wiksells. 1966.

*Brown, M.S. and Goldstein, J.L. How LDL receptors influence cholesterol and atherosclerosis. *Scientific American*, pp. 58-66. Nov. 1984.

Clinical Pearls. Hamilton, K. (ed) Sacramento CA. ITS Services. 1990, 1991, 1992.

Composition of Foods: raw, processed, prepared, Washington, DC, *Agriculture Handbook* No. 8., USA Dept. of Agriculture. 1963.

CP Currents. Hamilton, K. (ed) Sacramento CA. ITS Services. 1991, 1992, 1993.

Enig, M.G. *Trans-fatty acid isomers in selected food items*. Thesis, University of Maryland. 1981.

Enig, M.G. *Trans-fatty acids in the food supply: a comprehensive report covering 60 years of research*. Enig Associates, Inc. Silver Spring, MD. 1993.

Fette, Seifen, Anstrichmittel (Fats, Soaps, Paints). Leinenfelden Echterdingen, W. Germany. Industrieverlag von Herrnhaussen. 1894 to present (5 changes in title).

*Holman, T.(ed) Essential Fatty Acids and Prostaglandins. In: *Progress in Lipid Research*. Vol. 20, 1981. Elmsford, NY. Pergamon Press.

Journal of Lipid Research. Bethesda, MD. 1959 to present.

Levy, P. *Vegetable Oil: the unsaturated facts*. Talking Food. Salem, Mass. 1977.

Lipids. Champaign, IL. American Oil Chemists' Society. 1966 to present.

Progress in Lipid Research. Holman, T. (ed) Elmsford, NY. Pergamon Press. 1978 to present.

Progress in the Chemistry of Fats and other Lipids. Holman, T. (ed) Elmsford, NY. Pergamon Press. 1951 – 1977.

Rath, M. & Pauling, L. Solution to the Puzzle of Human Cardiovascular Disease. *Journal of Orthomolecular Medicine*, Vol. 6, 3&4, pp.125 - 146. 1991.

Report of the Ad Hoc Committee on the Composition of Special Margarines. Ottawa, Canada. Supply and Services Canada. 1980.

Schreiber, J. and Fillip, J. *Edible Oils: the cold facts on 'cold-pressed'*. Whole Foods Magazine. 1978.

Lipoprotein (a) in Heart Disease. *Scientific American*, June, 1992.

Vaughn, L. Getting the Most of the F complex. *Prevention*, pp.48-54. Sept. 1984.

Vaughn, L. The Fish Oil Factor: healthy-heart gift from the sea. *Prevention*, pp. 64-69. March 1984.

Industrial uses of fats and oils

Anderson, A.J.C. *Refining of Oils and Fats*. Williams (ed). Elmsford, NY. Pergamon Press. 1962.

Baldwin, A. *Proceedings: World Conference on Emergent Technologies in the Fats and Oils Industry*. Champaign, IL. AOCS. 1986.

Emken, E. & Dutton, H. *Geometrical and Positional Fatty Acid Isomers*. Champaign, IL. AOCS. 1979.

Function and Biosynthesis of Lipids. *Advances in Experimental Medicine and Biology*, Vol. 83. New York, NY. Plenum Publishing Co. 1976.

Kirschenbauer, H.G. *Fats and Oils. An outline of their chemistry and technology*. 2nd Ed. New York, NY. Van Nostrand Reinhold. 1960.

*Swern, D. (ed) *Bailey's Industrial Oil and Fat Products*. 3rd Ed . New York, NY. Wiley and Sons. 1964.

*Swern, D. (ed) *Bailey's Industrial Oil and Fat Products*. 4th Ed. Volumes I and II. New York. Wiley and Sons. 1979.

*Weiss, T.J. *Food Oils and their Uses*. 2nd Ed. Westport, CT. Avi Publishing Co. 1983.

442

Physics, chemistry, biochemistry, physiology

Brady, J.E. & Humiston, G.E. *General Chemistry,* 4th Ed. New York, NY. John Wiley & Sons. 1986.

Campbell, P.N. and Smith, A.D. *Biochemistry Illustrated.* New York, NY. Churchill-Livingstone. 1982.

da Silva, J.J.R.F. & Williams, R.J.P. *The Biological Chemistry of the Elements: the inorganic chemistry of life.* Oxford, U.K. Clarendon Press. 1991.

Eckert, R. and Randall, D. *Animal Physiology: mechanisms and adaptions.* San Francisco, CA. Freeman Book Co. 1983.

*Gurr, M.l. and James, A.T. *Lipid Biochemistry.* 3rd Ed. London, England, Chapman and Hall. 1980.

Graedon, J. *The People's Pharmacy.* New York, NY. Avon Books. 1976. Vol. 2, 1980.

Guyton, A.C. *Textbook of Medical Physiology,* 7th Ed. Philadelphia, PA. W.B. Saunders Co. 1986.

Halliday, D. & Resnick, R. *Fundamentals of Physics,* 3rd Ed. New York, NY. John Wiley & Sons. 1988.

Keeton, W.T. & Gould, J.L. *Biological Science,* 4th Ed. New York, NY. Norton & Co. 1986.

Lide, D.R. (Ed in Chief). *Handbook of Chemistry and Physics,* 73rd Ed. Boca Raton, FL. CRC Press. 1992.

Masoro, E.J. (ed) *Physiological Chemistry of Lipids in Mammals.* Philadelphia, PA. Saunders.

Memmler, R.L. and Wood, D.L. *Structure and Function of the Human Body,* 3rd Ed. Philadelphia, PA. Lippincott, 1983.

The Merck Index. 10th Ed. Merck & Co. Rahway, NJ. 1983.

Pryde, E.H. (ed) *Fatty Acids.* Champaign, IL. American Oil Chemists' Society. 1979.

Smith, L.H. and Thir, S.O. *Pathophysiology: The Biological Principles of Disease.* Philadelphia, PA. Saunders, 1981.

Stryer, L. *Biochemistry,* 3rd Ed. New York, NY. W.H. Freeman & Co. 1988.

Tortora, G.J. and Anagnostakos, N.P. *Principles of Anatomy and Physiology.* New York, NY. Harper & Row Publishers. 1981.

Varder, A.J. et al. *Human Physiology: the mechanisms of body function.* New York, NY. McGraw-Hill. 1985.

Vollhardt, K.C.P. *Organic Chemistry.* New York, NY. W.H. Freeman and Co. 1987.

West, J.B. (ed) *Best & Taylor's Physiological Basis of Medical Practice,* 11th Ed. Baltimore, MA. Williams & Wilkins. 1985.

*Zubay, G. (ed) *Biochemistry.* Reading, MA. Addison-Wesley. 1983.

Index

About the Author

Udo Erasmus was born in Poland during the second world war to parents from Latvia and Estonia escaping from communists. His family fled to West Germany at the end of the war, and emigrated to Canada when he was 10 years old.

His parents, having endured the first world war and the bolshevik revolution during their childhood, and having lived through the depression during adulthood only to be caught in the middle of the second world war, moved to northern Canada where Udo and his four siblings grew up on 112 acres of bush land. Without television, telephone, or radio, nature was both his teacher and entertainer.

At 16, Udo began university studies in the sciences – math, physics, chemistry, and biology. Eventually, he settled on zoology and psychology as his fields of study, and specialized in genetics and biochemistry. His papers in genetics were published in the peer review journal *Mutation Research*.

At 25, Udo found the direction science was taking unacceptable – it was increasingly used to control people rather than to help or free them, and geneticists talked about cloning super-races. Udo left the University of British Columbia and went in search of his mission. "I traveled, looked around for several years, and did all sorts of different jobs to get to know more about my society and the world. Eventually, I was poisoned by pesticides and, in search of self-help, re-discovered a childhood passion for health and healing."

He resumed studies, now focused on nutrition, health, and human nature. The first edition of this book *(Fats and Oils)* was his PhD thesis in nutrition. His M.A. thesis in counseling psychology, entitled *The Nature of Human Nature*, will also be published in book form, "when I'm satisfied with my understanding of the details. I want to let my experience of this topic mature a little longer."

Udo pioneered our understanding of the effects of fats, oils, and cholesterol on human health at a time when other writers were quoting wrong information from outdated sources. The result of his painstaking assembly of relevant research resulted in this landmark book, seminal in the field.

His technological innovations include: development of custom-made parts for existing oil presses to protect the oils being pressed from damage caused by light, oxygen, and heat; use of opaque containers for fresh oils to protect them from light; refrigeration or freezing of oils during transport to slow deterioration; and shelf-dating of oils to warn consumers about old oils. The use of the name *flax* oil (to distinguish the fresh, unrefined oil made with human health in mind from *linseed* oil, which comes from the same seed but is a paint-grade, refined, rancid, industrial product previously offered for human consumption) was Udo's suggestion.

Udo has worked with professionals (doctors, pharmacists, dieticians, osteopaths, naturopaths, nutritionists, chiropractors, massage therapists, other healing professionals, educators, veterinarians, and researchers); consumer health organizations; individuals who want to become more educated in nutrition and health; manufacturers who want help formulating high quality products; and developers of machinery and processes for making products with health in mind.

As an authority on fats, oils, cholesterol, essential fatty acids, technology for pressing healthy oils, complete nutrient programs for human health, and other health topics, Udo has been invited to tour throughout North America and Europe. Since 1987, he has reached an estimated five million viewers, listeners, and readers. He is particularly appreciated for his detailed, precise, clear, and non-technical style.

Services Provided

Udo Erasmus BSc (Zoology, Psychology); Graduate Studies (2 years Genetics, Biochemistry); **MA** (Counseling Psychology); **PhD** (Nutrition)
Researcher, author, educator, and consultant specializing in fats and oils, cholesterol control, essential fatty acids, omega 3s, flax, natural therapies for degenerative conditions, nutrient enrichment, detoxification, and human health.

1. Educational Services:
You can use Udo's website www.udoerasmus.com to educate yourself, get answers to your questions, obtain information about products, find out where to go for help, explore the nature of health, and check his tour itinerary.

2. Product Services:
Udo's Choice ® Line of Products are available at all fine health food stores and natural product pharmacies.
- Udo's Choice Oil Blend   (essential fatty acids)
- Udo's Choice Beyond Greens
- Udo's Choice Wholesome Fast Food Fibre Blend   (fibre product)
- Udo's Choice Digestive Enyzmes
- Udo's Choice Probiotics (age specific probiotics)

Complete product information can be found at www.udoerasmus.com/productmain.htm. For store locations in the USA and Canada or to locate an International distributor near you, please go to www.florahealth.com You may also contact Flora Health at:

In Canada:	In the USA:
Flora Manufacturing and Distributing Inc.	Flora Inc.
1-888-436-6697	1-800-446-2110
www.florahealth.com	www.florainc.com

More Great Books from Canada's Leading
Publisher of Natural Health and Nutrition Books

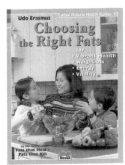

Choosing the Right Fats

Udo Erasmus

Following Udo Erasmus' groundbreaking work Fats that Heal is Choosing the Right Fats—a new alive Natural Health Guide that belongs on every bookshelf. In it, Udo distills decades of nutritional research and development into an informative and accessible form.

This book provides clear answers to various pressing questions, including: What happens when we don't get enough essential fatty acids? How much healthy oil should we take daily? Which is better—flax, sunflower, or sesame oil? Can these fats really help burn calories? There are also useful instructions for using fats to boost athletic performance and to treat conditions such as hair loss, dandruff, and skin inflammations in dogs, cats, horses, and other pets.

This guide is indispensable for helping us integrate these healthy fats into our diet. Delightful soup, pasta, fish dishes, and salad dressings provide a great opportunity for creatively blending the healing oils and putting the right fats on your plate.

$10.95 Cdn/$ 9.95 US

Fantastic Flax

Siegfried Gursche

Who better to tell us about flax than Siegfried Gursche, the man responsible for the introduction of dietary flax products to this country? Drawing upon the author's considerable experience, Fantastic Flax provides a fascinating discussion of flax, a nutritional powerhouse high in fibre, lignans, proteins, vitamins, minerals, and beneficial fats.

Long recognized for its healing properties, flax is now used to develop preventative and therapeutic treatments for cancer, high blood pressure, high cholesterol, digestive problems, and ulcers. Gursche also shows off flax's tasty side with his family recipes for Flax and Vegetable Soup, Flax Muffins with Chocolate Chips, and more.

$10.95 Cdn/$ 9.95 US

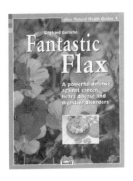

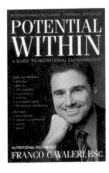

Potential Within

Franco Cavaleri, BSc

A Guide to Nutritional Empowerment

Today's world is contaminated with old diseases, fraught with ever proliferating new diseases, environmental hazards and food so adulterated that it fails to deliver the nutrients necessary for optimum health. Against this
backdrop, the *Potential Within* teaches appropriate food choices and nutritional supplementation that leads to healthy hormonal cascades and metabolic activity for healthy fat loss, reverse Type II diabetes, ameliorate Type 1 diabetes and heighten physical health and athletic performance.

553 pages, softcover
$29.95 Cdn / $21.95 US
ISBN 0-9731701-0-7

The Raw Gourmet

Nomi Shannon

Nomi Shannon opens a door onto a refreshing new world of food preparation that will make a raw gourmet of even the most die-hard baker, boiler, and fryer!

This is a complete guide to one of the world's fastest-growing nutrition and health movements— the living foods diet.

224 pages, softcover
Over 70 full-colour photos
$29.95 Cdn / $24.95 US
ISBN 0-920470-48-3

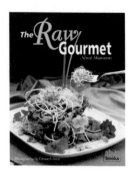

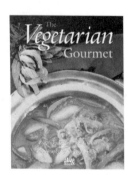

The Vegetarian Gourmet

Dagmar von Cramm

More than just a recipe book, *The Vegetarian Gourmet* provides information on nutrients, food combining, diets, and cooking methods. It includes practical charts on cooking for weight loss, cooking solo, peak season calendar for fruit and vegetables, menu suggestions for special events, and invaluable information for going vegetarian.

246 pages, softcover
Over 200 full-colour photographs
$29.95 Cdn / $24.95 US
ISBN 0-920470-80-7

The Breuss Cancer Cure

Rudolph Breuss

Fasting has long been used in Europe as a preventative measure, as a cure, particularly for degenerative conditions, and to purge the body of impurities and toxins. Knowledgeable in this tradition, Rudolph Breuss developed a 42-day juice fasting program to nourish the body but to starve cancer.

He also provides naturopathic and sometimes unusual treatment suggestions for a wide range of conditions from leukemia to rheumatism, and infertility to cramps. As his book reflects a lifetime of practice, it is well worth consideration.

Translated from the original German into eight languages, this book has sold over one million copies worldwide, and gives hope to many who previously have not had access to Breuss' simple, yet effective cures.

112 pages, softcover
$15.95 Cdn / $12.95 US
ISBN 0-920470-56-4

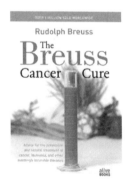

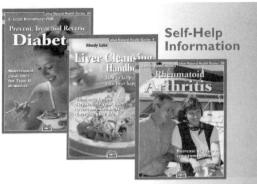
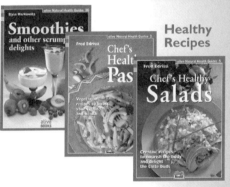
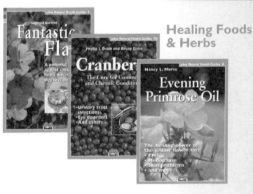
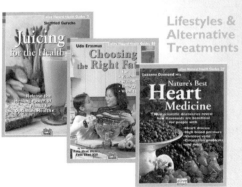

	Natural Health Guides	**CDN $10.95 US $9.95**
1	**Fantastic Flax** by Siegfried Gursche	
2	**Chef's Healthy Pasta** by Fred Edrissi	
3	**Juicing for the Health of It** by Siegfried Gursche	
4	**Liver Cleansing Handbook** by Rhody Lake	
5	**Chef's Healthy Salads** by Fred Edrissi	
6	**Evening Primrose Oil** by Nancy L. Morse, BSc, CNPA	
7	**Natural Alternatives to Vaccination** by Zoltan Rona, MD, MSc	
8	**Nature's Own Candida Cure** by William G. Crook, MD	
9	**Chef's Healthy Desserts** by Fred Edrissi	
10	**Cranberry** by Phyllis I. Dales and Bruce Dales	
11	**Healing with Water** by Giselle Roeder	
12	**Natural Relief from Asthma** by C. Leigh Broadhurst, PhD	
14	**Papaya, The Healing Fruit** by Harald W. Tietze	
15	**Boosting Male Libido** by Zoltan Rona, MD, MSc	
16	**Osteoarthritis** by Zoltan Rona, MD, MSc	
20	**Fighting Fibromyalgia** by Zoltan Rona, MD, MSc	
21	**Super Breakfast Cereals** by Katharina Gustavs	
22	**Health Hazards of White Sugar** by Lynne Melcombe	
23	**Menopause – Normally and Naturally** by Zoltan Rona, MD, MSc	
24	**Prevent, Treat and Reverse Diabetes** by C. Leigh Broadhurst, PhD	
25	**Good Digestion** by Ken Babal, CN	
26	**Rheumatoid Arthritis** by Zoltan Rona, MD, MSc	
27	**Nature's Heart Medicine** by Suzanne Diamond, MSc	
28	**Health and Healing with Bee Products** by C. Leigh Broadhurst, PhD	
29	**Attention Deficit Disorder** by Nancy L. Morse, BSc, CNPA	
30	**Sprouts** by Kathleen O'Bannon, CNC	
31	**Whole Foods for Seniors** by Kathleen O'Bannon, CNC	
32	**Sauna, The Hottest Way to Good Health** by Giselle Roeder	
33	**Choosing The Right Fats** by Udo Erasmus	
35	**Making Sauerkraut** by Klaus Kaufmann & Annelies Schöneck	
36	**Smoothies and other Scrumptious Delights** by Elysa Markowitz	

These Guides are available through your local book retailer, health food store or by contacting alive at 1-800-663-6580.

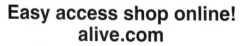

Easy access shop online!
alive.com

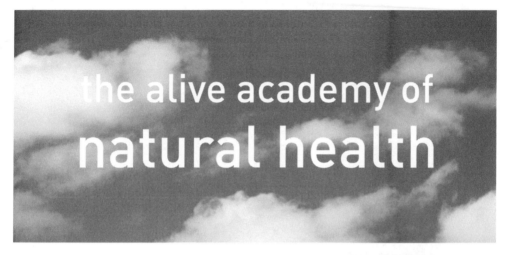
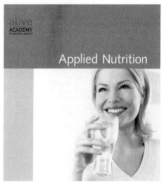
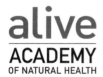

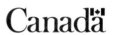